Ethical Considerations and Health Policy

Dr. Susan B. Matt

NURS 5010/6010

Seattle University College of Nursing

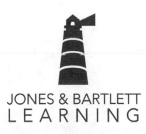

JONES & BARTLETT
LEARNING

World Headquarters
Jones & Bartlett Learning
5 Wall Street
Burlington, MA 01803
978-443-5000
info@jblearning.com
www.jblearning.com

Jones & Bartlett Learning books and products are available through most bookstores and online booksellers. To contact Jones & Bartlett Learning directly, call 800-832-0034, fax 978-443-8000, or visit our website, www.jblearning.com.

This book is produced through PUBLISH – a custom publishing service offered by Jones & Bartlett Learning. For more information on PUBLISH, contact us at 800-832-0034 or visit our website at www.jblearning.com.

Disclaimer
This publication is sold with the understanding that the publisher is not engaged in rendering medical, legal, accounting, or other professional services. If medical, legal, accounting, or other professional service advice is required, the service of a competent professional should be sought. The authors, editor, and publisher have designed this publication to provide accurate information with regard to the subject matter covered. However, they are not responsible for errors, omissions, or for any outcomes related to the use of the contents of this publication and make no guarantee and assume no responsibility or liability for the use of the products and procedures described, or the correctness, sufficiency, or completeness of stated information, opinions, or recommendations. Treatments and side effects described in this publication are not applicable to all people; required dosages and experienced side effects will vary among individuals. Drugs and medical devices discussed herein are controlled by the Food and Drug Administration (FDA) and may have limited availability for use only in research studies or clinical trials. Research, clinical practice, and government regulations often change accepted standards. When consideration is being given to the use of any drug in the clinical setting, the health care provider or reader is responsible for determining FDA status of the drug, reading the package insert, and reviewing prescribing information for the most current recommendations on dose, precautions, and contraindications and for determining the appropriate usage for the product. This is especially important in the case of drugs that are new or seldom used. Any references in this publication to procedures to be employed when rendering emergency care to the sick and injured are provided solely as a general guide; other or additional safety measures might be required under particular circumstances. This publication is not intended as a statement of the standards of care required in any particular situation; circumstances and the physical conditions of patients can vary widely from one emergency to another. This publication is not intended in any way to advise emergency personnel concerning their legal authority to perform the activities or procedures discussed. Such local determination should be made only with the aid of legal counsel. Some images in this publication feature models; these models do not necessarily endorse, represent, or participate in the activities represented in the images.

Cover Image: © AbleStock

6048
Printed in the United States of America
21 20 19 18 17   10 9 8 7 6 5 4

Contents

1 Philosophical Foundations of Applied and Professional Ethics

Pamela J. Grace
From: *Nursing Ethics and Professional Responsibility in Advanced Practice by Pamela J. Grace* 1

2 Nursing Ethics

Pamela J. Grace
From: *Nursing Ethics and Professional Responsibility in Advanced Practice by Pamela J. Grace* 42

3 Professional Responsibility, Social Justice, Human Rights, and Injustice

Pamela J. Grace
From: *Nursing Ethics and Professional Responsibility in Advanced Practice by Pamela J. Grace* 91

4 To Engage or Not Engage: Choices Confronting Nurses and Other Health Professionals

Nancy Aries
From: *Policy and Politics for Nurses and Other Health Professionals by Donna M. Nickitas; Donna J. Middaugh; Nancy Aries* 125

5 Public Health Policy: Promotion, Prevention, and Protection

Mary Mincer Hansen; Mary Jones
From: *Policy and Politics for Nurses and Other Health Professionals by Donna M. Nickitas; Donna J. Middaugh; Nancy Aries* 147

6 The History of Health Insurance in the United States

Leah Curtin; Franklin A. Shaffer
From: *Policy and Politics for Nurses and Other Health Professionals by Donna M. Nickitas; Donna J. Middaugh; Nancy Aries* 176

7 Health Services Research

Donna M. Nickitas; Keville Frederickson; Jonathan Small
From: *Policy and Politics for Nurses and Other Health Professionals by Donna M. Nickitas; Donna J. Middaugh; Nancy Aries* 201

8 Conclusions: A Policy Toolkit for Healthcare Providers and Activists

Roby Robertson; Donna J. Middaugh
From: *Policy and Politics for Nurses and Other Health Professionals by Donna M. Nickitas; Donna J. Middaugh; Nancy Aries* 219

9 Photo Credits

Donna M. Nickitas; Donna J. Middaugh; Nancy Aries
From: *Policy and Politics for Nurses and Other Health Professionals by Donna M. Nickitas; Donna J. Middaugh; Nancy Aries* 245

10 Index 245

Philosophical Foundations of Applied and Professional Ethics

Pamela J. Grace

Believe those who are seeking the truth. Doubt those who find it.
—ANDRE GIDE,
So Be It, or, The Chips Are Down (Ainsi Soit-Il, ou, Les Jeux Sont Faits), 1959

Introduction

For the purposes of this text, the term "APN" is used to denote any and all nurses who are working in expanded roles, regardless of their country of practice. This chapter explains that the roots and strength of advanced practice nurses' (APNs') professional responsibilities are in philosophical understandings about what constitutes good human action and why. From this foundation, it is possible to trace the development and nature of professional responsibility to the population served by the nursing profession. A clear argument is presented about why membership in a profession that provides an important service to individuals and society involves stronger obligations to further the human good than exists in civilian life. Finally, an exploration of the appropriate roles of philosophical skills, theories, and principles in decision making about good action provides a basis for examining the complex issues encountered by APNs. This is an important first step for developing and enhancing APNs' confidence in their ethical decision-making skills.

Groundwork

The Problem of Professional Responsibility

Most nurses and allied health professionals understand that the privilege of professional healthcare practice is accompanied by both moral and legal accountability for professional judgments and resulting actions. However, many are not confident that they are adequately equipped to address obstacles to good practice or the complex ethical problems that can arise in direct care or supervisory situations. Nevertheless, good patient care requires the following essential clinician characteristics: knowledgeable, skillful, and experienced; perceptive about inadequacies in the care-giving environment; willing to focus on the individual needs of the patient in question; and motivated to resolve problems at a variety of levels as necessary. Professionals also need to understand the limits of their knowledge and be willing to draw on the expertise of others. These characteristics are important for obvious reasons and are discussed in more detail in Chapter 2, but less obvious is the idea that those in need of healthcare services are often not knowledgeable about what is required to meet their current or future health needs; they are not qualified to evaluate the quality of the services offered and/or they cannot advocate effectively to receive the care they need (Newton, 1988). Unmet or even unrecognized health needs make people more than ordinarily vulnerable to the ups and downs of life. The effects of unaddressed health needs on human functioning and flourishing make it crucial that healthcare professionals can be trusted to maintain their primary focus on individual and societal healthcare needs, even when faced with economic, institutional, or time pressures.

FIDUCIARY RELATIONSHIPS

Many scholars have argued that the healthcare professional–patient relationship is fiduciary (Grace, 1998; Pellegrino, 2001; Spenceley, Reutter, & Allen, 2006; Zaner, 1991). That is, it is based on trust. People with healthcare needs are forced to rely on clinicians to understand, anticipate, and provide what is needed. Yet in questioning professionals about their responsibilities, how strong or binding these are, or about the basis for claiming that professionals are responsible for good practice, answers are varied and inconsistent; sometimes clinicians even express bewilderment that the question is being raised. Chambliss (1996), in the course of his study of nurses working in institutional settings, noted that when nurses see themselves as powerless

2

to influence change in a setting where there are problematic practices, they can become numbed to the ethical content involved and fail to address it. Others have also documented the problems of nurses feeling powerless. In addition to ceasing to respond to unethical practices when they feel powerless, some nurses leave the setting or seek other types of employment and/or can experience lasting unease, also called *moral distress* (Corley, 2002; Corley, Minick, Elswick, & Jacobs, 2005; Gallagher, 2011; Jameton, 1984; Mohr & Mahon, 1996). Additionally, there is reason to believe that some nurses do not understand the ethical nature of daily practice (Grace, Fry, & Schultz, 2003). Thus, recognition of the fiduciary nature of practice responsibilities requires the nurse to reflect on practice in an ongoing fashion in order to avoid becoming anesthetized to recurrent problematic situations that at best fail to focus on optimal care and at worst are detrimental to patients. Throughout this text, reasoning and support are provided for the idea that professional responsibility exists to address both immediate problems and more deeply rooted systemic or societal obstacles to practice. APNs are ideally prepared and situated to see their responsibilities broadly and influence change, whether this is within their immediate environment or the social contexts of care delivery, the education and supervision of others, or empowering patients and patient populations to get their needs met.

GOOD PRACTICE

From a philosophical stance, *good practice* is equivalent to ethical practice. *Ethical practice* is the use of disciplinary knowledge, skills, experience, and personal characteristics to conceptualize what is needed either at the level of the individual or of society. Ethical professional practice uses the goals and perspectives of the given profession to direct action. Although it is true that various healthcare professions share common goals such as promotion of health, cure of disease, and relief of suffering, they nevertheless have different practice philosophies and draw on different knowledge bases to achieve these goals.

Even when professionals understand the strength of their responsibilities, many factors can interfere with accomplishing good care. This is especially true in contemporary healthcare settings, where competing interests can make it difficult to provide good patient care to individuals even when the clinician's judgment about what is needed is sound. Barriers to autonomous practice are frequently encountered and can include economic interests, institutional priorities, interpersonal communication difficulties, or provider conflicts of interest. Some obstacles to practice are recurrent and arise out of underlying contextual or societal conditions that disadvantage groups of people and thus require a broader understanding of professional responsibility as relating to individuals, institutions, and society (Ballou, 2000; Grace, 2001; Grace & Willis, 2012; Spenceley et al., 2006).

As noted, this and the next three chapters are designed to provide a firm basis for APNs, master's- or doctor of nursing practice (DNP)-nurses, and those from other countries practicing in expanded roles, to understand the origins, scope, and limits of their responsibilities to patients and society. The text provides the APN and equivalent with the knowledge, tools, and skills for ethical practice. Included in the necessary skill set is an understanding of the language of clinical ethics. This is because all nurses—but especially APNs—collaborate with others on behalf of their patients and need a common language for articulating their concerns about the ethical issues they face in practice.

Philosophy, Professional Responsibility, and Nursing Ethics: What Is the Connection?

Nursing ethics and *professional responsibility* are equivalent concepts. However, one cannot merely say this is so and expect to be met with acceptance; the assertion has to be supported by discussion and evidence. This is one of the techniques of philosophical argumentation. As a starting place, it is important to grasp that the idea and possibility of ethical practice lie in philosophical understandings about human beings and their relationship to the world in which they live.

To trace the development of the concept "professional responsibility"—or the obligations of a profession's members toward the population served—from its origins in philosophy, it is helpful to rely on an analogy commonly seen in primary care settings, that of a family tree. The tree and its branches are traced here to give an overview, and then pertinent aspects are discussed in more detail. A word of caution: The branches are made distinct for the purposes of clarity, but there are often areas of overlap or shared space.

PHILOSOPHY'S FAMILY TREE
The discipline of philosophy is the starting point where all theorizing about the nature of the world and our place in it begins. There are several branches of the parent philosophy. These branches represent particular areas of philosophical inquiry: "aesthetics, ethics, epistemology, logic, and metaphysics" (Flew, 1984, p. 267), as shown in **Figure 1**. They all share some common

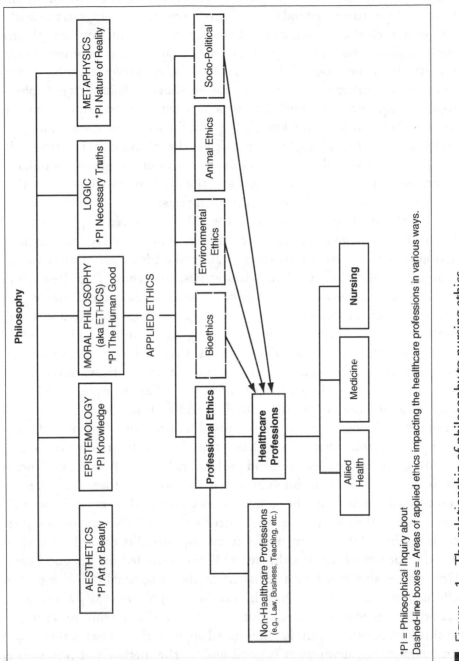

*PI = Philosophical Inquiry about
Dashed-line boxes = Areas of applied ethics impacting the healthcare professions in various ways.

■ Figure 1   The relationship of philosophy to nursing ethics

characteristics. They all use questioning and reasoning (the methods of philosophy) to try to understand the relationship of human beings to the world. However, their themes or focuses of inquiry are different. For example, *aesthetics* is philosophical inquiry about art or beauty. *Ethics* is philosophical inquiry about the good and is also called *moral philosophy* (everyday definitions of *ethics* differ from this, as discussed shortly). *Epistemology* is philosophical inquiry about knowledge—what it is, what we can know, who is the knower, how reliable is the knowledge, and for what purposes. *Ontology* is another branch of philosophy; it investigates the meaning of an entity's existence. Nursing's ontology, then, results from inquiry by nursing scholars—informed by practice environments and the needs of society—about what nursing is, what nurses do, and why nursing exists.

For present purposes, our interest is in Ethics viewed as philosophical inquiry about the good. Philosophical inquiry about what is good in human action branches further into areas of applied ethics. *Applied ethics* are the practical applications of theoretical ethics. Branches of applied ethics include *eco-* or *environmental ethics* (what is good human action with regard to the environment?), *animal ethics* (how should we treat animals and why?), *bioethics* (what are the implications of biological advances and how should they be used?), and *professional ethics* (what is the nature of a given profession's services, and what are the implications of this for those served?).

As noted earlier, there are areas of overlap. For example, bioethics is inquiry about the impact of biological and technological advances on humans and what actions are permissible, prohibited, or mandatory. Professional ethics related to healthcare professions has to do with understanding what is required for good professional action. Because healthcare professionals often use technology to provide good care, these areas overlap. A bioethical question might be "How do we decide who gets the one available heart of the four people who urgently need it?" Nursing ethics questions might be "What is my professional responsibility toward my patient whether or not he receives the heart? What is needed for his good care? How do I ensure that he gets what he needs for optimal well-being or to alleviate his suffering?" When Ethics or philosophical inquiry about good action is coupled with an area of human practice of some sort, for example, health care, business, or the law, it is called applied ethics. That is, theoretical understandings about what is good and/or the methods of philosophy (analysis and reasoning) are brought to bear upon a situation to both understand it and, if necessary, resolve it.

ETHICS: A FEW NECESSARY DISTINCTIONS

For the most part, in daily life when people discuss *ethics* they mean something very different from *ethics* as the word is being used here. In common language, *ethics* can merely mean how persons act in their daily lives and whether these actions accord with community values. In professional practice, *ethics* are sets of rules or standards, developed within the profession, that guide the actions of the professionals while working in their professional capacity. The American Nurses Association's (ANA) *Code of Ethics for Nurses with Interpretive Statements* (2001) is an example of this latter meaning of ethics. Nursing ethics scholars have recently provided more in-depth interpretations of the Code's interpretive statements (Fowler, 2010). These senses of *ethics* might be grasped more easily if a modifying term is added. For example, *personal ethics* is related to personal conduct, *nursing ethics* is related to the conduct of nurses as they engage in practice, *medical ethics* has to do with the conduct of physicians, and *bioethics* is concerned with the use of technological advances (and so might include a variety of health professionals, researchers, and technology professionals involved in using or propagating these).

Additionally, many people make a distinction between ethics and morals. They view *morals* as personal conduct that reflects personal values, whereas ethics is associated with critical reflection of the values (Weston, 2002). In fact, the root meaning of both terms is the same: "customs, mores, . . . conventions, institutions, laws" (Bahm, 1992, p. 8). For this text's purposes—considerations of professional judgment and action—the terms *ethical* and *moral* are used interchangeably to mean those actions most likely to further the goals of the profession.

Philosophy

The term *philosophy* can be used in a variety of ways. It can simply mean a personal view of a particular thing, as in "What is your philosophy about always telling the truth?," or, "What is your philosophy on balancing leisure and work?" Philosophy can also mean a group's view of the nature and purposes of its work; for example, there are a variety of philosophies of nursing practice. Philosophies of practice use the tools of philosophy to answer important questions about that practice. Florence Nightingale wrote hers as early as 1859 in *Notes on Nursing*. She believed that nurses attended to the patient's environment, making it conducive to natural healing. However, for the purposes of this discussion, *philosophy* means the overarching discipline, under which more specific philosophies belong.

Philosophy as a discipline encompasses the centuries-old endeavors of thinkers and scholars to find answers to the questions of existence. Philosophy, in this sense, has been concerned with a "search for wisdom about the universe and its workings," as well as the place and role of humans within the universe (Grace, 2004c, p. 280). The pre-Socratic (meaning before the time of Socrates) Greek philosophers such as Thales, Heraclitus, and Parmenides (around the 6th century B.C.) are considered the first philosophers (Russell, 1972). It is thought that before this time period people relied on mythological explanations for the mysterious and seemingly unpredictable workings of nature. The pre-Socratics, however, sought explanations using reason and observation.

For the purposes of this discussion, the discipline of philosophy uses reason and analysis to examine questions that are not answerable or not completely answerable by empirical science. As Nagel (1987) noted, "The main concern of philosophy is to question and understand very common ideas that all of us use every day" (p. 5) but often without giving much thought to their meanings. As an example, empirical science investigates the causes and effects of heart disease in the interests of both prevention and cures. Philosophical inquiry, however, would be concerned with questions such as "Is it possible to have a stable definition of health? Is health measurable?" If the answer to the question of "What is health?" is at all dependent on a subjective interpretation by a given individual, then it is not measurable by science.

Another way to look at this is to say philosophical inquiry highlights what cannot be true but does not necessarily give us truths. In fact, one major question of philosophy is "What is truth?" The main methods of philosophy are thinking and questioning. Reason is used to formulate and pose questions, seek out and examine possible answers, anticipate what objections could be made to the answers, or question whether counterexamples exist that would reveal a theory to be false. Philosophy also helps in understanding the limits of our knowledge.

The discipline of philosophy, then, can be seen to be the enterprise of inquiry itself. The major subareas of philosophical inquiry were presented earlier. The branch of philosophy most pertinent to the current discussion of healthcare professional responsibility is that of moral philosophy, also known as Ethics. From now on, when referring to that branch of philosophical inquiry that is concerned with human good, the terms *moral philosophy* or *Ethics* with a capital *"e" will be used* to distinguish it from the definition of ethics as rules or standards for action.

Moral Philosophy: The Study of Ethics

Ethics, as a term used to describe the area of philosophical inquiry concerned with what it means to say something is good, bad, or neutral in human activity, is also often referred to as moral philosophy. As explained earlier, this is a different view of ethics from that apparent in the term's use in everyday language. Philosophical inquiry is a theoretical endeavor; therefore, Ethics is also a theoretical endeavor. Ethics or moral philosophy is concerned with understanding human values. In fact, moral philosophy as a field of study often leads to the development of theories of value.

Value theories, often also called *moral theories*, try to answer such questions as "What do we mean when we say something is good, bad, praiseworthy, or blameworthy? What makes something, someone, or some action good or bad? Is something good because it is in line with divinely given rules using certain people as intermediaries (for example, Moses and the 10 commandments), or because it helps humans live a satisfying life? Are qualities of goodness and badness inherent in human nature? Are there some things that are absolutely right or wrong? Or are the understandings we have about right and wrong, good and bad, just conventions developed over the years to make it easier for humans to live in relative harmony with others?" Moral philosophers have different answers to these questions. The answers they give are meticulously thought through and provide important insights into the meaning and purposes of human life. It is, however, important to remember that these insights are always necessarily influenced by the lives and political times in which the philosophers engaged in their analyses, as well as by the philosophers' conscious or unconscious motivations for making sense of the world. Different theories can give conflicting directions related to a given situation depending on their premises and assumptions. Moral theories, then, are not capable of giving concrete direction in healthcare settings, because they are mostly theories about the conditions of living together within a society. Moreover, different moral theories give different answers to complex problems. Thus, what is considered "right" depends on which fundamental underlying premise is relied on to assert what is good for humans to strive for and why. In health care, however, the goal is to further the health and well-being of given persons or populations in the context of a particular goal. Moral theories serve to help explain the possible "considerations." They can provide clarity about a given situation, but they do not provide definitive answers. It might be desirable to have the comfort of relying on a particular theory for ethical decision making, but theories cannot serve this function. The following paragraphs are some examples of moral theories, along with critiques of their roles and limits in healthcare decision making.

Applied Ethics

As noted, the term m*oral philosophy* is synonymous with Ethics viewed as a theoretical endeavor—the larger sense of ethics. When philosophical and theoretical concepts, suppositions, and skills are applied to practices or human action, the tendency is to refer to this as applied ethics rather than applied moral philosophy, although there is no particular reason for this—it is simply a convention. Applied ethics uses the theoretical knowledge and assumptions gained as a result of ethical theorizing, as well as the skills and tools of moral philosophy (analysis), to solve difficult problems of living. Applied ethics, as its name implies, is the application of moral philosophy to actual situations where it is important to determine good or appropriate actions and where a person or group can be held responsible for these actions. Thus, branches of applied ethics are many and varied and include such entities as ecoethics (good human actions related to the ecosystem), animal ethics, bioethics, and professional ethics.

The appropriate ethical conduct of a profession such as nursing is determined by a synthesis of philosophical inquiry about the ontology of the profession (what nursing is, why it exists, and what its goals are), what constitutes good practice for the discipline (moral philosophy), and what is the force of the responsibility of the profession, both as an organized body and via its individual members, to engage in actions that further its goals (applied or practice ethics). The result of this synthesis is *nursing ethics*. Nursing ethics is an applied ethics. It is the study of what constitutes good nursing practice, what obstacles to good nursing practice exist, and what the responsibilities of nurses are related to their professional conduct. Nursing ethics can be exploratory, descriptive, or normative (also called prescriptive). These distinctions and their importance are discussed in detail in later chapters.

Moral Reasoning in Health Care: Tools

"Ethics as a field of inquiry studies the foundation for distinguishing good from bad and right from wrong in human action" (Grace, 2004a, pp. 299–300). "The theoretical interest is concerned with knowing; the practical interest is concerned with doing" (Melden, 1967, p. 2). Thus, moral reasoning in health care uses theoretical understandings, reasoned assumptions, and proposals about what is the good for humans and applies these theoretical explanations to problematic or complex situations where it is not clear what actions should be taken. In addition to the tools of philosophy, personal characteristics and abilities are needed to apply theory to particular cases. The purpose of this section is to describe the scope and limits of various philosophical approaches in resolving ethical issues in healthcare settings. This section is designed to familiarize APNs with the language and techniques of ethics in the interest of facilitating communication and collaboration on behalf of their patients or patient groups.

An important point that is emphasized throughout this book is that nursing goals serve as the linchpin for decision making and are related to different aspects of promoting health and human functioning as determined by the specialty practice focus and/or the leadership, supervisory, educational, and policy roles of the DNP, nurse practitioner (NP), clinical nurse specialist (CNS), or other expanded nursing role. The tools of applied ethics, then, facilitate an understanding of what is required to promote professional goals. In this sense, the question, "What is the good?" has already been answered by nursing's scholars and theorists. Unlike the larger unanswered or unanswerable philosophical question "What is the ultimate good for human beings?" the nursing profession has an answer related to its practice and existence. Nurse scholars and practitioners have determined what constitutes the profession's good.

The four main types of philosophical tools that apply to morally ambiguous healthcare situations are moral theories, moral perspectives, moral principles, and analytic techniques. Additionally, skills of mediation are increasingly recognized as a way to keep moral spaces open (Blackall, Simms, & Green, 2009; Dubler & Liebman, 2011; Fiester, 2012; Walker, 1993). That is, mediation allows the voices of everyone involved to be heard in an unbiased fashion and in the interest of a mutually satisfactory resolution. An extensive discussion of ethical theory and principles is not possible (or desirable) here—whole books are devoted to any one of the theories or principles, and further books are dedicated to the critiques of these. However, a comprehensive summary of those aspects of previous work in moral theory that are important for our contemporary understanding of moral authority and responsibility follows.

Moral Theory

What is moral theory? The simple answer is that it is a systematic justified explanation of what good means in terms of how human beings *do* or *should* seek to live their lives. That is, it may be either a descriptive (this is what people do or seem to believe) or prescriptive theory (this is what people *should do if the precepts and assumptions of the theory are right*). The author of the theory has tried to formulate an answer to the unsolved question "What is the meaning of good as it relates to human lives and human living?" The theorist, using reasoning, observation, and questioning, formulates a hypothesis and systematically justifies it, all the while trying to anticipate and address possible objections that could be raised by critics of the theory or by those holding different views. Because one of the tasks of philosophy is to show what cannot logically be true (the logic branch of philosophy), every moral theory has many philosopher critics.

Theorizing about human lives and the nature of good has been a human pursuit since the times of the ancient Greek philosophers such as Socrates (circa 450 B.C.), Plato, and Aristotle. There has been an ongoing quest to find systematic explanations and/or unchangeable, irrefutable truths about what is valuable in human lives. One reason this has been seen as important is the human desire for stability, the need to dispel uncertainty about action, and also the need for clarity and direction about how people should live. As stated earlier, moral theory may sometimes be referred to as value theory because its subject matter has to do with what is taken to be valuable, or what should be valued. That is, if it is possible to know what is good for humans to pursue, what sorts of lives are good to live, and which human characteristics are good to develop, and humans have sound reasoning, then society can feel it has a relatively firm footing from which to move forward.

THERE IS NO THEORETICAL AGREEMENT ABOUT THE ULTIMATE GOOD

No theorist, however, has found a flawless answer to the question, "What is good?"; neither have any developed theories that can completely withstand critique. Contemporary thinkers argue that this quest to find the highest good for human beings, or in Latin the *summun bonum*, is misbegotten. In fact, Dewey (1980), a philosopher of the American Pragmatist School, noted the reason that philosophers have struggled so hard and long for answers is that "man who lives in a world of hazards is compelled to seek for security" (p. 3), but the nature of human life is such that it cannot be found. Thus, a paradox exists.

When relatively cohesive theories have been proposed, they often made sense because of the contexts and time periods in which the particular philosopher lived, but these same theories may not remain relevant in current times or may not be relevant in all situations. Additionally, moral theories for the most part come up with different answers to similar questions, as noted earlier.

> The ultimate "good" for persons (or that which persons should or do strive for as an end in itself) has been conceptualized variously as happiness (Bentham, 1789/1967; Mill, 1863/1967), duty (Kant 1785/1967; Ross, 1930), the cultivation of virtue (Aristotle, trans. 1967; MacIntyre, 1984), or something else. This variation is the result of fundamentally contrasting beliefs about the nature of human beings and their place and purpose in the world. (Grace, 2004a, p. 299)

Thus, it is not surprising that there will be many different answers to the hard questions of life. Significant time is not devoted here to discussing the different moral theories because nurses do not tend to rely on one or another of them in clinical or healthcare settings although, from my experiences in teaching ethics, it is evident that people often *want* to use a moral theory to frame a question or justify action. This desire arguably stems from the mistaken idea that theories such as utility or Kantian deontology are authoritative—there is security in "right" answers and "right" actions. However, people can only ever be *reasonably* sure that their actions will have good consequences.

Moral theories can be useful in clarifying an issue or highlighting underlying assumptions. They may provide the structure with which to examine an issue, but nurses—especially APNs—must always be clear about why they think a theoretical perspective is pertinent to use for the task at hand. That is, it is necessary to understand the limits of the theory and what its flaws are, rather than uncritically relying on theories to answer difficult issues in health care.

More frequently, people use ideas from an assortment of moral theories to help clarify their thinking. These ideas are referred to as *principles*. Principles that are particularly pertinent to use in health settings are discussed shortly. However, as noted earlier, the goals of decision making in advanced practice situations are usually concerned with the well-being of a patient, or patient group, directly in the APN's sphere of practice. This is true even when APNs are in supervisory, collaborative, or consultative relationships with other providers—decisions are ultimately being made with the interests of the patient in mind. Finally, the tools of moral reasoning also prompt APNs to ask questions about underlying conditions that give rise to the problems in front of them and help APNs to recognize the wide scope of professional responsibilities.

DESCRIPTIVE VERSUS NORMATIVE THEORIES

Moral theories such as David Hume's (1777/1967) are based on observations of what people seem to believe with regard to good actions and what reasons they give for their decisions or actions. Such theories do not prescribe what people ought to do. They are observational and explanatory rather than having any moral force. They make no claims about the existence of some universal underlying purpose that human beings should strive to fulfill but rather aim to describe human action. Lately, a number of research studies have looked at how nurses practice, what they think is good care, what characteristics are important, and/or how they address obstacles (Corley et al., 2005; Doane, Pauly, Brown, & McPherson, 2004; Hardingham, 2004; Pavlish, Brown-Saltzman, Hersh, Shirk, & Rounkle, 2011; Peter, Lunardi, & Macfarland, 2004; Varcoe et al., 2004). These result in *descriptive* conceptions of ethical practice. That is, they do not say what is right or wrong, but rather what people think is right and wrong and the reasons they give for their actions.

Normative theories, on the other hand, direct action. "They are either, reasoned and logically explored explanations of the moral purpose of human interactions, or they are divinely revealed truths about good action (religious ethics)" (Grace, 2005, p. 102). Essentially they argue that because this or that is the ultimate good for human beings, then humans should pursue that good; there is a responsibility to do so. For example, although the ANA's *Code of Ethics for Nurses with Interpretive Statements* (2001) is not a theory as such, it is a normative document. It tells nurses how they ought to practice and what their behavior or conduct should be. It has moral force.

NORMATIVE MORAL THEORIES: SOME EXAMPLES

Two types of normative moral theory familiar to most people are (1) consequentialist, that is, good consequences are the focus of action, and (2) duty based or deontological, where what matters more than actual consequences is that a person acts according to his or her duty. Perhaps the best known consequentialist theories are those of the utilitarians. Jeremy Bentham (1748–1832) and John Stuart Mill (1806–1873) both were instrumental in the development of utilitarianism. Both were social reformers reacting to the injustices of the time period in which they lived. The Industrial Revolution, which started around 1760 according to Ashton (1961/1997), caused oppression of the new working classes and mass poverty—it resulted in vast inequities in wealth. A few industrialists held all the power and wealth (Engels, 1845/1987).

Bentham was heavily influenced by Hume's descriptive moral theory, which proposed that most human values are socially constructed and stem both from intrinsic human characteristics such as the ability to sympathize with others and the pleasurable effects of benevolent acts as enacted, experienced, or observed (this is a greatly simplified explanation of Hume's work). Hume is credited with introducing the idea of a utility principle into the English language. It represents the idea that human responses are fortified in relation to perception of the usefulness of their actions to others and the pleasure gained from this (Hume, 1748/1963).

Bentham, a peer and friend of John Stuart Mill's father, James Mill, further developed the principle of utility, presenting it as one having moral force. That is, if it is true that humans desire happiness and shun pain and suffering, then that is the good toward which human beings *should* strive. Giving these ideas moral force allowed the social reformers to criticize inequities caused by the Industrial Revolution and to push for reform. Many reforms, "legal, political, social, and educational" (Flew, 1984, p. 41), did occur as a result of utilitarian ideas. As Melden (1967) notes, "Hume's principle of Utility was transformed [by Bentham] with unwavering consistency into 'the greatest happiness principle'" (p. 367).

Following Bentham, Mill (1861/1965) wrote that "pleasure and freedom from pain are the only things desirable as ends . . . all other desirable things (which are as numerous in the utilitarian as in any other scheme [*sic*]) are desirable either for the pleasure inherent in themselves, or as a means to the promotion of pleasure and the preventions of pain" (p. 281). Pleasure was characterized as qualitative in nature in Mill's view, so he distinguished between mere physical pleasures and higher level intellectual ones. Further, in his view the goals of action were to maximize overall happiness for a society and minimize overall pain or suffering. Each person's happiness is equally important; in this sense, the theory presents an impartial view. "Because of their focus on overall good, there are implications to these theories that many would find troubling" (Grace, 2004a, p. 300) and not in tune with common intuitions about good actions. For example, according to this approach, it would be permissible to cause harm to one innocent person if it would relieve 100 other sufferers from pain. However, when any one person becomes a means to achieving the good of another or others, all persons are in danger of becoming that person whose worth is being discounted. There are other critiques of utilitarianism, but the most salient for this text's purposes is that APNs are interested in the well-being of each patient, and this requires understanding who the patient is. Context and details, the *"who"* of nurses' patients, are important. Utilitarian considerations might require nurses to ignore individual details, deferring to an obligation to provide an overall good. Nevertheless, in social policy and justice settings, the ideas behind utilitarianism are important. People do not tend to think that social arrangements need benefit only a few when the majority is living in poverty. In healthcare settings, APNs obviously do think that the possible consequences of their actions are crucial considerations in planning actions—however, particular consequentialist theories do not provide a stable framework for APNs because of their flaws.

Deontologic or duty-based theories are also unsuitable as blanket frameworks for decision making in health care. Immanuel Kant's (1724–1804) moral philosophy is deontologic. It focuses on the idea that something other than consequences is the most important consideration in decision making. That something is duty. The main philosophical assumption underlying Kant's (1785/1967) theory is that human beings are rational animals. Humans have the ability to reason and therefore the capacity for self-governance. Indeed, "the hallmark of human beings is their innate reasoning ability" (Grace, 2004a, p. 300). Because humans have this capacity, Kant went further to say that people have a duty to do the action that their reason tells them is the most rational. How do we do this? We ask ourselves whether in all similar circumstances we would agree that people could act in the same way that we are proposing to act and whether we would be willing to support a rule to this effect. If the answer is yes, then it is permissible to act in this way. If the answer is no, then duty forbids the action. Duty forbids us because it would be irrational for us to act in a way that we would not wish others to act. Kant called this principle the Categorical Imperative because it is unwavering in its moral force. People must act from duty, regardless of consequences. For Kant, interestingly, it was this capacity of human beings to determine right from wrong actions that made them, in his eyes, worthy of respect as individuals; this capacity underlies the principle of autonomy, which will be discussed in more detail shortly.

Other versions of duty-based theories are derived from religious traditions. Kant's exquisitely argued and detailed theorizing was an attempt to avoid the criticisms leveled at religious theories by basing the idea of moral duties on the human capacity to reason. For Kant (1785/1967), then, there were absolute rules, such as truthfulness. He wrote that deviating from the truth even when it might not be convenient is irrational because if people cannot rely on the sincerity of others with whom they are conversing, then meaningful communication becomes impossible. Interestingly, Kant did not think that women and children had the same capacity for reasoning as men.

Criticisms of duty-based theories include: (1) The rules are too abstract to apply in practice; for example, how specific should we be in determining whether a situation is similar to another? What is truth telling and does it include withholding information that might be unpleasant to us and yet not necessary for us to know? (2) What if telling the truth might cause harm to another? Yet reason (Categorical Imperative) dictates that people should not harm each other. How do people decide between equally compelling duties?

Ethical Principles

It is clear that although moral theories exist as attempts to describe how human beings act or propose how human beings should act, and additionally provide justification for the soundness of the theory, they should not be treated as authoritative frameworks for action in healthcare settings. Nevertheless, they do provide some important insights about human values and characteristics: utilitarianism for its ability to critique social injustices, and deontology for its implications that there are general rules that all people can rationally agree on.

The APN's job is to determine both what are good professional actions in situations that require attention to nuance and particularities and what is needed to identify and address more entrenched problems related to inadequacies in the healthcare system. A key point is that certain principles

17

derived from moral theories, together with analytic philosophical techniques, have proved helpful in healthcare settings for separating out aspects of complex situations, illuminating hidden assumptions and factors, and revealing gaps in information. Also, they are helpful in assisting clinicians as they reflect on why they feel uneasy about certain situations. It is important for collaboration and communication that the implications of certain principles are understood. Yet there is often confusion about the origins, definition, and implications of a given ethical principle. The next section explores some important principles in a little more depth, and in later chapters the principles are discussed relative to specialty practice problems.

WHAT ARE ETHICAL PRINCIPLES?

Ethical principles are rules, standards, or guidelines for action that are derived from theoretical propositions (different moral theories) about what is good for humans. Important principles emerge over time as their usefulness in imposing order on a situation, highlighting important considerations in solving complex issues, locating the proper object of decision making, or enhancing social harmony is realized. They reflect philosophical, cultural, religious, and societal beliefs about what is valuable. Thus, what are considered priority principles in one society may not be taken as important in another society. In Western cultures, particularly in relation to problems of healthcare delivery, several principles have retained importance over the last few decades. The most prominent examples of Western principles that are pertinent to healthcare settings have been explored and described in detail by Beauchamp and Childress (2009) and include autonomy, nonmaleficence, beneficence, and justice. These "four clusters of principles derive from considered judgments in the common morality and professional traditions in healthcare" (p. 25). APNs are charged with determining which, if any, apply in a given situation and whether clarity or insights about a dilemma or ethical issue can be gained by using these principles to explore the problem. Put another way, in healthcare practice professional judgment is still needed to determine whether a given principle applies and, if it does, how it will be honored. For example, most people understand that respect for another's autonomy is an important ethical principle, and that, all things being equal, this respect is likely to serve another's good. However, if the issue that the APN encounters is related to an incompetent colleague, then the pertinent principle to use as a guide is nonmaleficence (or how to prevent a patient from being harmed by an incompetent colleague).

In nursing practice, advocacy, caring, engagement with the patient, and knowing the patient within his or her context are also important principles derived from the profession's philosophies of practice, goals, and the roles of nurses. These principles are explored further in the next chapter.

USEFULNESS AND LIMITS OF ETHICAL PRINCIPLES

Ethical principles are useful in helping APNs identify salient issues, clarify important factors, uncover hidden assumptions, and affirm appropriate actions. However, the goals of nursing drive the principles used rather than the other way around. For example, the principle of beneficence (in general) exhorts APNs to provide a good, but the goals of nursing describe what that good is (e.g., promotion of health or relief of suffering), and nursing knowledge, skills, and experience provide the recipe for achieving the good. Motivation provides the impetus for action.

It is critical to understand that principles alone cannot solve healthcare problems because two or more principles pertinent to a situation can give conflicting direction. Additionally, principles tend to be too abstract and nonspecific to be practical. For example, no one is ever completely autonomous; everyone is influenced by conscious and unconsciously experienced pressures—so, what degree of autonomy is acceptable and how is this determined? Principles are not always sensitive to context. For example, what does *autonomous choice* mean when the patient is from a culture where family, not individual, decision making is the norm, or when a controlling relative is pressuring the patient? Finally, human decision making and the actions that flow from this process involve conscious and subconscious values and emotions as well as reasoning, so these are also considerations. In the next few paragraphs, the four major principles highlighted by Beauchamp and Childress (2009) are explored in more detail, as are other perspectives that serve as useful tools in clinical and practice ethics. Beauchamp and Childress's book is recommended for those who want to delve in some depth into a detailed analysis of the implications of these principles and their use in healthcare decision making. However, the unquestioning use of principles to analyze everyday as well as dilemmatic ethical issues in healthcare practice has been criticized by many ethicists as not giving a full enough picture of the issues at hand (Clouser & Gert, 1990; Engelhardt, 1996; Evans, 2000; Fiester, 2007; Gert, Culver, & Clouser, 2006; Macklin, 2003). Fiester (2007) argues that "the Principlist Paradigm is a tool that can only flag certain types of issues and considerations as morally salient in a case, and it leaves many others undetected" (p. 4). The next section will highlight both helpful and problematic aspects of these principles when used in nursing or healthcare practice settings. Other philosophical perspectives that can aid APNs in solving practice problems include feminist ethics, caring ethics, narrative ethics, and virtue ethics. These approaches can remind APNs to ask questions of the situations that permit the uncovering of hidden aspects. In later chapters, these concepts are illustrated in the specialty cases and case analyses.

THE PRINCIPLE OF AUTONOMY

If 20 people were randomly polled and asked about their understanding of the term *autonomy*, there would probably be several related but different answers. Autonomy is a term that is susceptible to a variety of interpretations. The word comes from Greek and literally means self-rule. It was originally used to describe the nature of governance in Hellenic cities (Beauchamp & Childress, 2009) rather than to describe individual capacities or rights. Subsequent understandings of autonomy are related to persons as individuals. Among the various meanings are self-determination, independence, freedom of the will, and a person's ability to regulate personal conduct using reason. It has become one of the more powerful moral principles in framing Western social and political systems and underlies ideas of universal human rights.

Because all of these different if overlapping meanings exist, it is important that clinicians clarify what definition of *autonomy* they are using when engaged in collaborative discussions or when presenting a patient's point of view. Transparency is necessary to avoid miscommunication. There are two main senses of the term *autonomy* as it is used in healthcare settings. In the first sense, autonomy means an attitude of respect for persons regardless of the incidental characteristics of any given human being. The principle charges people to respect all other persons as equally worthy of moral concern, simply because that person is a human being. This principle is justified by several different philosophical and theological arguments (it is beyond the purposes of this text to detail each argument). However, one branch of arguments asserts that the individual importance of human beings is derived from a divine, God-given or innate purpose. A second more secular string of arguments posits that all human beings share interests in being alive and flourishing, and thus all have a right to expect equal moral treatment. When individuals or groups of individuals are treated differently, it actually puts all persons at risk from a change in attitudes that then allows anyone to be treated as less than fully human, which in turn lessens the prohibition against being treated as a means to someone else's ends. For example, slavery treated a whole group as if it did not warrant the same respect as other groups of persons—slaves were a means to the economic and agricultural ends of the slave owners and possessed no individual rights. Autonomy as respect for persons, then, means that regardless of socioeconomic status and intellect, all people will receive equal consideration with others in social arrangements and interactions.

In the second sense, autonomy is the right to make personal decisions; historical arguments for this are based on the idea that human beings have the ability to reason and decide for themselves what actions are best, whether on behalf of themselves or in interactions with others. In current healthcare practice, the recognition that patients have rights to self-determine both acceptable treatment and with whom information may be shared is derived from the ethical principle of autonomy. However, autonomy is often interpreted by nurses and others as the right to make bad healthcare decisions. This is a distorted view of the concept and its use in healthcare settings. Honoring autonomy means the professional is responsible for evaluating what the person needs in the way of information and assisting the person to interpret all available knowledge in light of his or her own projects and desires.

Philosophical Theories of Autonomy

Immanuel Kant (1724–1804) is perhaps the best known proponent of autonomy as a moral principle. He wrote that because human beings have the capacity to reason, decide, and act, they should be free from the interference of others, at least as far as personal decision making is concerned. Moreover, "reason is the ruler of our will" (Kant, 1785/1967, p. 322). Our will is good in and of itself. This was evident to Kant because of "the common idea of duty and moral laws" that is evident in social life (p. 319). Kant gave the example that people know lying is wrong—they can reason this out for themselves—because lying works against social interests in being able to communicate and interact. Thus, it was self-evident to Kant that morality is an a priori condition, inherent in people. What he meant by this is that human beings are born with a capacity (and therefore are purposed) to determine what are moral actions and to carry these out. Kant believed that because man has the inherent capacity for moral decision making, he should never be used as a means to an end but always respected as having dignity and being equally worthy of moral consideration as any other man.

As previously mentioned, Kant did not view women and children as having the same capacity to reason as men.

For Kant there were two aspects to autonomy. Men, at least, are (1) capable of making their own decisions using reason, and (2) have the inherent structure to permit them to act morally (create moral rules) using the Categorical Imperative described earlier. Like Kant, "John Stuart Mill also argued that human beings—women included—have the capacity and the right to make their own decisions" (Grace, 2004b, p. 33). For Mill, diversity and creativity were to be welcomed. Freedom, he believed, is in the interests of society—it allows people to flourish and makes for better societies. Indeed, for Mill the only conditions under which it was permissible to interfere with the actions of persons was when their actions posed a serious threat of harm to another person, including restricting the other person's freedom. Mill did not believe that restricting an individual's actions for that person's own good was permissible. In healthcare settings, both theoretically and ideally, the proscription against overriding the autonomy of another cannot and does not go to this extreme. There are occasions when the ethical action is to stop a person who is at risk for serious harm from an action, at least until the APN can determine whether the person's act is informed, reasonable, and in line with his or her own values and preferences. Whether in actuality the APN always intervenes when there is ambiguity about a patient's decision-making capacity is a different issue that is discussed later in this book in relation to obstacles to good practice.

Contemporarily, there is agreement among moral philosophers that the reasoning process of human beings is never completely free from the influence of such things as culturally determined beliefs, emotions, lack of information, or other environmental conditions (Grace, 2004b). Autonomy is always a "more or less" condition: the more powerful and complex the influences we are subjected to, the less likely we are to be able to exercise our autonomy effectively. Decisions may seem to be autonomous when in actuality they are heavily influenced by overt or hidden influences. Recent research in cognitive, behavioral, and moral psychology highlights a more powerful role of subconscious mechanisms than previously recognized and accounted for in moral decision making (Doris, 2010; Eagleman, 2011). All people suffer from cognitive biases that prevent them from thinking as logically as they think they do (Kahneman, 2011). Therefore, people do not possess even the potential for the sort of detached reasoning that Kant theorized was inherent to human nature.

People are more or less capable of logical reasoning but never have absolute freedom to exercise reasoning that is divorced from unconscious, emotional, or powerful external influences.

Nevertheless, it is generally accepted that most people know themselves and their preferences better than other people can, and thus given certain conditions they have the right to exercise this freedom without interference. After all, they will live with the consequences of decisions made. Indeed, this moral right has been legislated as a legal right under the Patient Self-Determination Act of 1991 (PSDA) in the United States and is acknowledged as a moral right in many other countries (European Patients' Forum, 2009). Patients have the right to decide whether they will accept or refuse health care, including treatment and interventions. The PSDA as well as European patient rights guidelines and those of other countries are discussed in later chapters. It is important to note that many follow the prescriptions of the Universal Declaration of Human Rights adopted by member states of the United Nations in 1948. Two questions related to autonomy in either sense, respect for persons or the right to make one's own decisions, arise here. First, and in addition to the possibility of overt and hidden influences on decision making, some people are not capable of autonomous decision making because they either lack the developmental or cognitive skills necessary. This lack may be temporary or permanent. What is the responsibility of healthcare professionals in such cases? The short answer is that where possible, a healthcare providers responsibility is to try to discover what is known about the person and what his or her wishes would most likely be, so that actions are still predicated on the individual and the way that person has lived his or her life. However, in cases where health professionals are not able to determine what a person would have wanted, the *"reasonable person"* standard can be used. The healthcare provider tries, as a proxy, to decide what a reasonable person would want under similar circumstances. This issue of proxy decision makers is discussed in later chapters and also as related to specialty practice. Proxy decision makers cannot be said to be making autonomous decisions in the sense of autonomy discussed earlier, however. The decisions they make are on behalf of another, not themselves. Proxy or substitute decision makers are, nevertheless, supposed to support the autonomy of their wards by representing as accurately as possible what they would likely want.

The second question relates to the shifting nature of factors influencing the exercise of autonomy. This is often also referred to as *decision-making capacity.* For APNs, related questions are (1) How do we decide when and under what circumstances a person might be deemed capable of autonomous decision making? and (2) What is necessary to facilitate autonomous decision making? Criteria have been proposed that facilitate judgments about whether a person has sufficient decision-making capacity to make a decision that is likely to serve his or her interests. These criteria present their own challenges, but they do provide a framework for judging and thus for addressing impediments to decision making.

The President's Commission (1982) formulated from the pertinent literature, commission members' expertise, and discussions a minimum set of capacities needed for competent decision making. These are as follows:

- Possession of a set of values and goals
- The ability to communicate and to understand information
- The ability to reason and deliberate about one's choice (President's Commission, 1982, p. 57)

This means that for a voluntary choice to be made, professionals need to evaluate the cognitive maturity and abilities of the person. They must assess what information the person needs and how best to provide this—thus, a process of informing (rather than a singular presentation of information) is often needed. An evaluation of influences that might interfere with information processing is important. Interfering influences could include any of the following: unconscious or conscious psychological pressures; physiologic factors such as hypoxia, fever, pain; or contextual issues such as economics (personal and institutional), provider pressures, or wishing to please a provider. Finally, the patient should be able to describe how a given course of action is likely to map on to his or her own life trajectory.

Perhaps the most important thing to understand is that patients who obviously do not grasp the implications of proposed actions for their own goals and future life are not in a position to act autonomously. Thus, respecting autonomy in health care does not simply mean letting a patient make his or her own mistakes. Finally, in respecting autonomy there is a tendency not to interfere with people's decisions if providers are sure these are informed and/or if the risks are low. However, if the risks of a proposed course of action chosen by a patient are high, then providers must make a more concerted effort to ensure that these are autonomous decisions. Overriding a person's autonomy is a serious business but is sometimes necessary to serve the patient's interests. The rationale for overriding a patient's decision is that this is most likely to serve the patient's own interests and preserve autonomy (if the person dies—then no further autonomy is possible in this life anyway).

THE PRINCIPLE OF NONMALEFICENCE

Of the ethical principle nonmaleficence, Beauchamp and Childress (2009) note that "in medical ethics it has been closely associated with the maxim *primum non nocere:* 'Above all [or first] do no harm'" (p. 149). Some scholars have said that nonmaleficence means to do no *intentional* harm. In healthcare practice, and especially in APN practice settings, nonmaleficence is a nuanced principle with several implications. Some scholars treat nonmaleficence as a subcategory of beneficence (the obligation to do good or provide a good). However, exploring it separately facilitates better conceptual clarity. Moreover, healthcare professionals, by virtue of their interventional and therapeutic roles, are often in a position to cause harm in the course of attending to a patient's needs. First, what is meant by harm? Does psychological, spiritual, or economic distress count as harm, or does only physical distress count? Beauchamp and Childress (2009) construe harm as "thwarting, defeating, or setting back some party's interests . . . (A) *harmful action* by one party may not be wrong or unjustified (*on balance), although acts of harming in general are prima facie wrong*" (italics as in the original) (p. 152). *Prima facie* means on first sight. Thus, harms that are generally forbidden may occasionally be justified. In civilian life, this means a robber may be harmed by incarceration, but this harm is justified by the wrong actions of the robber and the robber's infringement on the rights of another. In healthcare settings, harms are not justifiable unless they set back the patient's interests temporarily to provide a longer term benefit. For example, inserting an intravenous catheter to provide fluids and antibiotics to someone in septic shock may be permissible even if the patient objects because not doing so risks irreversible damage, and APNs do not have time to evaluate the person's decision-making capacity.

For the purposes of this discussion, it is best to think of harm as either any avoidable distress caused to the patient in the course of providing care, or avoidable distress that is observed by the professional and/or experienced by the patient and brought to the attention of the professional but that is ignored or left unaddressed. Thus it is clear that harm can be caused both by actions and by inaction. APNs can do harm in several ways; most are *unintentional* but nevertheless often avoidable:

- APNs might fail to adequately understand a patient's needs and thus not protect him or her from preventable harms related to unmet needs.
- An APN's skills and competence might be inadequate to care for the patient's recognized needs, yet the APN fails to seek qualified assistance.
- The APN can neglect to anticipate foreseeable harmful effects from a proposed course of action.
- The APN can fail to intervene to protect a patient against the actions of an impaired, incompetent, or careless colleague.
- The APN can fail to assist the patient manage pressures from others that result in him or her accepting unwanted treatment.

In advanced practice roles, nurses can also cause harm by referring patients to inappropriate colleagues or not adequately training or supervising others who are caring for the patient under an APN's direction. Patients can also be harmed by ongoing interventions that are not likely to achieve desired effects (for example, chemotherapy that can only minimally prolong life and causes suffering in the process). Nonmaleficence, then, is closely aligned with ideas of accountability for the APN's own practice and for practice actions. Accountability means that care providers take responsibility for trying to anticipate foreseeable harms so that these can either be minimized or are balanced against the good that the actions are intended to achieve. Moreover, the effects on the nurse of causing or not preventing harms include moral distress, as noted earlier. Because moral distress can lead to a nurse distancing himself/herself from patients or even to leaving the profession, more diffuse harms to patients may result from the loss to the profession of experienced caring nurses. The APN can inadvertently cause harm through ignorance, incompetence, or failure to understand the patient's unique needs and desires. Harm can also be caused to patients when the APN cannot get them optimal treatment.

Additionally, nurses can cause harm indirectly. The principle of nonmaleficence provides what in legal terms would be called a duty of due care. "Due care is taking sufficient and appropriate care to avoid causing harm, as the circumstances demand of a reasonable and prudent person" (Beauchamp & Childress, 2009, p. 153). Another implication of this principle is that APNs are responsible for balancing the risks of interventions and treatments with the likely benefit. As illustrated with the chemotherapy example, within acute care settings harm can be caused by continuing life-sustaining treatments when the chances of recovery are minimal.

THE PRINCIPLE OF BENEFICENCE

For healthcare professionals the principle of beneficence might be viewed as a more active principle than nonmaleficence because it is the duty to provide a good or to benefit persons. In a sense the very reason for the existence of the healthcare professions is beneficence. These professions exist to provide a service that requires specialized training and skills. In public life, *beneficence* "connotes acts of mercy, kindness, and charity" toward others (Beauchamp & Childress, 2009, p. 166). It concerns the duty one person has to provide benefit to another. Certain moral theories, such as utilitarianism, have as their singular underlying premise the idea that people have a duty to maximize the good in society. Beneficence is unlike nonmaleficence in that it is not morally required of societal members except in special circumstances such as parents or guardians toward their wards. "Whether beneficence is viewed as a moral requirement of societal members very much depends upon [the] philosophical beliefs," culture, and values of the individual or prevalent societal values (Grace, 2004a, p. 317). Although beneficent actions may not be morally required, they do serve a purpose in maintaining the cohesiveness of society. In Western countries at least, and to greater or lesser extent in other countries, people tend to think that if they can easily help someone who is struggling then they should. This is the basis for charitable actions.

In healthcare settings, though, beneficence is viewed as the duty to maximize benefits and minimize harm to patients. It is morally required of the clinician acting as clinician, whether they are physicians, nurses, physical therapists, respiratory therapists, and so on. The goals of healthcare professionals are beneficent—they are inherently for the patient's good, and more broadly, to further societal health. As argued earlier, healthcare professions exist because they provide a critical good for persons. Therefore, beneficence underlies all actions of the professional while engaging in role-related activities.

Paternalism

Paternalism is often taken to be a derogatory attitude that connotes one person's attempts to control another or condescension toward another. However, in its original or legal sense, the principle of paternalism is both an ethical and legal principle that protects the interests of one who cannot be self-protective. The principle is derived from the term "parens patriae," or the state's interests in protecting the vulnerable in society from neglect or abuse. There are extensive philosophical and political debates about whether and when legislative or governmental paternalism is permissible (for the collected arguments see Coons & Weber [2013], *Paternalism: Theory and Practice*). However, in healthcare settings paternalistic actions are ethically permissible or even obligatory—depending on the circumstances—if they serve an incapacitated person's best interests. A person is incapacitated when he or she is unable to make a substantially informed decision as described under the principle of autonomy. Paternalistic actions, then, are beneficent actions. They promote the good for a person who is unable, whether because of cognitive or developmental status, to advocate for his or her own best interests. These best interests can be served by using the person's own history, values, and beliefs where possible. However, in the case of a person who has never had capacity or whose history is unknown or unknowable, the standard used is that of a "reasonable person." Beauchamp and Childress (2009) define paternalism as "the intentional overriding of one person's known preferences or actions by another person, where the person who overrides justifies the action by the goal of benefiting or avoiding harm to the person whose preferences or actions are overridden" (p. 208). Thus, the patient's own interests are the main focus of paternalistic actions. In viewing paternalism this way, it becomes clear that knowledge of the patient in context and as an individual with a life history, beliefs, and values, where this is possible, is a crucial goal of paternalism. Beauchamp and Childress (2009) propose five criteria for justifying paternalistic actions:

1. A patient is at risk of a significant preventable harm.
2. The paternalistic action will probably prevent the harm.
3. The projected benefits to the patient of the paternalistic action outweigh its risks to the patient.
4. There is no reasonable alternative to the limitation of autonomy.
5. The least autonomy-restrictive alternative that will secure the benefits and reduce the risks is adopted. (p. 216)

To summarize, paternalism is sometimes understood differently in healthcare settings than warranted by a fuller understanding of the principle. It has assumed negative connotations in many instances. Some people, nurses and others, have used it to label the condescending, arrogant, or even self-interested behavior of healthcare providers toward patients who they think are making bad decisions. Patients may be persuaded to accept certain treatments, important information may be withheld from them, or a competent patient may have his or her decision overridden. Understanding the real nature of paternalistic actions as both beneficent (patient's best interests) and supportive in the long run of autonomy (restoring the patient to a state where autonomy can be exercised) keeps the focus on the needs of the patient and away from the lure of expediency or other conflicts of interest.

CONFLICTS BETWEEN BENEFICENCE AND AUTONOMY

Sometimes ensuring beneficence seems to be in conflict with the principle of autonomy. For example, a patient with impending sepsis refuses to have a cannula inserted so that treatment with fluids and antibiotics can begin. At first sight, it seems as if there is a dilemma: honor her autonomy or override it and give the fluids because this is what will save her life. The conflict, however, may be false. If the patient does not meet all of the criteria for voluntary informed consent, then she is not capable of exercising her autonomy. She is not adequately aware of the risks and benefits of refusal. Thus, the beneficent action is to treat but to minimize the harms that may stem from overriding her decision. She may, for instance, feel disrespected or that her trust was undermined. Additionally, beneficence supports the idea that as soon as the patient regains decision-making capacity, she resumes her right to make her own decisions, as long as these are adequately informed and align with her own life values and goals. Beneficence does not, as some have assumed, mean that providers know what is best for the patient, but rather that decisions are made based on the individual patient and his or her values, beliefs, and what is known about the patient's life and preferences. In overriding a person's autonomy, health professionals are still charged with formulating actions that accord with an understanding of the patient as an individual with unique characteristics.

THE PRINCIPLE OF JUSTICE

Several different conceptions of justice exist. In Western societies, *retributive justice* has to do with punishment for problematic actions; *restorative or compensatory justice* has to do with restoring to people what they lost in being harmed by another or others. These two forms can be considered noncomparative stances or perspectives. They both are concerned with "seeing to it that people receive that to which they are entitled, that their rights are recognized and protected" (Munson, 2008, p. 774). *Comparative justice*, on the other hand, has to do with how the benefits and burdens of living in a social context—where people are dependent on one another for certain goods and services—should be distributed across a society. For health care and healthcare delivery purposes, distributive justice can also be conflated with *social justice*. It is an important ethical principle in times or circumstances of limited resources.

Philosophical theories of justice try to show what are or would be sound justifications for the rules of distribution. In this sense, comparative justice is social justice. Theories try to delineate which formal social systems will result in the fairest conception of deciding who should get what in terms of social goods such as education, food, shelter, and health care. Buchanan (2000) reports that social justice has been an important concept for centuries and continues to be "central to human understandings of socially significant values" (p. 155).

> There are two broad socially oriented ideas regarding justice. One perspective views justice as being based on deserving it—those who are more worthy of merit or who contribute more are viewed as deserving of better social benefits. The other perspective views justice as equalizing benefits across society regardless of merit. This latter view is "justice as fairness." (Grace, 2005, p. 120)

In the literature related to health care, the predominant accounts are of justice as fairness. The principle of equality underlies accounts of justice as fairness. Justice is impartial in the sense that each person is considered initially as equally worthy of concern. Underlying the various theories is a basic principle that "similar cases ought to be treated in similar ways" (Munson, 2008, p. 774). The conception of distributive justice that is probably most often cited contemporarily is that of John Rawls. His work, *A Theory of Justice* (1971), is a systematic look at the sort of social structures that would need to exist for justice as fairness to prevail. Rawls takes as a starting point Kant's ideas about people as rational and able to divine which actions are morally permissible, obligatory, or forbidden. Rawls's method is a hypothetical device. That is, he wants to show what the underpinnings of a just social system would be and what just institutions would look like. Because man is his own lawmaker, as we have seen from the idea of the Categorical Imperative (the right action is the one that I could agree everyone else *should* take in similar circumstances—that is, it is ethically sound), the design of the system will be dependent on a "group of persons" in the "original position" (Rawls, 1971, p. 12) who do not know their standing in society, or what physical characteristics or material goods they would possess, nor what their "natural assets, and abilities" (p. 12) would be. The hypothesis is that such a group would come up with the rules and standards necessary for the initiation and arrangement of institutions that would ensure everybody is served fairly. That is, if one did not know whether one would be rich or poor, one would be more likely to build in remedies for those who are the least well off even if that did somewhat disadvantage those who are well endowed with worldly goods.

Rawls identifies two rules of justice that he believes would emerge from a group's deliberations taking place behind this "veil of ignorance" about their individual states and traits (Rawls, 1971, p. 136). "First: each person is to have an equal right to the most extensive liberty compatible with a similar liberty for others. Second: social and economic inequalities are to be arranged such that they are both (a) reasonably expected to be to everyone's advantage, and (b) attached to positions and offices open to all" (Rawls, 1971, p. 60).

As might be expected, Rawls's theory is subject to a variety of criticisms, including that the nature of human beings is such that this would not eliminate jockeying for power and advantage and thus upset any ethical system initiated. However, the salient aspects of the theory for the purposes of this discussion are that justice in this sense means being alert to inequities and being willing to address them. Any inequities within a society's arrangements should be slanted toward benefiting the least well off. In contemporary U.S. health care, most would agree that justice as fairness might be accepted in spirit but not in reality. Nevertheless, for APNs the ideas behind justice as fairness cohere with the premises of the ANA's (2003) *Social Policy Statement* and its *Code of Ethics for Nurses with Interpretive Statements* (ANA, 2001). Therefore, it is among APNs' professional responsibilities to promote justice in health care because without this, the most vulnerable will remain most at risk for not receiving good care.

Justice is an important concept related to research, managed care, and health disparities. The important thing to keep in mind about justice as fairness is that it is an impartial look at inequities. It might be a requirement of justice as fairness that the special needs of a disadvantaged group are considered, but each member of the group is impartially and equally accorded that consideration. The nature of justice in health care, then, is that in some circumstances it might give rise to tensions for the APN. For example, a nurse's clinical judgment leads her to believe that her patient needs an expensive drug that is not on formulary, perhaps because of prior sensitivities to other drugs or because current drugs are detrimental in some other way. She feels that she must advocate for her patient to get this drug and that other patients might also benefit but not to the same degree. In advocating for this treatment, resources may be diverted away from others in her care.

Others have argued that although justice as fairness is meant to ensure equal consideration for like cases, in practice people who are perceived as the most meritorious sometimes receive priority over those with a higher need. For example, celebrities seem to get moved up the waiting list for organs more rapidly that others who may be in more immediate need or have fewer resources (Simmerling, 2007).

The justice as fairness perspective in healthcare settings also tends to be directed toward the allocation of scarce resources in terms of technologically or biologically based innovations and interventions and as arising within the healthcare institution or as a result of the types of insurance or funding available. The disease model of health care predominates in the United States in a way that it does not (or not so much) in other countries with universal healthcare coverage. This sometimes directs attention away from looking for inequalities as arising from the "fabric of society" (Grace & Willis, 2012). Therefore more than just redistribution of resources is necessary to rectify injustices and to promote health and healing. In a recent article in *Nursing Outlook* my colleague Danny Willis and I (2012) critiqued the problem that social justice viewed as fairness does not necessarily facilitate looking for the source of intractable injustices in the fabric of societal institutions and arrangements. Moreover, injustices can seriously affect health or the ability of persons to heal. We used an alternate conception of social justice to look at the problem of child abuse and its long-range effects on health. Powers and Faden's (2006) model takes the job of social justice as being concerned with ensuring a basic minimum level of six essential dimensions of well-being needed for living a "minimally decent" life (Grace & Willis, 2012). This conception matches the responsibility of the nursing profession for individual and societal health as outlined in the nursing code of ethics for various countries, including the ANA (2001) and the International Council of Nurses (ICN, 2012). Chapter 4 on human rights and responsibilities expands on the discussion of justice presented here. For the purposes of this text, it is necessary to have a foundational understanding of justice in order to optimize health, both for individuals and the larger society.

THE PRINCIPLES OF VERACITY AND FIDELITY

These two principles, while not achieving the same status in healthcare ethical decision making as Beauchamp and Childress's framework of the four ethical ideals discussed earlier, are nevertheless important in professional ethics. They represent professional characteristics or intents that support the realization of autonomy, beneficence, nonmaleficence, and even justice. Veracity is about the duty to be truthful. The term has its origins in the French *véracité* and medieval Latin *veritas* and means "the quality or character of speaking the truth . . . truthfulness, honesty, trustworthiness" (Brown, 1993, Vol. 2). A related principle is that of fidelity. Fidelity means "loyalty, faithfulness, unswerving allegiance" to another (Brown, 1993, Vol. 1).

Veracity

Although it might seem that veracity is a simple concept—of course APNs should be truthful in their dealings with patients, families, and others—this is not always so easy to accomplish, especially in light of trying to honor the principles of beneficence and nonmaleficence. What does it mean to be truthful? Truthfulness is generally thought to be supportive of autonomy, but is it always? Beauchamp and Childress (2009) note, "[v]eracity in the health care setting refers to comprehensive, accurate, and objective transmission of information, as well as to the way the professional fosters the patient's or subject's understanding" (p. 289). But stark veracity can be harmful to some patients in certain circumstances. Additionally, APNs do not always know what interventions work under what circumstances. How then can APNs decide when, if ever, the standard of veracity should be bent for the good of the patient? Sissela Bok (1999), in her seminal work, *Lying: Moral Choice in Public and Private Lives*, pointed out "the lack of a theory of moral choice which can help in quandaries of truth-telling and lying" (p. xxxi). How do APNs determine what and how much information accomplishes professional goals of providing for patient good? Bok (1989) delineates three arguments that are generally given to support less than full disclosure to patients: "truthfulness is impossible; that patients do not want bad news; and that that truthful information (can cause) harms (to patients)" (p. 129). Each of these stances is susceptible to argument. During the course of the book, the issue of using ethically supportive clinical judgment in decision making is illustrated via cases. The extent and intent of veracity, nuances of veracity, and exploring the permissibility, nature, and role of deception are explored in more detail also in later chapters. In giving honest information the delivery and extent of information are necessarily tailored to the knowledge of the patient, who he or she is, and what he or she wants to know, as far as this is possible. All of the following can be used in determining how to use truthfulness to benefit the patient and uphold his or her autonomy: clinical judgment, collaboration, evidence, knowledge of the patient including cultural needs, and a clinical decision-making framework. Self-reflection related to biases and prejudices as well as reflection on practice are important elements of decision making related to the continuum of veracity. In general, veracity supports trust in the professional, other professionals, and the institution.

Fidelity

The duty of allegiance to the patient is closely aligned with the idea that healthcare professional relationships are fiduciary or trust relationships, as discussed earlier. Provision 2 of the ANA's *Code of Ethics for Nurses with Interpretive Statements* (2001) states "The nurse's primary commitment is to the patient, whether and individual, family, group, or community." Element 1 of the ICN's (2006) *Code of Ethics for Nurses* asserts, "[T]he nurse's primary professional responsibility is to people requiring nursing care." There are many opportunities for nurses and other healthcare professionals to be sidetracked from this priority. Nurses working within institutions and practices may experience pressures to follow the wishes of their employers, supervising physicians, or administrators. There are many other conflicts of interest that arise within healthcare settings that must be negotiated. Additionally, for providers who work within the prison system or the armed forces, there may be overt priorities that work in opposition to a focus on the good of the patients.

Other Approaches

Several other helpful approaches can assist in ethical decision making. These are discussed briefly in the following section. They are not theories; rather they are added dimensions that permit looking more deeply into the underlying conditions that give rise to practice problems. They help clarify the dimensions of an issue or dilemma.

FEMINIST ETHICS AND THE ETHICS OF CARE

Over the past few decades, feminist philosophers have criticized analytic philosophical theory and its methods as they are applied in healthcare settings (Donchin & Purdy, 1999; Tong, 1997; Warren, 2001). They suggest that in addition to moral theory and reasoning, ethical decision making in health care requires the "unearthing of buried assumptions about the influence of power in relationships and situations" (Grace, 2004a, p. 302). *Feminist ethics*, then, is not a singular approach but an assortment of perspectives. "A feminist approach is defined by taking as its starting point the experience of women, by acknowledging that this experience is characterized by oppression and domination" (Peter & Liaschenko, 2003, p. 33). Feminist ethics approaches do not limit themselves only to the concerns of women but address oppression and domination wherever they occur. Other issues of concern are "race, class, class, disability, sexual orientation, and so forth" (Peter & Liaschenko, 2003, p. 37).

This is different from the focus of many of the theories explored thus far. The traditional moral theories tend to view persons as isolated individuals with the right to have their autonomous actions protected or to pursue happiness. Davis, Aroskar, Liaschenko, and Drought (1997) note that Gilligan's research on moral development revealed women's moral concerns to be focused more on "care and responsibility in relationships rather than on the application of abstract principles such as respect for individual autonomy and justice" (p. 58). This is an important insight for nurses because their work is most frequently with individuals and the goals of the profession include caring for the individual as a unique being in all of his or her complexity. Good nursing care involves engagement with the patient and a willingness to focus on the whole person in context. This means that nurses understand the place and importance of significant others in the patient's life.

Feminist perspectives are also helpful in looking at the contexts within which nurses work. Feminist ethics supports the idea that "moral decision-making must include an investigation of both hidden and overt power relationships implicit in ethical problems" (Grace, 2005, p. 105). Questions to pose from a feminist perspective, when involved in ethically challenging situations, include: What are the power structures—social, institutional, or interpersonal? Is there an imbalance? Who has an interest in keeping a power imbalance? How is this affecting the patient or the decision making?

How can we change the focus of power or empower the person who is the primary focus of the issue?

NARRATIVE ETHICS

Narrative ethics represents another contemporary approach to addressing ethical issues. Narratives are stories of people's lives or situations told with rich detail and often from different perspectives. They are most frequently used either in a teaching/learning environment or as an after-the-fact exploration of a difficult case. In narrative ethics, stories are used to explore hidden facets of morally worrisome cases. They may portray the experiences of different persons involved in the story, giving fuller dimensions than usually available in a clinical case presentation. Narrative explorations permit the fleshing out of nuances in a given situation as well as stimulating further questions to be asked. Stories also permit people to vicariously engage in the experience of another from their own subjective stance. This can enhance empathy and compassion, which in turn facilitates understanding of how the person or situation got to a certain point in time. Stories are attentive to context and evolve over the time period of the narrative rather than being a static time slice. Narrative ethics is also a way of learning from situations that have already occurred. Criticisms of narrative ethics include the problem that it is difficult to apply ethical norms or determine what the good action would be.

Summary

This chapter systematically introduced the idea that professional nursing practice is intimately related to philosophy, moral philosophy, and applied ethics. Theories and principles of ethics were discussed in light of their uses, scope, and limits for good decision making in healthcare settings. These ideas will be elaborated on, put into context, and become more familiar as they are used to explore or analyze cases in this text. The following discussion questions are designed to help you understand your own professional values. There are no right or wrong answers, only thoughtful and interesting ones.

Discussion Questions

1. Preventive ethics is the anticipation of potential problems, followed by actions taken to stop their further development. For critically

or chronically ill patients, inadequate consideration of end-of-life options can give rise to patients receiving care and treatments they do not want or not receiving the care and treatments that they do want.

Mrs. Durant is a 75-year-old patient who has experienced a return of breast cancer that was successfully treated 20 years earlier. She now has bone metastases. She is eligible for a chemotherapy protocol that may extend her life for up to a year, but it is not expected to be curative. As an oncology nurse specialist, you are charged with discussing options with Mrs. Durant.

In what ways do the principles and concepts explored in this chapter permit gaining clarity about the situation and thus facilitate preventive ethics? The goal of preventive ethics is to facilitate good patient care and prevent the development of dilemmas or ethical crises.

2. Virtue ethics is another approach. In virtue ethics, the idea is that a person can cultivate a good character. The argument is that "a person of good character will engage in good actions." Thus, the actions of a good nurse would necessarily be good.

Do you think a good character can be cultivated?
Does the nurses' code of ethics from your country or the ICN code support this idea?
What is a good person?
What is a good nurse?
Would a good nurse necessarily be a good person?
What characteristics would a good nurse possess?

Present counterexamples (examples that would point to flaws in virtue ethics theory) and discuss these with your peers.

3. How has this chapter changed your understanding of nursing or healthcare ethics?

4. Knowledge of theories and principles is necessary for dialogue and collaboration with other professionals in the interest of good care for the patient. Do you agree with this statement or not? Defend your answer.

References

American Nurses Association. (2001). *Code of ethics for nurses with interpretive statements.* Washington, DC: Author.

American Nurses Association. (2003). *Social policy statement*. Washington, DC: Author.

Aristotle. (1967). The Nichomachean Ethics, Books I, II, III (chapters 1–5), VI & X. In A. I. Melden (Ed.), W. D. Ross (Trans.), *Ethical theories: A book of readings* (2nd ed., pp. 88–142). Englewood Cliffs, NJ: Prentice Hall. (Date of original work uncertain.)

Ashton, T. S. (1997). *The Industrial Revolution, 1760–1830*. New York, NY: Oxford University Press. (Original work published in 1961.)

Bahm, A. J. (1992). *Why be moral?* (2nd ed.). Albuquerque, NM: World Books.

Ballou, K. A. (2000). A historical-philosophical analysis of the professional nurse obligation to participate in sociopolitical activities. *Policy, Politics, & Nursing Practice, 1*(3), 172–184.

Beauchamp, T. L., & Childress, J. F. (2009). *Principles of biomedical ethics* (6th ed.). New York, NY: Oxford University Press.

Bentham, J. (1967). An introduction to the principles of morals and legislation. In A. I. Melden (Ed.), *Ethical theories: A book of readings* (pp. 367–390). Englewood Cliffs, NJ: Prentice Hall. (Original work published in 1789.)

Blackall, G. F., Simms, S., & Green, M. J. (2009). *Breaking the cycle: How to turn conflict into collaboration*. Philadelphia, PA: American College of Physicians.

Bok, S. (1989). Lies to the sick and dying. In P. Y. Windt et al. (Eds.), *Ethical issues in the professions* (pp. 127–133). Englewood Cliffs, NJ: Prentice Hall.

Bok, S. (1999). *Lying: Moral choice in public and private life* (2nd ed.). New York, NY: Random House.

Brown, L. (Ed.). (1993). *The new shorter Oxford English Dictionary*. New York, NY: Oxford Clarendon Press.

Buchanan, D. R. (2000). *An ethic for health promotion*. New York, NY: Oxford University Press.

Chambliss, D. F. (1996). *Beyond caring: Hospitals, nurses, and the social organization of ethics*. Chicago, IL: University of Chicago Press.

Clouser, K. D., & Gert, B. (1990). A critique of principlism. *Journal of Medical Philosophy, 15*, 219–236.

Coons, C., & Weber, M. (2013). *Paternalism: Theory and practice*. New York, NY: Cambridge University Press.

Corley, M. C. (2002). Nurses' moral distress: A proposed theory and research agenda. *Nursing Ethics, 9*(6), 636–650.

Corley, M. C., Minick, P., Elswick, R. K., & Jacobs, M. (2005). Nurse moral distress and ethical work environment. *Nursing Ethics, 12*(4), 381–390.

Davis, A. J., Aroskar, M. A., Liaschenko, J., & Drought, T. S. (1997). *Ethical dilemmas and nursing practice* (4th ed.). Upper Saddle River, NJ: Appleton & Lange.

Dewey, J. (1980). *The quest for certainty: A study of the relation of action knowledge and action*. New York, NY: Perigee Books. (Original work published in 1929.)

Doane, G., Pauly, B., Brown, H., & McPherson, G. (2004). Exploring the heart of ethical nursing practice: Implications for ethics education. *Nursing Ethics, 11*(3), 240–253.

Donchin, A., & Purdy, L. (Eds.). (1999). *Embodying bioethics: Recent feminist advances*. Lanham, MD: Roman & Littlefield.

Doris, J. M., & the Moral Psychology Research Group. (2010). *The moral psychology handbook.* New York, NY: Oxford University Press.

Dubler, N., & Liebmann, C. B. (2001). *Bioethics mediation: A guide to shaping shared solutions.* Nashville, TN: Vanderbilt University Press.

Eagleman, D. (2011). *Incognito: The secret lives of the brain.* New York, NY: Random House.

Engelhardt, H. T. (1996). *The foundations of bioethics.* New York, NY: Oxford University Press.

Engels, F. (1987). *The condition of the working class in England.* (Edited with an introduction by V. Kiernan.) Middlesex, UK: Penguin Books. (Original work published in Germany in 1845.)

European Patients' Forum. (2009). Patients' rights in the European Union. Retrieved from http://www.eu-patient.eu/Documents/Projects/Valueplus/Patients_Rights.pdf

Evans, J. H. (2000). A sociological account of the growth of principlism. *Hastings Center Report, 30*(5), 31–38.

Fiester, A. (2007). The principlist paradigm and the problem of the false negative: Why the clinical ethics we teach fails patients. *Academic Medicine, 82*(7), 684–689.

Fiester, A. (2012). Mediation and advocacy. *The American Journal of Bioethics, 12*(8), 10–11.

Flew, A. (1984). *A dictionary of philosophy* (2nd ed.). New York, NY: St. Martin's Press.

Fowler, M. D. M. (2010). *Guide to the code of ethics for nurses: Interpretation and application.* Silver Spring, MD: ANA.

Gallagher, A. (2011). Moral distress and moral courage in everyday nursing practice. *Online Journal of Issues in Nursing, 16*(2). doi: 10.3912/OJIN.Vol16No02PPT03

Gert, B., Culver, C. M., & Clouser, K. D. (2006). *Bioethics: A systematic approach.* New York, NY: Oxford University Press.

Gide, A. (1959). *So be it, or The chips are down (Ainsi soit-il; ou, Les jeux sont faits).* New York, NY: Knopf.

Grace, P. J. (1998). *A philosophical analysis of the concept 'advocacy': Implications for professional–patient relationships.* Unpublished doctoral dissertation. University of Tennessee, Knoxville. Retrieved from http://proquest.umi.com. Publication number AAT9923287, Proquest Document ID No. 734421751.

Grace, P. J. (2001). Professional advocacy: Widening the scope of accountability. *Nursing Philosophy, 2*(2), 151–162.

Grace, P. J. (2004a). Ethics in the clinical encounter. In S. K. Chase (Ed.), *Clinical judgment and communication in nurse practitioner practice* (pp. 295–332). Philadelphia, PA: F. A. Davis.

Grace, P. J. (2004b). Patient safety and the limits of confidentiality. *American Journal of Nursing, 104*(11), 33, 35–37.

Grace, P. J. (2004c). Philosophical considerations in nurse practitioner practice. In S. K. Chase (Ed.), *Clinical judgment and communication in nurse practitioner practice* (pp. 279–294). Philadelphia, PA: F. A. Davis.

Grace, P. J. (2005). Ethical issues relevant to health promotion. In C. Edelman & C. L. Mandle (Eds.), *Health promotion throughout the lifespan* (6th ed., pp. 100–125). St. Louis, MO: Elsevier/Mosby.

Grace, P. J., Fry, S. T., & Schultz, G. (2003). Ethics and human rights issues experienced by psychiatric-mental health and substance abuse registered nurses. *Journal of the American Psychiatric Nurses Association, 9*(1), 17–23.

Grace, P. J., & Willis, D. G. (2012). Nursing responsibilities and social justice: An analysis in support of disciplinary goals. *Nursing Outlook, 60*(4), 198–207.

Hardingham, L. (2004). Integrity and moral residue: Nurses as participants in a moral community. *Nursing Philosophy, 5,* 127–134.

Hume, D. (1963). *An enquiry concerning human understanding and other essays.* New York, NY: Washington Square Press. (Original work published in 1748 by A. Millar, London.)

Hume, D. (1967). An enquiry concerning the principles of morals. In A. I. Melden (Ed.), *Ethical theories: A book of readings* (pp. 273–316). Englewood Cliffs, NJ: Prentice Hall. (Original work published in 1777.)

International Council of Nurses. (2012). *Code of ethics for nurses.* Geneva, Switzerland: Author.

Jameton, A. (1984). *Nursing practice: The ethical issues.* Upper Saddle River, NJ: Prentice Hall.

Kahneman, D. (2011). *Thinking fast and slow.* New York, NY: Farrar, Straus & Giroux.

Kant, I. (1967). Foundations of the metaphysics of morals. In A. I. Melden (Ed.), *Ethical theories: A book of readings* (pp. 317–366). Englewood Cliffs, NJ: Prentice Hall. (Original work published in 1785.)

MacIntyre, A. C. (1984). *After virtue: A study in moral theory* (2nd ed.). Notre Dame, IN: University of Notre Dame Press.

Macklin, R. (2003). Applying the four principles. *Journal of Medical Ethics, 29*(5), 275–280.

Melden, A. I. (1967). On the nature and problems of ethics. In A. I. Melden (Ed.), *Ethical theories: A book of readings.* Englewood Cliffs, NJ: Prentice Hall.

Mill, J. S. (1965). *Mill's ethical writings.* (Edited with an introduction by J. B. Schneewind.) New York, NY: Macmillan. (Original work published in 1861.)

Mill, J. S. (1967). Utilitarianism. In A. I. Melden (Ed.), *Ethical theories: A book of readings* (pp. 391–434). Englewood Cliffs, NJ: Prentice Hall. (Original work published in 1863.)

Mohr, W. K., & Mahon, M. M. (1996). Dirty hands: The underside of marketplace health care. *Advances in Nursing Science, 119*(1), 28–37.

Munson, R. (2008). *Intervention and reflection: Basic issues in medical ethics* (8th ed.). Belmont, CA: Wadsworth.

Nagel, T. (1987). *What does it all mean?* New York, NY: Oxford University Press.

Newton, L. H. (1988). Lawgiving for professional life: Reflections on the place of the professional code. In A. Flores (Ed.), *Professional ideals* (pp. 47–56). Belmont, CA: Wadsworth.

Nightingale, F. (1859). *Notes on nursing: What it is and what it is not.* London, England: Harrison. (Reprint Philadelphia, PA: Lippincott)

Pavlish, C., Brown-Saltzman, C., Hersh, M., Shirk, M., & Rounkle, A. (2011). Nursing priorities, actions, and regrets for ethical situations in clinical practice. *Journal of Nursing Scholarship, 43*(4), 385–395.

Pellegrino, E. D. (2001). Trust and distrust in professional ethics. In W. Teays & L. Purdy (Eds.), *Bioethics, justice, and health care* (pp. 24–30). Belmont, CA: Wadsworth. (Reprinted from *Ethics, trust, and the professions: Philosophical and cultural aspects,* by E. D. Pellegrino, R. M. Veatch, & J. P. Langan, Eds., 1991, Washington, DC: Georgetown University Press.)

Peter, E., & Liaschenko, J. (2003). Feminist ethics. In V. Tschudin (Ed.), *Approaches to ethics: Nursing beyond boundaries* (pp. 33–44). New York, NY: Butterworth-Heinemann.

Peter, E., Lunardi, V. L., & Macfarland, A. (2004). Nursing resistance as ethical action: Literature review. *Journal of Advanced Nursing, 46*(4), 403–413.

Powers, M., & Faden, R. (2006). *Social justice: The moral foundations of public health and health policy*. New York, NY: Oxford University Press.

President's Commission for the Study of Ethical Problems in Medicine and Biomedical and Behavioral Research. (1982). *Making health care decisions*. Washington, DC: U.S. Government Printing Office. 33. PB83236703.

Rawls, J. (1971). *A theory of justice*. Cambridge, MA: Harvard University Press.

Ross, D. (1930). *The right and the good*. Oxford, England: Oxford University Press.

Russell, B. (1972). *A history of Western philosophy*. New York, NY: Simon & Schuster.

Simmerling, M. (2007). Beyond scarcity: Poverty as a contraindication for organ transplantation. *Virtual Mentor, 9*(6), 441–444.

Spenceley, S. M., Reutter, L., & Allen, M. N. (2006). The road less traveled: Advocacy at the policy level. *Policy, Politics, and Nursing Practice, 7*(3), 180–194.

Tong, R. (1997). *Feminist approaches to bioethics: Theoretical reflections and practical applications*. Boulder, CO: Westview Press.

Varcoe, C., Doane, G., Pauly, B., Rodney, P., Storch, J. L., Mahoney, K., . . . Starzomski, R. (2004). Ethical practice in nursing: Working the in-betweens. *Nursing Philosophy, 45*(3), 316–325.

Walker, M. U. (1993). Keeping moral spaces open: New images of ethics consulting. *The Hastings Center Report, 23*(2), 33–40.

Warren, V. L. (2001). From autonomy to empowerment: Health care ethics from a feminist perspective. In W. Teays & L. Purdy (Eds.), *Bioethics, justice, and health care* (pp. 49–53). Belmont, CA: Wadsworth.

Weston, A. (2002). *A practical companion to ethics* (2nd ed.). New York, NY: Oxford University Press.

Zaner, R. M. (1991). The phenomenon of trust and the physician–patient relationship. In E. D. Pellegrino, R. M. Veatch, & J. P. Langan (Eds.), *Ethics, trust and the professions: Philosophical and cultural aspects* (pp. 45–67). Washington, DC: Georgetown University Press.

Nursing Ethics

Pamela J. Grace

The professional must respond . . . if practices in his field are inadequate at any stage of the rendering of the service: if the client the ultimate consumer is unhappy; if he is happy, but unknowing, badly served by shabby products or service; or if he is happy and well served by the best available product but the state of the art is not adequate to his real needs.

—L. H. NEWTON, "Lawgiving for Professional Life: Reflections on the Place of the Professional Code," 1988

Let whoever is in charge keep this simple question in her head (not, how can I always do this right thing myself, but) how can I provide for this right thing to be always done?

—FLORENCE NIGHTINGALE, *Notes on Nursing: What It Is and What It Is Not*, 1946

Introduction

The purposes of this chapter are several. The primary intent is to reinforce advanced practice nurses' (APNs') understanding of the different senses of nursing ethics, its conceptual origins, its relationship to practice, and the importance of this understanding for good patient care. It locates the foundation of APN responsibilities securely within the goals of the profession and the responsibilities of human service professions to individuals and society. An understanding of how and why professions developed and what purposes they served and now serve provides a basis for grasping the importance of contemporary professions to individual security and the relatively smooth running of societies. While the authors' contexts of practice are mostly within the U.S. healthcare system, implications for nurses practicing in advanced roles internationally have been researched and are highlighted when evidence was available. Some characteristics and concepts that have

42

gained importance in professional nursing and in nursing ethics are discussed. Finally, a decision-making heuristic (helpful device) is applied to a deceptively simple case to demonstrate how all of the following are essential elements in meeting nursing goals of good patient care. These essential elements include nursing knowledge, a basic understanding of the language of ethics, certain personal characteristics (discussed later), personal and professional experiences, and the philosophical tools of exploration, analysis, and clarification. The goals of nursing have been articulated in terms of responsibilities "to promote health, to prevent illness, to restore health and to alleviate suffering" (International Council of Nurses [ICN], 2012, p. 2). Additionally, Willis, Grace, and Roy (2008) recently synthesized from nursing literature an implicit central unifying focus for the discipline that gives nursing its unique perspective. This focus, "facilitating humanization, meaning, choice, quality of life and healing in living and dying" (p. E28), provides a basis for clinical/ethical judgments and action and is aligned with the principle of beneficence.

Table **1** describes some habits that are vital for critical appraisals both of practice situations and reading material. Many readers will have already acquired such habits as a result of life and practice experiences; if so, these tips will serve as a refresher, and hopefully as reinforcement. The first task, though, is to be clear about what is meant by the term *nursing ethics*. This is necessary because, although the term is used widely in the nursing literature, it is not always clear from the topic or content discussed exactly what is meant.

Two Senses of Nursing Ethics

For many people working in health care, the term *ethics* has come to be associated with bioethical dilemmas or with other extremely difficult situations. A dilemma is a special sort of problem that requires a choice to be made between two or more equally undesirable options. The origin of the term is in the Greek *di*, meaning two, and *lemma*, meaning premises or assumptions (Brown, 1993). One reason for the association between bioethics and dilemmas is that the sorts of problems typically brought to public attention are those raised by technological or biological innovations. Nurses may well be involved in decision-making situations involving dilemmas; however, these situations are far from the most common issues that they face in daily practice.

■ Table 1 Habits of Critique

Questioning Authority	**Assumptions:** Authorities are human beings. Authoritative texts are the interpretations of human beings. The orders of superiors, managers, and leaders can be mistaken or misinformed. Important details of a situation can been missed, time may be an issue, or conflicts of interest may supplant goals.
	Case: The chief nursing officer (CNO) is under pressure to cut costs and urges her clinical nurse specialists (CNSs) to limit the time spent mentoring new staff in favor of completing more administrative work. The CNSs understand that in the long run spending the time to mentor staff will result in better patient outcomes and be more likely to meet professional goals.
	Actions: CNSs should ask themselves what assumptions the CNO is making in proposing the plan and whether these are supportable given available data, not supportable for other reasons, or require more data. CNSs must gather needed data and present the data to the CNO. They should consider eliciting peer support, weighing the risks and benefits of this.
Self-reflection	It follows that the APN's authority and expertise are also subject to critique. Thus a second important (and sometimes painful) habit is that of genuine self-reflection. Genuineness refers to willingness to recognize and admit that a person's position may not be the only valid one, that others may have equally valid positions, even if they radically differ. It is possible to learn from listening carefully to these alternate perspectives. Asking what is underlying these perspectives provides further insights.
	Many people believe themselves to be self-reflective although actually they are more interested in molding the facts and details to fit their original belief (rationalization).
	Self-reflection allows a person to both assume that biases and prejudices exist and try to discover what these might be in relation to a particular situation in the interests of controlling for them.

(continues)

■ Table 1   Habits of Critique (*continued*)

Logical Critique	Throughout this text reasoned argument is used to support positions taken. A reasoned argument is not a dispute; it is the presentation of concept, or an assertion that results from a chain of reasoning about a specific entity. It entails questioning underlying assumptions, discarding irrelevant information, and ensuring that the tentative conclusion can be supported by facts, logical reasoning, and/or sound assumptions. Sound assumptions are those that have stood up to critique and for which no counterexample can be given. There is an area of philosophy that actually studies the logic of arguments. When the premises of a logically sound argument are true, a conclusion derived from the premises will be true. A simple example of a sound argument is this: Premise: Human beings need nutrition for survival. Premise: Mr. Jones is unable to eat and refuses to take in nutrition by any other route. (*Assuming this is true . . .*) Conclusion: Mr. Jones will not survive. Sometimes, however, in the course of presenting an argument, a person discovers that an important aspect has been overlooked or that an assertion is made that is not true of all situations. In this example, if some persons were known to have survived without nutrition, it would not be possible to conclude that Mr. Jones would not survive.
Reading Critically	As you read, ask yourself, "Does this ring true?" If it does not, then try to isolate what is troubling. Are there counterexamples that would disprove the statement being made? Is the author missing some important facts? Discuss your thoughts with your peers. Refuse to take anything at face value. There are no moral experts in health care. No group of professionals has superior ethics knowledge; someone might have superior technical or content knowledge, but this is no preparation for ethical reasoning.
Living with Nuance	There will always be some uncertainty in ethical decision making because of the complex nature of human beings. Absolute security in having the right answer is not possible. Dewey's (1929/1980) insight is, "The distinctive characteristic of practical activity, one which is so inherent that it cannot be eliminated, is the uncertainty which attends it" (p. 6).

Keeping Professional Goals in Mind	However, nursing ethics assumes that the application of nursing judgment and action can positively influence patient well-being and reduce the likelihood of harm.
	A basic foundation for ethical professional action is the knowledge developed by the practitioner's discipline and/or knowledge from other sources that is then filtered through the discipline's lens and modified to meet the discipline's goals. Additionally, the possession or development of certain characteristics is important to good practice. In nursing, these include the willingness to be self-reflective, reflect on practice, and engage with patients as individuals whose needs differ in important ways from those of others. The process of furthering nursing's goals often also requires willingness to tackle difficult systemic problems arising from unjust societal healthcare arrangements. Thus, the political skills of negotiation and collaboration are also crucial to hone.

Professional responsibility and nursing ethics may be understood as equivalent concepts. This statement requires some further explanation. The term *nursing ethics,* like the term *ethics* can represent either a field of inquiry about nursing's responsibilities or nurses' actual practice-related actions (that is, those actions nurses undertake in the role of nurse and the extent to which these both flow from nursing knowledge and are anchored in nursing goals). Nursing ethics as a field of inquiry and nursing ethics as rules of professional conduct are, of course, closely related and inform each other. Here is a common example—if an intensive care nurse is asked to provide care for three critically ill patients during the same shift, each of whom realistically requires the attention of one nurse, he or she cannot fulfill nursing goals for all or, probably, for any of the patients. No matter how experienced a nurse, the situation is impossible. The best the nurse can do is to try and head off disaster. He or she cannot give what is considered good or optimal care to each patient. How is Nursing Ethics as a field of inquiry helpful in this situation? It investigates what a nurse's options are for the immediate circumstances and what changes might need to be made in the environment so that such problems do not recur. Nursing Ethics as inquiry, then, seeks to understand the following: What is an individual nurse's responsibility in such situations, and how should such problems be addressed so that the conditions that gave rise to it are changed or removed? Additionally, the profession's collective responsibility to address underlying or accompanying environmental concerns is the subject of critique and investigation by Nursing Ethics, when viewed as a field of study. Fry (2002) succinctly summarized the main concerns of Nursing Ethics as being about "describing the characteristics of the 'good' nurse, and identifying nurses' ethical practices" (p. 1). Implicit in this definition is the further political task of critiquing environments of practice and describing the necessary educational strategies to prepare ethical nurses. However, for the nurse involved in the example situation given, nursing ethics is her professional responsibility to recognize the ethical nature of the problem while trying to minimize possible harms and maximize patient good using available resources and within the limits of the immediate situation. It may also mean working after the fact (probably in concert with others) to address the conditions that led to this patient care problem.

In Nursing Ethics as a field of inquiry, the situation described explores why the nurse is being asked to do the seemingly impossible, what this means to the nurse, what this means to individual patients and society, and what the legitimate avenues of response are. These are questions for nursing's philosophers, scholars, and other interested parties to address (with input from practice). In contrast, nursing ethics, viewed as professional responsibility to further nursing's goals of practice in individual situations, pertains to the nurse being and acting within the context of actual practice or perhaps in the interests of actual practice (for example, political action to change inadequate practice settings as discussed in Chapter 4). This may also be termed *professional advocacy* (Grace, 1998, 2001). Professional advocacy is the nurse's responsibility both to address immediate situations of inadequate practice and to be active in addressing the environmental conditions that give rise to practice problems. (Professional advocacy is addressed in more detail later in this chapter.)

This chapter uses the convention of capitalizing the term Nursing Ethics when referring to the field of inquiry and will leave in lowercase the term nursing ethics when discussing the ethical conduct of nurses. Nursing Ethics, then, is a field of study involved in theorizing about, or researching, what nursing practice is, what good it provides, and how nurses should or do act. It has exploratory, descriptive, and prescriptive interests. The exploratory task of Nursing Ethics includes philosophical and theoretical investigations about professional goals and ways to further these. The descriptive task involves the use of research or observation to understand how nurses act in practice, what nurses think are good ways of acting, and how they recognize and address problems. Finally, the prescriptive or normative aspect provides guidelines for nurses about what actions are expected of the nurse. For example, the American Nurses Association's (ANA, 2001) *Code of Ethics for Nurses with Interpretive Statements* (**Table 2**) or the ICN's (2012) *Code of Ethics for Nurses* (**Table 3**) both provide guidelines for ethical conduct that are derived from disciplinary goals. More recently, the European Council

■ Table 2 American Nurses Association *Code of Ethics for Nurses*

Content removed due to copyright restrictions

■ Table 3 The International Council of Nurses' *Code of Ethics for Nurses*

Section of the Code	Text
Preamble	Nurses have four fundamental responsibilities: to promote health, to prevent illness, to restore health and to alleviate suffering. The need for nursing is universal. Inherent in nursing is a respect for human rights, including cultural rights, the right to life and choice, to dignity and to be treated with respect. Nursing care is respectful of and unrestricted by considerations of age, colour, creed, culture, disability or illness, gender, sexual orientation, nationality, politics, race or social status. Nurses render health services to the individual, the family and the community and coordinate their services with those of related groups.
Element 1 Nurses and People	■ The nurse's primary professional responsibility is to people requiring nursing care. ■ In providing care, the nurse promotes an environment in which the human rights, values, customs and spiritual beliefs of the individual, family and community are respected. ■ The nurse ensures that the individual receives accurate, sufficient and timely information in a culturally appropriate manner on which to base consent for care and related treatment. ■ The nurse holds in confidence personal information and uses judgement in sharing this information. ■ The nurse shares with society the responsibility for initiating and supporting action to meet the health and social needs of the public, in particular those of vulnerable populations. ■ The nurse advocates for equity and social justice in resource allocation, access to health care and other social and economic services. ■ The nurse demonstrates professional values such as respectfulness, responsiveness, compassion, trustworthiness and integrity.
Element 2 Nurses and Practice	■ The nurse carries personal responsibility and accountability for nursing practice, and for maintaining competence by continual learning. ■ The nurse maintains a standard of personal health such that the ability to provide care is not compromised.

Section of the Code	Text
	■ The nurse uses judgement regarding individual competence when accepting and delegating responsibility. ■ The nurse at all times maintains standards of personal conduct which reflect well on the profession and enhance its image and public confidence. ■ The nurse, in providing care, ensures that use of technology and scientific advances are compatible with the safety, dignity and rights of people. ■ The nurse strives to foster and maintain a practice culture promoting ethical behaviour and open dialogue.
Element 3 Nurses and the Profession	■ The nurse assumes the major role in determining and implementing acceptable standards of clinical nursing practice, management, research and education. ■ The nurse is active in developing a core of research-based professional knowledge that supports evidence-based practice. ■ The nurse is active in developing and sustaining a core of professional values. ■ The nurse, acting through the professional organisation, participates in creating a positive practice environment and maintaining safe, equitable social and economic working conditions in nursing. ■ The nurse practices to sustain and protect the natural environment and is aware of its consequences on health. ■ The nurse contributes to an ethical organisational environment and challenges unethical practices and settings.
Element 4 Nurses and Co-workers	■ The nurse sustains a collaborative and respectful relationship with co-workers in nursing and other fields. ■ The nurse takes appropriate action to safeguard individuals, families and communities when their health is endangered by a co-worker or any other person. ■ The nurse takes appropriate action to support and guide co-workers to advance ethical conduct.

Source: Courtesy of the International Council of Nurses—Four Elements of the ICN *Code of Ethics for Nurses* © 2012. Geneva, Switzerland: Author.

of regulatory bodies and competent authorities for nursing (FEPI) formed in 2004 and has proposed a *European Code of Ethics and Conduct* (FEPI, 2012) aimed to provide consistency in standards across the increasingly fluid nursing work boundaries of the European Union. The development of a code of ethics is one of the hallmarks of a contemporary service profession and is an especially important characteristic of what are often called crucial professions (Windt, 1989), or those that address an important societal need such as health care. These codes of ethics and their implications for APNs internationally are discussed again later.

Nursing as a Profession

Characteristics of Professions

For the purposes of this text on ethical issues associated with advanced practice roles, nursing is characterized as a profession. The responsibilities of a profession's members are more extensive than those of a technical occupation or vocation. Although nursing has not reached the level of profession in many developing countries (for reasons given shortly), in those countries where the nursing role includes responsibility and accountability for professional judgment and action and/or has expanded as a result of advanced education and skills, it can be considered a profession. What does it mean to say that nursing is a profession? Why is this an important point? These questions can be answered through a brief review of what professions are and what purposes they are supposed to serve. In everyday circumstances almost any vocational group may refer to itself as a profession. For example, dry cleaning businesses advertise themselves to be professional, and in the business section of any phone book there are many instances of plumbers, carpenters, and others all advertising their professional status. Historically, however, the term *profession* meant something very specific, and contemporarily this meaning remains important for individuals and society. This is especially true of those disciplines that provide crucial human services; services that individuals do not have the knowledge, skills, or capacity to provide for themselves but that are necessary for both existing and flourishing.

The earliest organized occupational groups were the craftsmen's guilds. They are noted to have formed in medieval times and perhaps earlier (Carr-Saunders & Wilson, 1933). They consisted of groups of technically accomplished artisans who banded together to hone and protect their skills and knowledge in order to make a living. Out of these beginnings some groups began to affiliate themselves with religious orders, which besides engaging in ministerial duties often also had educational and intellectual aims. Much university education in medieval times and later was ecclesiastical in origin.

The original professions were ministry, medicine, and the law. These three disciplines often required members to take a vow to be accountable for actions, to profess their sincerity, abilities, and/or motivations. These Church-affiliated groups supposedly had altruistic motivations behind their educational endeavors and a service focus. They were less inclined toward substantial monetary awards and more inclined toward developing virtues than many other occupational groups (Carr-Saunders & Wilson, 1933). Thus, a distinction evolved that separated the artisan or tradesman from the professional. Gradually professions such as medicine and law withdrew from their theological origins, yet they maintained their service goals and mission.

Contemporary professions emerged from this background. Perhaps the most well-known attempt to describe the essential characteristics and purposes of professions emerged from Flexner's (1915) extensive study of medical education in the United States and Germany, which resulted in major reforms in medical education in the United States and elsewhere. Flexner, an educator, proposed that professions have an extensive and specialized knowledge base, take responsibility for developing and using their knowledge, have a practice or action orientation that is used for the good of the population served, and autonomously set standards for and monitor the actions of their members.

Following Flexner, further attempts have been made to identify essential characteristics of professions. Kepler (1981) notes that "professions are organized . . . [and] a high level of education is necessary to provide knowledge not readily available or capable of being understood by all. Professions normally interact with clients for whom they provide services rather than goods" (pp. 17–18). The profession is also self-reflective so that it can adapt to changing needs. It is, however, the possession of not readily available knowledge that persuades societies to grant a certain level of prestige and autonomy to professions (Grace, 1998). Perhaps the aspect of contemporary professions that is both the most important to those served and to the membership is the explicit formulation of codes of conduct or ethics.

In reviewing historical accounts of the traditional professions—ministry, law, medicine, and later the professoriate—less noble accounts of their purposes emerge. Some have argued that professions are self-serving and deliberately protective of their knowledge in order to benefit their memberships. My doctoral dissertation (Grace, 1998) investigates such claims in more detail than there is room for here. However, a synthesis of the literature reveals that, though historically some disciplines were protective of their power and prestige, modern helping professions do not see their goals as being primarily self-serving. Nor do they view themselves as engaged in promoting the interests of their membership. Rather it is evident from their published codes of ethics that they view themselves as existing for the primary purpose of serving the public good via their areas of knowledge, skills, and expertise.

CODES OF ETHICS

The codes of ethics of contemporary healthcare professions in essence represent the discipline's promises to society (Grace, 2004b). These codes were developed over time and are periodically revised by the profession's leadership, with membership input, in response to how well they continue to address professional goals and the evolution of societal needs. Although they tend to be abstract rather than specific (the exception to this is lawyers' codes of professional conduct, which are more specific and directive), they provide general direction and guidance to their membership related to professional conduct and the scope of practice. Some, such as the ANA's *Code of Ethics for Nurses with Interpretive Statements* (2001), are accompanied by interpretive statements that provide more detailed explanations of each provision or tenet.

Importantly, professions and their members can be held accountable by the public through such agencies as professional licensure boards for the promises made (Grace, 2004b, p. 284). Curtin (2001) notes that historically "codes of ethics came into being—as did almost all early laws—to protect the vulnerable from the powerful; the unwary from the unscrupulous" (p. 1). However, the public is typically not cognizant of the existence, never mind the content, of professional codes of ethics. Nevertheless, were these to be broadly publicized, they could serve as a potent tool for political action. (This idea is discussed in more detail later.)

Helping Professions and the Public Good

Codes of ethics, formulated as they are from within a profession, also serve as a profession's check on what it expects of its members related to the primary focus of actions. For example, the preamble to the American Medical Association's *Principles of Medical Ethics* (2001) asserts that "a physician must recognize responsibility to patients first and foremost, as well as to society." The ANA's (2001) and ICN's (2012) codes of ethics for nurses likewise assert that nurses' primary interest is the service of individual and societal well-being. The relatively new *Code of Ethics and Conduct for European Nurses* was thought necessary for "the establishment of ethical and deontological principles [that could be] shared throughout Europe [and] would give better protection to European citizens and enhance professional development" (Sasso, Steviano, Jurado, & Rocco, 2008, p. 821). The National Association of Social Workers (1999) in its preamble promises, "A historic and defining feature of social work is the profession's focus on individual well-being in a social context and the well-being of society."

In an earlier work, I noted that "the philosophical roots of the helping professions are imbedded in the idea that humans are not solely self-interested individuals but also have the capacity for altruism" (Grace, 2004b, p. 283). *Altruism* is the ability to understand that others have aims, projects, and life ambitions just as we do and to feel sympathy for someone who is suffering as a result of being unable to fulfill his or her own needs. Humans understand that others sometimes require assistance in achieving their aims and are willing to assist, even if doing so does not necessarily result in a direct gain or primary benefit (Nagel, 1970). That is, the philosophical aims of the helping professions are directed not primarily at furthering the needs of the professional to make a living (as they might be in retail or business settings) but toward the well-being of the individuals served (of course, it is also important that nurses are able to achieve a reasonable standard of living). This is one meaning of altruism. It has been extensively documented as well as supported in the research literature that what draws many people to a profession such as nursing is the desire to contribute to the well-being of others.

Societal Importance of Professions

As has already been pointed out, nursing, medicine, and other professions such as law and education provide services that are crucial in some way to the functioning of individuals and the societies in which they live. Looking at the relationship of what Windt (1989) terms a crucial profession to the population served might shed some light on the persistent importance to society of having professions, given the existence of ongoing debates about what exactly these are and what groups qualify for the designation.

The explanation for the importance of professions hinges on the idea of human vulnerability. Crucial professions serve a specific human need that left unserved would make people, as Sellman (2005) terms it, "more-than-ordinarily vulnerable" to the environment in which they live. Moreover, this vulnerability is widespread. Lack of education (teaching profession) disadvantages people in all sorts of ways. An inability to hold people accountable for infringing on the property or other rights of people (law) would cause security and safety problems for civilians, and everyone is susceptible to ill health or less than optimal functioning. Healthcare professions, such as nursing and medicine, supply services that promote human functioning and flourishing, albeit they have different perspectives on this.

Society should be able to trust professions to provide the services that they profess to be capable of delivering (see the discussion in Chapter 1 related to trust and fiduciary relationships). The existence and privileges of certain professions are sanctioned by society in exchange for their specialized services. In return for these services, society awards professions and professionals a certain standing. It places a high value on the information and skills that professionals contribute and supports the education of professionals (often) by subsidizing their training costs. Professionals are trusted to provide what they promise in exchange for financial or other types of compensation. In return, professionals are held to standards of practice that support the betterment of society as a whole (Grace, 2004b, p. 284).

Some philosophers, sociologists, and political commentators have expressed concern about the dangers to society should crucial professions lose their professional status. This phenomenon has been termed *deprofessionalization* (Bruhn, 2001; Dougherty, 1990; Sullivan, 1999). In deprofessionalization, the professions lose the ability and right to control their own practice—two of the most essential aspects of professions. These are essential aspects for many reasons, but most especially because professionals understand what is needed to meet individual and societal goals. Professional goals are focused on a good that is not primarily economic or business oriented, and the results of inadequate services are generally more immediately perceived and more concerning to the professional than to others with commercial rather than service interests.

The current global financial crisis, healthcare delivery reform in the United States, and cost-containment initiatives in other countries that have varying methods of healthcare financing have led or may lead to the focus of healthcare delivery being diverted away from patients and society and toward cost containment and/or profit making. In addition, the contemporary disease focus fails to adequately account for the roots of ill health in societal conditions. Many scholars and critics in the United States have pointed to problems for society when business models are used to structure healthcare delivery (Fineberg, 2012; Reid, 2009; Relman, 2007). Although many other countries do not rely on business models to structure their healthcare systems and do not have profit as a driving force, nevertheless there is a trend toward cost containment and away from patient-centered or societal concerns in recent initiatives. These issues as well as the question of whether health and thus healthcare are human rights are taken up again in Chapter 4. Market and/or cost-containment forces tend to work against professional autonomy. What this means is that persons other than healthcare professionals make decisions about who needs what in terms of protecting and promoting health. However, for a professional to be held accountable for his or her clinical judgments and the actions that follow from them, there must be a choice of action. If someone else is dictating what will or can be done, and what cannot, then it is not reasonable to hold the professional responsible for performing impossible actions. That is not to say that the profession has no further ethical responsibilities, but it does shift the focus of responsibility toward the systemic, economic, or political issues that are constraining clinical judgment.

In philosophical circles this is termed the problem of "ought implies can," meaning that, if it is dictated that someone ought to provide the appropriate care for a patient, then the care needed must be available. It is unreasonable to hold someone responsible for carrying out an impossible task. However, a professional who does not attempt to locate and remedy the source of a problem after the fact might be held responsible. What it boils down to is that although sometimes health professionals do not have a choice of action in a problematic situation, they must still try to work with others after the fact to ensure that better options are available in the future. For example, in the case of the critical care nurse who is asked to care for three patients, the nurse must do what he or she can until reinforcements arrive; however, the nurse also has a responsibility to try to change the underlying conditions that led to this current situation. The idea is that professionals, perhaps especially healthcare professionals, understand the end results and implications of poor care for their population, perhaps better than any other group.

The Status of Nursing as a Profession

CONCERNS

Why should nurses be concerned with the quality and intent of all clinical judgments and the actions that follow from them? Is it not true that some actions are purely routine? Why should everything about nursing practice be subject to ethical appraisal (nursing ethics)? The answer lies partly in the idea that nursing is one of those professions that caters to the sorts of human needs that left unmet make subjects more than ordinarily vulnerable to their environments and partly in the idea that all actions are in some way directed toward the care of a human individual with unique needs. Thus, even tasks that at first glance seem simple, such as giving an intravenous (IV) medicine or taking a blood pressure, will have a different meaning for that patient than for any other. APNs are responsible for responding to patients as unique individuals with unique needs. And when circumstances do not allow for this, for whatever reason, nurses are responsible for recognizing the ethical nature of the obstruction to what they know to be good care. In addition, problems that have often been assumed to be out of the purview of nurses, such as institutional obstructions to patient care, inadequate staffing, poor inter- and/or intradisciplinary communication about a patient, all have ethical aspects for the same reason: they obstruct efforts to provide good care.

Therefore, in addition to responsibilities related to direct care, there is logical support for the idea that nurses have broader societal responsibilities as outlined in the ICN's (2012) and ANA's (2001) codes of ethics and in the ANA's (2010) *Social Policy Statement*. Furthermore, individuals on entering a profession and achieving professional status are implicitly promising to fulfill the goals of the profession. The profession's code of ethics applies to the practice of each professional. It supersedes all other institutional policies and cannot be negated by other professions, by administrators, or by the demands of the workplace (ANA, 1994). In advanced practice settings, where APNs so often find themselves working side by side and on a par with colleagues from other disciplines, they may find it hard to resist the "pull" of the other profession's particular aims, or of economic interests, and lose sight of the importance to individual and societal health of prioritizing nursing goals (Bryant-Lukosius, DiCensio, Browne, & Pinelli, 2004; Hagedorn & Quinn, 2004). Additionally, nurses working in research and correctional facilities may experience pressures to prioritize the goals of research or of the prison system over nursing goals.

Therefore, it is critically important that APNs understand that advanced practice, although it may bring with it augmented responsibilities, is nevertheless specific to nursing practice, and they must be able to articulate what this means. One way to think about this is that further education enables nurses to meet professional goals of good patient care more comprehensively because they are then able to provide for a wider array of patient needs. This lessens the fragmentation that can occur with multiple providers attending to different problems or systems and makes it easier to elicit the real needs of patients both for care and information.

Finally, some have noted the problem of dual loyalties arising for professionals working in certain circumstances such as military service (Gross, 2010; Williams, 2009). The question revolves around primary duties. Is the military nurse a nurse first—subject to the nursing code of ethics—or a member of the armed forces first and subject to military rules as a priority? The practical answer is probably that military service (unlike correctional service) provides an exception to the rules of professional (medical, nursing, or allied healthcare) conduct. A military nurse is bound first by military ethics rules and nursing ethics rules second. Moreover, the military nurse is not free to change her job and is subject to different legal sanctions than civilian nurses. The problem of military nursing and divided loyalties has not been sufficiently explored in the philosophical or ethics literature. Nevertheless, the ethical decision-making tools provided throughout this text provide strategies for military nurses to practice well in spite of their sometimes conflicting loyalties.

Changes in Contemporary Healthcare Settings

Changes in contemporary healthcare settings both in the United States and elsewhere, resulting from a shift of emphasis to the economic bottom line and expediency and away from the patient and/or societal good, lend urgency to the need for all professional nurses to understand that the basis for their work is firmly attached to the goals of their profession. Unless this is taken seriously, the goals of other professions or institutions will dominate nursing work at all levels—this is a problem for the reasons given in more detail shortly but mostly because nursing serves a distinct purpose and has a distinct perspective that is crucial to the well-being of individuals and for societal health. Should nursing merge with another healthcare profession or its goals become subsumed under the goals of another profession, the gains that have been made over the last century in professional autonomy, and thus the ability to directly influence nursing care, will be lost.

Not only do contemporary healthcare delivery systems both in the United States and elsewhere present a danger that nursing will lose its hard-won autonomy, but the autonomy of other professions is also at risk. Thus it is more vital than ever that the healthcare professions in general, including nursing, retain their societal status as professions—they are, arguably, the last line of defense against the political and/or business interests of contemporary health care and other major shifts that have been projected in healthcare delivery internationally (Anscombe, 2008; Bruhn, 2001; Dougherty, 1992; Mechanic, 1998).

Interdisciplinary work and action are becoming more common because collaboration is often needed to address or research complex health issues. The danger is that a blurring of professional boundaries will occur. Nursing is perhaps more vulnerable to this than other professions, yet nursing's perspective is important because of its unique emphasis on the person as contextual and continuously evolving.

Ambiguity About Nursing as a Profession

The question of whether nursing is a full-fledged or mature profession is still somewhat open for debate. Achieving generally accepted professional status within a society is important because it is accompanied by a certain amount of control or autonomy of practice. In some countries nursing is accorded professional status and with that status the ability to regulate itself. In some countries other more established professions have ignored or are unaware of nursing's particular knowledge about, and contributions to, the health of persons and the larger society. The troubled history of nursing as a female profession, the progress of which "has echoed the status of women in society" (Grace, 2004b, p. 285) as an oppressed group, is well documented (Andrist, Nicholas, & Wolf, 2006; Group & Roberts, 2001). Nursing as a predominantly female discipline has been subject to "gender discrimination" (Andrist et al., 2006, p. 1), lessening its ability either to realize its political potential or be taken seriously by others as a political force. Wuest (2006) highlights the paradox that a key factor of professions historically is that they excluded women. When women did enter professions such as nursing, their motivations did not tend to include the acquisition of power. This has led to relatively easy domination by other groups working within the same environments, such as physicians and administrators. This statement is not intended to denigrate the significant contributions of some eminent members of the profession who managed Herculean tasks of nursing and healthcare reform, but rather to highlight the idea that nurses as the largest workforce within most healthcare systems could have significant power to improve the lot of individuals and society related to health.

Multiple Entry Levels

A further problem for the development of the nursing profession, in the United States at least, is lack of internal cohesiveness caused in part by the multiple levels of entry and multiple grades of practice. A registered nurse in the United States, for example, may have completed a 2-year associate's degree program, a 3-year diploma program, a baccalaureate degree, or have entered nursing as a second-career nurse with degrees in another field. This lack of a unified entry level is suspected to have contributed to the delayed progress of nursing as a driving force for change in health care. Additionally, specialization has tended to cause the formation of special interest groups, the focus of which is addressing concerns that arise within those practice areas or settings. Nursing's scholars and leaders continue their struggle for disciplinary unification. By using insights from nursing's history, the feminist movement, sources of nursing knowledge development, and a changing professional body with its increasingly more highly educated membership, it is hoped nursing will be more equipped to meet its goals related to the health of individuals and society. Arguably, an important unifying force for the good of individuals and society is recognition of the profession's social responsibilities to further its shared goals.

NURSING POSSESSES THE ESSENTIAL CHARACTERISTICS OF A PROFESSION

Although no agreement has been reached about the precise nature of professions, there is nevertheless a general consensus that professions serve an important purpose in democratic societies and that they have certain characteristics in common. The discipline of nursing possesses these characteristics and thus fits the description of a profession. Professions have responsibilities to society that should not be circumvented by economic or business interests. Professions direct and monitor their own activities independent of those who might wish to subvert professional goals. The loss of professional status would not bode well for the population nursing serves, for reasons highlighted later. And yet there is great concern among nursing scholars that nursing, instead of realizing its potential for societal good, is in danger of becoming weakened by lack of attention to, or concern for, the philosophical and theoretical work that draws upon and contributes to nursing practice (Fawcett, Newman, & McAllister, 2004).

The Relationship of Nursing's Goals and Nursing Ethics

In the preceding discussion, not much distinction was made between medicine and nursing in regard to goals because the greater point of focus was the importance of certain professions to individuals and society. This section concentrates more on laying out the distinct nature of nursing goals and nursing perspectives as they have developed over the last century or so.

There is an inevitable relationship between nursing's goals and nursing ethics that has not always been as well recognized as it is currently. Nursing's philosophers and scholars over the past 150 years or so have been diligently involved in trying to determine and describe what the purpose of nursing is, who is served, what knowledge is needed for addressing these goals, and the responsibilities of nursing's membership in keeping these goals as the focus of their endeavors. This quest to define nursing and its unifying purpose is well documented in nursing literature (Donaldson & Crowley, 1978; Milton, 2005; Newman, Sime, & Corcoran-Perry, 1991; Packard & Polifroni, 1992, Willis et al., 2008) and represents the self-reflective nature of the discipline. Interestingly, medicine as a discipline has not been so self-reflective—much of what has been written about the nature and goals of medicine has come from philosophers and historians who for the most part are not physicians.

Fowler (1997) draws attention to the fact that ethics has "been at the foundation of nursing practice since the inception of modern nursing in the United States in the late 1870s" (p. 17). Fry (1995) has documented the development of nursing ethics. She describes its evolution as "paralleling the development of nursing as a profession" in that early nursing ethics resembled rules of etiquette and duties that included such things as "neatness, punctuality, courtesy, and quiet attendance to the physician" (p. 1822).

It is clear that nursing ethics in the early days was less about nurses' autonomous actions than it was about good personal conduct in carrying out physician orders. Part of the reason for this was that a hierarchy existed. Nurse educators in the United States and elsewhere were drawn from an elite group of privileged women from the higher classes. They were influenced by Florence Nightingale's ideas about nursing as a virtuous activity. Coburn (1987) notes that it was difficult to attract the numbers of refined women to institutional nursing that were needed. Working-class women were attracted because they had limited work options. Thus, nurse educators attempted to instill in the women from the lower classes the characteristics thought necessary for the care of the sick.

On a personal note and in support of the historical account, my own mother, who was from a working-class family in Manchester, England, told her family that she wanted to become a nurse. She was 18 years old at the time. Her parents refused to sanction this because of the long working hours (72 hours per week) and the arduous nature of the work. So, for 4 years she worked as a secretary in a factory, at which point she applied for nurse training; she was accepted in 1942, and graduated in 1945. Later she became a midwife (perhaps the earliest version of advanced practice nursing). Anecdotal accounts of her training period echoed historical accounts.

The reason that ladylike characteristics were promoted, nevertheless, was directly related to the interests of the patient. It was thought that quiet diligence and competence in the tasks of caregiving would provide the most beneficial environment for a patient's recovery. This view of nursing conduct was heavily influenced by Nightingale's (1859/1946) theory of good nursing. As evidenced in her writings, she believed that the right environment was crucial to the healing process and nursing's job was to manage the environment to facilitate healing.

Since Nightingale's era, the nature and substance of nursing ethics literature has, not surprisingly, closely followed developments in the profession and in nursing education. As nursing has evolved and become increasingly differentiated from medicine in terms both of goals and of practice autonomy, the subject matter of Nursing Ethics has evolved and nurses' understanding about what constitutes good practice actions (nursing ethics) has developed.

Evolution of Nursing and Consolidation of Nursing Goals

IMPORTANT QUESTIONS

What is nursing's particular knowledge base and how does this differ from that of other professions? The question of whether nursing has a unique knowledge base continues to be argued in contemporary nursing literature. Many scholars believe the question has been answered; however, many more practicing nurses remain unsure of the theoretical bases for their practice. This is a problem at all levels of nursing but most especially at the level of advanced practice. Cody (2006) notes, "The practice of nursing at an advanced level requires a deep understanding of theory and the ability to apply theory effectively in providing healthcare services to people. Indeed, if such understanding and ability is not found within a given nurse, in any specialty whatsoever, his or her practice *cannot* be considered to be advanced at all" (p. ix).

The acceptance and proliferation of advanced nursing roles in the United States, parts of Europe and Scandinavia, and certain Eastern countries such as Korea, Japan, Taiwan, and Thailand (Chiang-Hanisko, Ross, Boonyanurak, Ozawa, & Chiang, 2008) makes an understanding of the particular and unique nature of nursing concerns ever more critical if individual and societal needs for holistic nursing care are to be met. The role of advanced practice nursing is crucial in "fostering better health around the world" (Chiang-Hanisko et al., 2008, para. 1). In the United States there was a concerted effort by the American Association of Colleges of Nursing (AACN) to move toward acceptance of a doctor of nursing practice (DNP) degree as the primary advanced practice qualification by 2015 (Cronenwett et al., 2011). This proposal has been tempered by several factors, including the economic downturn and its effects on education. Nevertheless, there is a proliferation of DNP programs in the United States (over 120 as of this writing), the contents of which are guided by the AACN's list of essential inclusions for the program (AACN, 2006). A lengthy discussion of the pros and cons of nursing practice doctorates is beyond the purposes of this text. The salient point is that all nurses, regardless of level of education, remain focused on the goals and purposes of nursing as a profession and use their advanced education to these purposes and not the purposes of other professions except where there are mutual goals. Nurses need to recognize that the profession's unique nature may become diluted or lost and guard against this (Dracup, Cronenwett, Meleis, & Benner, 2005; Silva & Ludwick, 2006). Concerns exist about the possibility that instead of advanced nursing practice, DNPs will be used to make up for shortages of physicians in both specialist and generalist medical settings. There are also worries that the control of these clinicians will fall under the department of medicine rather than belong to nursing's services. Although the central unifying focus of the discipline has been identified and highlights nursing's unique perspective on patient and society needs, it will, nevertheless, take a concerted effort for nurses to keep nursing perspectives and goals at the core of their work, regardless of the level and type of their preparation. It remains to be seen how doctorally prepared nurse clinicians augment the nursing profession and support professional goals—there is a growing but immature body of literature that can provide insights.

> Contemporary developments in nursing and the movement of nursing toward professional maturity have occurred partly because nursing's scholars, theorists, and even researchers have been willing to ask the hard questions about nursing. They have been willing to ask, "What is it we are doing when we are doing nursing? How is what we do different than what other professionals do? What is our unique purpose?" (Grace, 2004b, p. 288)

Present-day APNs, regardless of their level of preparation, will have an important role in keeping and promulgating a nursing perspective. Most readers engaged in higher nursing education are exposed to nursing's conceptual bases for practice and will have had courses or modules that trace and critique the theoretical works of nursing's scholars. This chapter does not explore these works in detail for that reason. However, a brief overview will help those who have not yet been exposed; it can also serve as a refresher for those who have and will facilitate an understanding of the inevitable link between theory development and the evolution of nursing ethics.

NURSING THEORY AND DISCIPLINARY KNOWLEDGE DEVELOPMENT

Florence Nightingale is generally considered the first person to have asked and answered the question "What is nursing?" In her *Notes on Nursing: What It Is and What It Is Not* (1859/1946), she clearly articulates her philosophy of nursing. Her philosophy embraced the idea that nurses, in appropriately manipulating the patient's environment, "put the patient in the best condition for nature to act upon him" (p. 75). She used previous knowledge, research, and current conditions to conceptualize good nursing actions. Thus, her particular focus proves very different from those followed by the medical and surgical establishments of the era. The focuses of the medical professions actually did very little to change conditions in spite of gains in empirical knowledge about disease and illness that were available. Nightingale's influence both on public health and on the education of nurses was significant and led to the development of schools of nursing in Europe and eventually the United States.

Nursing, for several decades after Nightingale, was vocational rather than professional. Cody (2006) writes that it was not until Hildegarde Peplau published *Interpersonal Relations in Nursing* as a theory of nursing in 1952 that a shift in the development of nursing into a more professional endeavor commenced in earnest. This development coincided with the post–World II implementation of tax-supported college education for veterans funded by the G.I. Bill of Rights of 1944. More opportunities arose for nurses to receive baccalaureate-level or higher nursing education.

In the 1950s and 1960s, "additions to the literature on philosophy and theory in nursing began to appear" (Cody, 2006, p. 2). The important idea that nursing was concerned with "the *whole person* and *health in all its dimensions*" (Cody, 2006, p. 2) emerged. In 1991, Virginia Henderson's definition of nursing was published by the ICN. She notes that the definition represents the crystallization of her ideas about nursing over a period of time.

> The unique function of the nurse is to assist the individual sick or well, in the performance of those activities contributing to health or its recovery (or to peaceful death) that he would perform unaided if he had the necessary strength, will or knowledge. And to do this in such a way as to help him gain independence as quickly as possible. (Henderson, 1991, p. 21)

In 1970, Rogers's account of human beings as consisting of more than the sum of their parts and inseparable from their environments was published. She termed this view of persons "unitary man." Cody (2006) points out that over the next 20 years or so "at least 20 significant frameworks intended to guide practice were published" (p. 3). Thus, he asserts, "The distinctiveness of nursing's disciplinary knowledge base is a reality that cannot be ignored" (p. 3). Nursing's knowledge base constitutes a science in this sense—that is, it is a developed body of knowledge about a phenomenon. The development of nursing's knowledge base has been directly informed by practice. Nursing's scholars and philosophers, almost all of whom have at some point been immersed in practice, have in turn used the questions and problems of practice to theorize about what it is that nurses do and how they might do it to meet professional goals more effectively.

"The (foundational) goal of the nursing profession is generally agreed to be that of promoting a 'good' which is health. Health may be variously defined depending on philosophical and theoretical perspectives guiding practice" (Grace, 2001, p. 155) and on the particular contexts of practice. Nevertheless, nursing has espoused a perspective of human beings that grounds the discipline's activity in the assumption that humans are contextual beings whose needs cannot be conceptualized in isolation from the larger contexts of their lives, histories, relationships, projects, and values. Additionally, many of nursing's philosophers have noted the importance of the nurse–patient relationship and engagement with patients to facilitate meaning-making in difficult and fluid circumstances. The relationship and engagement are important even in cases of those who have profound cognitive challenges that prevent the individual's direct input.

Some have criticized nursing's perspective, noting that certain allied professions could also lay claim to this perspective. Indeed, in the past 20 years or so, some physicians have moved to adopt what they call the "new medicine" or an "integrative medicine" approach to patient care (Blumer & Meyer, 2006). This is good for patients. Even so, the new medicine fails to draw on the copious previous work done in nursing, and "new medicine" practitioners cannot necessarily be found in all the disparate settings where nurses practice in advanced roles, and they do not stand in the same relationships to patients. Additionally, it is doubtful that many physicians see integrative medicine as a realistic approach, given the limits of current healthcare environments and their emphasis on cure, along with a narrow view of what constitutes a good outcome. Still, it is an encouraging movement and one where nurses are well equipped to provide leadership.

REVISITING NURSING ETHICS AS PROFESSIONAL RESPONSIBILITY

In light of the preceding discussion, it is clear that an examination of nursing ethics is appropriately addressed "via the explications of nursing's theorists and scholars" (Grace, 2006, p. 68). In turn, nursing's theorists and scholars can realistically be called nursing philosophers because their theories or thoughts emerge from their philosophical attempts (informed by practice experiences) to find reasonable answers to the following questions: What is nursing? Why is nursing necessary? How can it best be done? What is needed to do it (including knowledge, characteristics, and skills required of practitioners as well as the environments in which it can be done)? Hence the two main goals of theorizing in nursing are (1) "To describe and explain (all levels of) nursing" (Grace, 2006, p. 68), and (2) to provide a structure or framework that facilitates practice, guides research endeavors aimed at expanding nursing's knowledge base, and underpins practitioner development and education.

The use of philosophies, models, and theories as guides for nursing practice and the reverse influence of practice experiences on theory development are factors critical to the development of nursing's knowledge base and thus to the maturation and evolution of the discipline. However, it is the discipline's explicit aim of contributing both to the health of individuals and the overall health of society that makes nursing itself a moral endeavor.

Flaming (2004) has argued that because theories of nursing say what nursing is (ontology), they represent ethical imperatives. Take, for example, the goal of nursing to promote an individual's health. Because nursing views of health all include the understanding that human beings are complex entities, inseparable from the environment in which they live and connected to countless important others in their lives, promoting health means taking into account the person in context. Failure to do so represents a failure of nursing ethics or, alternatively stated, a failure of professional responsibility. Willis and colleagues (2008) synthesized a central unifying focus of the discipline that is implicit in almost all theoretical and philosophical nursing works and that gives nurses a way to articulate their work. This focus, as noted earlier, is facilitating humanization, meaning, choice, quality of life, and healing in living and dying. The central theme evident in the historical nursing literature is that nurses facilitate humanization for patients and patient groups. "Nursing facilitates humanization by engaging experiential human beings [persons who experience life and its events] in practice and modeling humane relating for other human beings. Humanization . . . is manifested when the nurse works with [any] human being [and views them as] relational, experiential, valuable, respectworthy, meaning-oriented, flawed, imperfect, vulnerable, fragile, complex, and capable of health and healing even if not capable of being cured" (p. E34).

Critical Questions

Given that there are quite a few nursing philosophers and theorists and as many philosophical, conceptual, or theoretical approaches to nursing knowledge development in the interests of nursing care, how does the APN know which perspective to follow to ensure professionally responsible care? The answer is that the perspective and knowledge brought to bear on a practice issue will, to a certain extent, depend on the nature of the problem, the patient or group involved, the nature of the practice setting, and the personal and professional characteristics and experiences of the clinician. The point is not so much that following a particular theory or perspective will result in ethical action, although having a structure to a nurse's practice definitely helps with consistency of data gathering and approach to care and so forth, but rather that much work has been accomplished in identifying nursing's goals, and that there is agreement among nursing scholars on certain key points.

There is implicit or explicit agreement that nursing's metaparadigm concepts, or the overarching concepts of the discipline, include person, environment, health, and nursing (Fawcett & Malinski, 1999). What this means, roughly, is that there is unity about the fact that "nursing has to do with assisting humans, who are viewed as complex individuals who interact with their environment and have health needs that nursing can address" (Grace, 2004b, p. 288).

THE GOALS OF NURSING

The authors of the current ANA *Code of Ethics for Nurses with Interpretive Statements* (2001)— informed by practicing nurses and contemporary societal developments—synthesized historical and current literature. In the preface to the code, the goals of nursing are stated as follows: "The prevention of illness, the alleviation of suffering, and the protection, promotion, and restoration of health." Similarly, the ICN affirms the goals of nursing in terms of the responsibilities of nurses and nursing "to promote health, to prevent illness, to restore health and to alleviate suffering" (ICN, 2012). These agreed-on goals of nursing should be kept in mind as the discussion moves to the skills and characteristics needed to practice ethically.

However, there are other factors that are important to ethical practice that apply regardless of what philosophical or theoretical approach to care is used. These factors include understanding the role of bias in data gathering or relationships, the boundaries of knowledge and skills possessed, moral development, and motivation to engage with patients and to act (refer to Table 1).

Nursing Ethics: State of the Science

THREE PHASES

To recap, the status of Nursing Ethics as a field of inquiry can be categorized into three phases, as described by Sara Fry (2002). The first phase covers the early days of nursing's formal development via training or apprenticeships in line with Florence Nightingale's vision. Fry (2002) notes that "during the early days of the 20th century, nursing ethics was understood as the articulation of the customs, habits and moral rules that nurses follow in the care of the sick" (p. 1). The transition to the second phase began after World War II. During this time, more nurses were able to gain access to university education, started to become more independent (from physicians) in their practice, and thus assumed more accountability for actions that resulted from their clinical judgments. "This new expectation of accountability created changes in how nurses' ethical duties and behaviours were understood"

(Fry, 2002, p. 1). Much earlier, nursing leaders had begun to recognize the need for a formalized code of ethics that would serve as a unifying guide for action. However, it took 53 years between recognition that a code was needed and the actual adoption of the 1950 *Code for Nurses* (Fowler, 1997). Following the ANA, in 1953 the ICN, a federation of nursing groups from several countries (now more than 128), also developed and published a document entitled *The Code of Ethics for Nurses* that reflected the "shared values of nurses" across borders (Curtin, 2001).

Finally, the current or third Nursing Ethics phase is concerned with exploration and analyzing contemporary nursing practice for its ability to meet nursing goals. The concerns of contemporary Nursing Ethics reflect the maturing of the discipline. Nursing Ethics explores the meaning of being a good nurse and good nursing practice in increasingly complex settings. This contemporary phase has seen an increase in research activities. See **Table   4** for a synopsis of nursing ethics research phases.

IMPORTANT CONCEPTS

Fry (2002) identifies four concepts that are important to contemporary practice and that apply also to advanced practice. These concepts are "co-operation, accountability, caring, and advocacy" (p. 2). These four related concepts are discussed in more detail in the following chapters. They are especially important in advanced practice because of the expanded nature of such practice and the leadership roles assumed by APNs. Briefly, cooperation and collaboration are responsibilities to work with others within and outside the profession to get what is needed for patient care on the individual as well as the societal levels. The problem for APNs in collaborative relationships is how to maintain their disciplinary perspective while taking into account other perspectives. That is, how do nurses ensure that the collaboration is egalitarian in view of nursing's history of subservience? Accountability was discussed earlier and refers to responsibility for one's professional actions. This discussion uses a modified conception of advocacy termed *professional advocacy* (Grace, 2001) to denote actions required to ensure good care at the level of the individual and at increasingly broader levels as necessary to demolish obstacles to good practice. This is a panoramic conception of advocacy that goes beyond mere protection of human rights. Many argue that the political activities required by conceiving the scope of professional responsibilities this way are not possible for most nurses, who do not possess the knowledge, skills, energy, or necessary supports.

■ Table 4   Phases of Nursing Ethics Empirical Research

Phase	Research Details
Earliest Nursing Ethics Research	In 1935 Rose Vaughan studied the diaries of student and graduate nurses related to ethical problems encountered for her dissertation (Fry & Grace, 2007).
1980s: Ethics Research Expands	Content related to nurses' ethical reasoning, judgments, and behaviors.
1990s: Nursing Ethics Research Focus	As in earlier phase, plus concepts such as advocacy, participation in end-of-life decision making, patient values, influence of education on moral reasoning, and nurses' experiences of ethical issues
1994 Nursing ethics research – dedicated publication venue	Inception of the *International Journal of Nursing Ethics* (Tschudin, 2006). Early issues featured research on advocacy, quality care, nurses' decision making, and ethical issues experienced by nurses. There was an increase in qualitative studies: reflective practice and experiences of moral unease and moral distress.
Contemporary Nursing Ethics Research	Qualitative and quantitative studies: Obstacles to care, the meaning of experiences, moral distress, nurse–patient relationships, characteristics of good nurses, patient decision making, collaboration, nurses engagement in preventive ethics, ethical decision making especially around end-of-life care, and political activity. Some studies on advanced practice: conflicts of interest, collaboration, specialty practice.

Finally, caring requires a little more discussion because contemporarily it has received a lot of attention both within and outside of the discipline. Indeed, nursing has been heavily criticized by feminists and other ethicists for framing caring as an ideal of practice. Defining caring in the nursing context provides an important foundation for the ensuing section.

Care and Nursing Practice: Ethical Implications

Care is a concept that highlights the relational aspects of human interactions. As an ethic of nursing practice, it has its origins in insights from feminist ethics and related research (Gilligan, 1982). These insights expose the idea that women consider context and relationships to be important in reasoning about ethically difficult situations. They do not rely purely on principle-based reasoning.

For example, a nursing home patient, Mr. Jones, wants to be allowed to walk to the bathroom unattended even though he is unsteady on his feet and has been evaluated as a falls risk. The adult nurse practitioner (ANP) reasoning about his autonomy and how best to facilitate this request would do a risk–benefit assessment and make a decision that balances protecting Mr. Jones's autonomy and the likelihood of a fall—this is the same assessment that would be made of any other patient whose autonomy was threatened. However, from a care perspective, the ANP is interested in knowing about Mr. Jones within this particular context, what it means to him to walk unaided, and how his wishes could be accommodated in a way that makes sense to him. The ANP would engage with Mr. Jones in the decision-making process. "The ethic of care means a responsibility to attend to the individual as individual in all of his or her complexities" (Grace, 2005, p. 105). Indeed the goals of nursing practice require that the clinician has, or cultivates, a predisposition to engage with the patient to understand that person's particular needs. Benner, Tanner, and Chesla (1996) note that care facilitates "the alleviation of vulnerability; the promotion of growth and health; the facilitation of comfort, dignity or a good and peaceful death" (p. 233).

Care as a facet of nursing requires engagement on the part of the nurse with the patient in a relationship that permits the meaning and context of the person's need to be exposed. This is not a purely emotional sense of care; it is not, for example, the same meaning as "I care about my friend." Rather, knowledge, skills, and motivation are all needed for an engaged knowing of the person. In their research, Benner and colleagues (1996) note that it appears as "the dominant ethic found in [nurses'] stories of everyday practice" (p. 233).

Of course, there are criticisms of the ethic of care. Nelson (1992), a bioethicist, notes the problem of moral predictability. That is, she wonders how to determine right actions from within the nurse–patient care relationship. Another criticism is that a care ethic does not permit a critique of morally suspect environments. Further, feminists have cautioned that adoption of an ethic of care as the dominant nursing ethic could further jeopardize nursing's power to effect change on behalf of patient care; nurses, they argue, could be manipulated by powerful patients. One other important criticism has to do with the fact that nurses have responsibility for more than one patient, so excessive care for one might disadvantage another.

These are all valid criticisms and represent worrisome issues if the ethic of care is taken to be the only important consideration in clinical decision making. However, an ethic of care is an important concept where knowledge of the patient as an individual is needed for the goals of the profession to be furthered. Ethical decision making, like sound clinical judgment, requires nurses to take into account both the larger context and the context of the individual. It includes determining which tools are appropriate to employ in identifying the ethical content of everyday practice.

Ethical Decision Making and Action for Good Care

Clinical and Moral Reasoning

So far, this chapter has traced the development of nursing into a profession and made the argument that membership in the profession leads to responsibility and accountability for practice actions and that all practice actions are subject to critique related to how well they are likely or able to fulfill the profession's goals as these have been developed over time. At this point, then, it is appropriate to gain clarity about practical applications. As articulated so far, the argument can be made that in many ways clinical and moral (ethical) reasoning are inseparable concepts. "Good or 'ethical' nursing practice results from the use of theoretical, conceptual, and practical knowledge in formulating clinical judgments, and evaluating ensuing actions for their ability to meet patient needs" (Grace, 2004a, p. 296). The "conceptual or theoretical knowledge may be derived from other disciplines as well as nursing" (Grace, 2004a, p. 296); however, this knowledge should still be filtered through a nursing lens (perhaps by asking "How will this facilitate the patient's good in the context of nursing practice?" or "How should I work to influence needed practice or societal changes?").

Clinically good actions, it can be argued, are synonymous with ethically good actions. It is even possible to go one step further and assert that when clinically good actions (those most likely to further the patient's good) are obstructed in some way, good clinical judgment would conceptualize what nonclinical actions are needed to circumvent or tear down the obstruction—these actions highlight what professional responsibility requires of nurses. Strategies for addressing obstacles are suggested and proposed throughout the following chapters. As synthesized from extant nursing, philosophical, and research literature, good or ethical practice requires all of the following:

- An ongoing focus on the goals of the discipline and the ethical nature of these goals
- Disciplinary knowledge and skills related to the practice setting and role assumed
- Adherence to the scope and limits of nursing or nursing specialty practice as well as a nurse's own knowledge and experience (entails knowing personal limits and being willing to seek assistance from knowledgeable or skilled others)
- Ability to communicate a nursing perspective using the language of ethics to convey a patient's or group's needs
- Understanding of personal and professional values (self-reflection and reflection on practice)
- Willingness and capacity to engage with patients where possible regardless of level of cognitive functioning (there may be some patients with whom a nurse cannot engage because of unresolved or unresolvable prior personal or life experiences; in this case, good practice permits turning care of the person over to another)
- Ability to make sound decisions
- Motivation to act
- Perseverance in carrying out ethical actions despite or in spite of obstacles

The next section explores in more detail the cognitive and affective processes that underlie ethically appropriate actions. Ethically appropriate means those actions that are required by nursing's goals and the role responsibilities of nurses.

Processes of Moral Action

James Rest (1941–1999) gleaned his views on the cognitive and affective processes that must underlie moral behavior from the contemporary theory and literature of disparate disciplines. He noted that there are at least four, but perhaps more, interrelated activities of a person's mind and ways of thinking that lead to that person acting to achieve a "good." This conceptualization of the "good" action is internal—it is not a predetermined good. That is, his theory does not presuppose that there is an ultimate good that only the most moral people are able to achieve or that there is some sort of factual principle that if followed would always lead to a good. There is no agreement about whether there is an "ultimate good" for humans to pursue, and many doubt that one exists. However, there is general agreement that human beings have interests in living a meaningful life without undue interference or obstruction from others (Weston, 2011).

Rest's theory of moral action is based in the idea that persons can be engaged in a process of considered intention to do good. His insights derived from accumulated research cohere, for the most part, with the list of attributes given earlier as synthesized from nursing and allied literature. Rest (1982, 1983), an educational psychologist, noted that research or inquiry about cognitive and affective processes underlying moral action is in its infancy. Approaches tend to be scattered or fragmented, often focused on only one of the following: moral thought, moral emotion, or moral behavior, but not the interfaces between these. Additionally, the different disciplines tend to be concerned only with their perspective, causing further fragmentation. Yet a coherent understanding of the processes of moral behavior is needed to know what can and cannot be fostered and what strategies are most likely to work. To be clear, Rest's quest was not about discovering absolute or universal truths; it was about the psychology of human action, that is, about what cognitive and affective factors are in play when a person acts morally, given some predetermined moral goal of action. More recently, Doris and colleagues (2010), in *The Moral Psychology Handbook*, describe the state of the science related to interdisciplinary research on human action. Unprecedented knowledge about how the human mind works is now available because of collaborative studies undertaken by disparate disciplines. Knowing more about human capacities and predispositions allows people to guard against certain errors of judgment that are common but not well understood. The assumption of all professional education is that it is, for the most part, possible to foster the sorts of characteristics needed for moral practice and moral decision making. That is, education can prepare professionals to achieve professional goals. Therefore, continuing to investigate how these processes are integrated or integral to each other is necessary for us to know more about how to foster moral behavior. Rest's assumption, derived from a thorough review of work done so far in a variety of sciences and disciplines, is that the processes are interrelated, and all are necessary for a moral action or moral behavior to result. A failure in just one area or one process may result in a failure to behave morally. Many disciplines have undertaken ongoing research related to moral behavior, including nursing (see Table 4 for examples of contemporary nursing ethics research). Although integrative approaches that look at the relationships of all processes are included, and work in moral and behavioral psychology as well as in the cognitive and physiological sciences has advanced our understanding, the state of the science remains immature.

Rest's tentative framework is also helpful in artificially delineating important aspects of moral action while understanding the necessary interdependence of these aspects. Appreciating that there are limits and hindrances to moral decision making and moral action alerts professionals to those factors that can interfere with their decision making and allows them to guard against these. Rest suggests four questions that have been partly addressed by contemporary philosophical and empirical research and that correspond to the probable internal processes behind moral decision making and action: "(1) How does the person interpret the situation and how does he or she view any possible action as affecting people's welfare? (2) How does the person figure out what the morally ideal course of action would be? (3) How does he or she decide what to do? and (4) Does the person implement what he or she intends to do?" (Rest, 1982, p. 29).

There are both affective (emotion) and cognitive (thought) components to these processes that may not be separable for the purposes of studying how people actually act. An implication is that good action results from all of these processes working together and that emotion and reason are both crucial elements. This is helpful in defining the characteristics of good clinicians. In **Table 5**, Rest's explanations of the nature of each process or aspect are modified by applying them to direct patient care situations to provide a clearer idea of what is meant. This illustrates how a nursing ethics course or book, together with group reflections on practice, might facilitate the development of or highlight already possessed attributes that are supportive of an APN's confidence in moral decision making and action. Table 5 also synthesizes the research and theoretical literature to present some factors that have been discovered to obstruct each process. The list of obstructing factors is not meant to be exhaustive.

Self-Reflection, Values Clarification, and Reflection on Practice

Gaining confidence in one's moral decision making is admittedly a slow process. My colleagues, Drs. Ellen Robinson (Project Director) and Martha Jurchak, Clinical Ethics Directors at Massachusetts General Hospital (MGH)

■ Table 5 Four Aspects of Moral Action and Interfering Factors

Rest's Processes (1982)	Practical Implications	Interfering Factors
1. **Interpretation of the situation**	APNs' understanding of the inherently ethical nature of any practice situation; APNs are responsible for their actions, and their professional actions are to facilitate the profession's goals directly or indirectly Assessment of this particular situation and what is needed to achieve optimal care for the person or persons in need	Personal troubles Energy level Time available Knowledge level No understanding of the inherently moral nature of practice Lack of connection with the patient/inability to engage Perception/sensitivity affected by age and life experiences Lack of self-reflection
2. **Discerning the morally ideal action—what ought to be done**	Using appropriate tools, methods, resources, and collaborations for decision making Identifying the beneficiary, the goal, appropriate actions	Level of moral development Level of independence Level and types of education Personal values conflict with patient/significant other/other professionals' values Lack of reflection on practice
3. **Deciding what to do**	Deciding among competing courses of action What ought to be done may not always be possible or consensus not reachable	Situational ambiguity Theoretical ambiguity Uncertainty about outcome Lack of institutional or peer support

(*continues*)

■ Table 5 Four Aspects of Moral Action and Interfering Factors (*continued*)

Rest's Processes (1982)	Practical Implications	Interfering Factors
4. Implementation and perseverance	Envisioning the steps and anticipating problems Addressing and overcoming problems and barriers Taking sociopolitical actions to get what is needed Keeping sight of the goal Reminding others of the goal	Too many obstacles Fear of personal consequences, peer/colleague disapproval Fatigue Frustration Lack of resources and supports

and Brigham and Women's hospital (BWH), respectively, and the Reverend Angelika Zollfrank, Director of Pastoral Education at MGH, have been working under a U.S. Department of Health and Human Services, Health Resources and Services Administration (HRSA) grant to build nurses' confidence and capacity in clinical ethics at the bedside. This is a 1-year program consisting of 8 hours per month of didactic, experiential (role play and simulation), and practice components—it is offered to select bedside nurses and APNs (N = 18–25 per year). The program is currently working with its third cohort. Data analysis of its efficacy in improving confidence and capability in addressing practice issues and speaking up on behalf of patients and families is ongoing. However, overwhelmingly nurses report verbally and in their course evaluations increased confidence in speaking up on behalf of good patient care and engaging in a variety of ethics-related projects such as organizing unit-based ethics rounds and participating in ethics committees and interdisciplinary ethics forums. Nurses unanimously note the importance of being able to discuss issues with others and the insights this permits, as well as gaining clarity about important aspects of the ethical crises and situations they face. Nursing research studies and scholarly literature reveal that many nurses at all levels of practice remain unsure of the validity or importance of their point of view in ethically difficult situations (Ceci, 2004; Dierckx de Casterlé, Izumi, Godfrey, & Denhaerynck, 2008; Dodd, Jansson, Brown-Saltzman, & Wunch, 2004; Duffy & Currier, 1999; Hardingham, 2004; Helft, Chamness, Terry, & Uhrich, 2011; Kelly, 1998; Pavlish, Brown-Saltzman, Hersh, Shirk, & Rounkle, 2011; Varcoe et al., 2004; Whitney et al., 2006). One explanation is the idea that ethics belongs in the realm of the obscure or difficult. There is a common belief that ethics in healthcare settings is about difficult dilemmas that require esoteric knowledge brought to bear by high-minded individuals. What I realized as a result of my studies in philosophy and medical ethics is that most ethical issues arise in daily healthcare practice and are the result of lack of focus on either the goals or the recipient of care. Thus, nurses, as the clinicians who tend to spend the most time with patients, are often the ones who have the most comprehensive version of the patient's story. Moreover, nurses probably have the best opportunity to diffuse situations that have the potential to develop into crises, in some cases simply by gathering important parties together to talk about goals in view of patient desires and preferences. APNs can serve as important resources both within institutional settings and in primary care settings.

CASE STUDY: MS. KNIGHT

Although this chapter clearly states that all practice actions, from the simple to the complex, are subject to ethical appraisal, that is, they can be judged good or bad according to whether they are focused on furthering nursing's goals, this slightly more complex case demonstrates how to approach moral decision making using the tools and skills described throughout the chapter, as well as in the accompanying tables. **Table** 6 lists some key factors in any healthcare decision-making process. However, there are many different frameworks available in the literature, and you may well find one of these is more in concert with your style of analysis. The important thing to remember is that there will never be enough information to unquestionably confirm that a decision is flawless, but it is possible to gain reasonable clarity on most situations by asking the questions posed in Table 6.

Ms. Knight

Ms. Jean Knight is an 80-year-old patient who was successfully treated for breast cancer 5 years ago. Her cancer has returned, however, and she now

**■ Table 6   Ethical Decision Making in Difficult Situations:
Important Considerations**

In the course of *daily practice,* what is needed for ethical action is the thoughtful exercise of knowledge, experience, and skill, together with a constant focus on the good of the patient or group in need of services and an understanding of the nurse's own biases.

In more *complex* situations, where what is good is not so clearly seen, a more in-depth analysis may be needed. This is not necessarily a linear process, nor will all of the following considerations always be pertinent. There are other decision-making models available, but all have similar considerations.

Steps	Questions
Identify the major problem(s)— relate these to professional goals.	■ What are the facts: clinical, social, environmental?
Pay attention to the "trigger"— you feel uneasy about a situation—try to discover why, what is bothering you. This is a good starting point for exploration.	■ What implicit assumptions are being made? ■ What ethical principles or perspectives are pertinent? Examples: autonomous decision making is in question, conflict of values among providers and patient/ significant others, economic versus patient good ■ Are there power imbalances? What are these? Who has an interest in maintaining them?
Identify information gaps.	■ Do you need more information? ■ From whom or where might you get this information?
Determine who is involved.	■ Who is the main focus? Is there more than one important party? Who has (or thinks they have) an interest in the outcome (relatives, staff, other)? Who will be affected by the outcome?
Decide what the prevalent values are.	■ Values held by patient, staff, institution ■ Are there value conflicts?—interpersonal, interprofessional, personal versus professional, patient versus professional.

■ Table 6 Ethical Decision Making in Difficult Situations: Important
Considerations (*continued*)

Steps	Questions
Determine if an interpreter is necessary (for cultural or language issues). Who would be the most appropriate interpreter (knowledgeable and neutral)? Often this is not the family member!	■ Are there cultural perspectives? Who can help with these?
Identify possible courses of action and probable consequences.	■ Which course of action is likely to be the most beneficial and the least harmful to those involved, including you? ■ Can safeguards be put in place in case of unforeseen consequences?
Implement the selected course of action. Conduct an ongoing evaluation.	■ Does the actual outcome correlate with the anticipated outcome? What was unexpected? Was this foreseeable given more data? ■ Do similar problems keep reoccurring? If so, why (requires a look at underlying environmental or societal issues perhaps)? Does this point to the need for policy changes or development at the site, institution, or societal level? What further actions might be needed? ■ Are there continuing staff provider education needs related to the issue?
Engage in self-reflection, reflection on practice (individually, in an interdisciplinary group debriefing session, or in a specialty group forum).	■ Could you have done things differently? What would you have liked to understand better? ■ Would a consultation with colleagues or an ethics resource person have altered your conception of the issue or the course of action taken? ■ What valuable insights did you gain that should be shared with others and may be applicable to the approach used for future problems?

has bone and liver metastases. She was admitted 2 days ago from a local nursing home, to Clarion, a medical floor, for pain management and pneumonia. She is being treated with IV antibiotics and fentanyl patches for her pain. She occasionally experiences breakthrough pain, for which she is prescribed oral hydromorphone. Her IV site has become obstructed and she is refusing to have a new IV inserted.

Gina Jenks is Ms. Knight's primary nurse. She has been working as a staff nurse for only 8 months and sometimes is not very confident in her skills. However, this is her second day with Ms. Knight, and she thought that she had developed a good rapport with her patient. She tries to reason with Ms. Knight about the importance of receiving the IV antibiotics, but Ms. Knight remained opposed to having the IV inserted.

Ms. Sandy Norton is the clinical nurse specialist (CNS) for this busy unit. Recently, Sandy Norton has been trying to encourage some of the newer nurses like Gina to take a more active role in presenting their patient's point of view to physicians, allied providers, and family members as needed. Gina seeks Sandy out to ask her advice. She tells her that Ms. Knight's exact words were, "I don't want any more medicines and I don't want any more fluids. I am ready to die. Just let me die, won't you?" Gina appears shaken.

Discussion

The decision-making considerations from Table 6 are italicized in the following discussion because, as with explorations of many difficult issues, they do not proceed in a linear fashion; rather, considerations or questions suggest themselves as the story unfolds. Not all considerations are pertinent in all cases; however, a cursory review of them permits relative confidence that no important aspect of analysis is overlooked.

The *main problem* seems relatively straightforward: Ms. Knight is refusing care that her providers deem to be in her best interests. Providing IV antibiotics is the standard treatment for her immediate medical problem of pneumonia and can also be used to give pain medicines if needed. The *underlying assumptions* being made are that (1) Ms. Knight will physically benefit from the IV antibiotics (beneficence), (2) without the antibiotics she will worsen and die (nonmaleficence), and (3) death is a bad outcome for Ms. Knight.

Although premise 1 is true, premises 2 and 3 are more questionable. Premise 2 depends on there being no alternative treatments for the pneumonia, and premise 3 requires more information about *Ms. Knight, her preferences, and values*. Additionally, Ms. Knight wants her autonomy respected. She appears to understand that she might die and, if her understanding is adequately informed as discussed in Chapter 1, she has both the moral and the legal right to decide for herself what treatments she will or will not accept.

However, nurses' responsibilities do not end even if a determination of decision-making capacity is made. *Professional goals* require that nurses find out more about how the patient feels and what alternatives are available that might be acceptable to her, thus not abandoning her to her autonomy. From the narrative it is not clear whether any overt *power imbalances* exist; however, implicit in most provider–patient relationships is an imbalance related to knowledge. The fact is that the provider serves as a gatekeeper for further care and interventions, and sometimes to setting. Power influences are likely present in the case of Ms. Knight, who is dependent on the nurses and institution to meet all of her other daily living needs. She has no relatives in the local area, and she has lost touch with many of her friends since entering the nursing home 2 years prior because of mild mobility issues. This power differential does need to be taken into consideration in communicating with her. The nurses must keep in mind that she might be susceptible to caregivers' influence if she thinks they will neglect her other needs, the most salient of which may be pain control.

Sandy (CNS) talks to *Gina (novice nurse)* about her feelings in the situation because Gina is visibly shaken by the event. Sandy's responsibilities as a CNS include staff support and education, both of which ultimately affect patient care. Gina says she is worried that Ms. Knight will deteriorate just when the nurses feel she is doing better. She hopes that there is something more that can be done—she does not want to "have to watch her die needlessly." Gina and Sandy must try to ascertain what Ms. Knight's understanding of the situation is, that is, what information gaps exist and how these could be filled in.

Gina and Sandy are charged with discovering whether Ms. Knight does actually have decision-making capacity. If decision-making capacity is impaired, her ability to understand the implications of the choices she makes will be limited. Autonomous action depends on her ability to take in information, digest it, and convey that what she understands and wishes is in line with her previous life choices and desires for the future. Sandy decides that the best way to proceed is to role model for Gina how such an assessment can be made, acknowledging the need for discussion later. First, she talks to Gina about her feelings, reassuring her they are normal, that she knows more than she thinks she does, and that increased experience in handling such situations will help her develop confidence in decision making.

Before approaching Ms. Knight, Sandy emphasizes the importance of first making sure that there are no obvious physiologic or psychological impediments to information processing. Gina reports that although Ms. Knight did have some confusion the previous day when her oxygen saturation levels were borderline and her temperature was 101.4°F, today she has been lucid and oriented. Additionally, her pain is being well controlled with the fentanyl patch, with only one additional dose of hydromorphone needed during the night. However, she did tell Gina that the management of her nursing home had changed and the residents were not getting the same quality of attention as they were previously. This made her very unhappy, and she was worried about the quality of her care on her return. Sandy asked Gina to consider how this information might be relevant to the current situation and something to investigate further.

Sandy and Gina approach Ms. Knight and find her crying. Sandy says, "Ms. Knight, Gina tells me that you don't want to have your IV reinserted. I am so sorry that you are experiencing these problems. I am here to help figure out what can be done to ensure that you are comfortable and your needs are taken care of. Tell me more about what you are thinking."

Ms. Knight accurately recounts what went on and in response to further questions admits that she does not *necessarily want to die but is not happy with her life lately*, is afraid that if she goes back to the nursing home she will not get her pain needs met, and thinks that if this is the way it has to be then she is prepared to die. She turns to Gina and says, "I am sorry I yelled—you have been so good to me—you didn't deserve it, but I am at the end of my rope. I really do not want any more IVs sticks—they always have trouble with my IVs."

Sandy talks to Ms. Knight about some of the *alternatives,* both to having the IV reinserted and to ongoing care in the nursing home. She also asks about her mood, suspecting that she may be depressed. They discuss the possibility of oral antibiotics and the need for Ms. Knight to drink plenty of fluids. Sandy also talks about other options that can be explored such as having hospice or palliative care services visit her at her nursing home. They can provide staff education related to pain management and the existential needs of a person facing death as well as extra patient care services. She suggests having a social worker come and talk to Ms. Knight so that arrangements can be made in advance of her discharge.

During the conversation, Ms. Knight stops crying and is agreeable both to the idea of oral antibiotics and a visit from the social worker. She admits to feeling "down what with the cancer coming back and everything, but isn't that to be expected?" Gina says, "Ms. Knight, I remember you talking to me about the pastor from your church and how she had visited you in the nursing home and been very helpful. Would you like me to contact her and ask her to visit?" Ms. Knight says, "Yes I would, I hadn't thought that she could come here to see me."

Back in Sandy's office, Sandy and Gina revisit the interaction. Sandy reassures Gina that her actions were appropriate, and that it was important that she recognized the limits of her experience and knowledge and sought appropriate advice, but that it was also apparent that she had her own resources to draw on—she indeed knew Ms. Knight better than anyone else. In Sandy's experience, events could have gone very differently if, for example, there had been an urgent need to restart the IV (for example, a dehydration issue) before anyone had talked to Ms. Knight about her preferences for care and interventions in the event of an emergency. Because the situation was not an emergency, Ms. Knight's wishes could be heard and conveyed to the physician. Gina said she would be comfortable phoning Ms. Knight's attending physician and explaining the situation, what had been discussed, and what Ms. Knight wanted. However, she thought that it would be helpful for the floor nurses to have a meeting to discuss the situation. Additionally, in her college classes they had discussed the problems of advance directives and how to talk to patients about their preferences should an emergency arise and thought this would be good time to reinforce the importance of these.

Summary

This chapter explores the status of nursing as a profession with its accompanying responsibilities. The relationship of clinical and moral reasoning was highlighted and supported. Finally, the exercise of clinical and moral decision making in advanced practice was exemplified by a case study and case analysis. An important facet of moral decision making in difficult situations is processing the event after the fact. This is a time when reflection and self-reflection can be crucial to the development of confidence in decision making and when the insights of others can broaden a nurse's perspective.

Yet, perhaps understandably, this is often the most neglected part of ethical practice. Time constraints, fiscal constraints, and the relative isolation of many advanced practice settings all conspire against collegial meetings of these kinds. Important tips for the conduct of such meetings include neutral settings, confidentiality, and sensitivity to the feelings of those presenting so that they are not made to feel that they "did it wrong." Rather, the emphasis should be on the idea that such sessions help further professional goals by facilitation of new tools, strategies, and approaches.

Discussion Questions

1. Does your country have its own code of ethics or does it rely on that of the ICN (over 130 member states)? What guidance is provided in your code of ethics or conduct related to restrictive contexts and environments? What are the responsibilities of the professional or professions?
2. Think of a simple case or situation you were involved in that left you feeling troubled. Explore this with colleagues using Table 6 or another decision-making heuristic (helpful framework). What new insights do you have? Would you have done things differently in light of what you learned in this chapter?
3. Preventive ethics is the process of anticipating and addressing potential problems before they arise. Many of the issues in health care that progress to the dilemma stage (choice between two or more equally bad alternatives) start off as minor communication problems. Think of one or more occasions from your practice when recognizing or addressing something early on would have defused an incipient difficult situation. For example, in my past experience with a patient critically ill with toxic shock syndrome, I believe that early honest conversations with her family would have prevented the loss of trust with its subsequent suspicion and anger.

References

American Association of Colleges of Nursing. (2006). *The essentials of doctoral education for advanced nursing practice*. Washington, DC: Author. Retrieved from http://www.aacn .nche.edu/publications/position/DNPEssentials.pdf

American Medical Association. (2001). *Principles of medical ethics.* Retrieved from http://www .ama-assn.org/ama/pub/category/2512.html

American Nurses Association. (1994). *Ethics and human rights position statements: The nonnegotiable nature of the ANA Code for Nurses with interpretive statements.* Washington, DC: Author. Retrieved from http://www.nursingworld.org/positionstatements

American Nurses Association. (2001). *Code of ethics for nurses with interpretive statements.* Washington, DC: Author.

American Nurses Association. (2010). *Social policy statement.* Washington, DC: Author.

Andrist, L. C., Nicholas, P. K., & Wolf, K. A. (2006). *A history of nursing ideas.* Sudbury, MA: Jones and Bartlett.

Anscombe, J. (2008). Healthcare out of balance: How global forces will reshape the health of nations. Report of A. T. Kearney Inc. Retrieved from http://www.atkearney.com /documents/10192/dced09b1-745b-4934-be20-3dec90d8195e

Benner, P., Tanner, C. A., & Chesla, C. A. (1996). *Expertise in nursing practice: Caring, clinical judgment and ethics.* New York, NY: Springer.

Blumer, R. H., & Meyer, M. (2006). *The new medicine.* Ashland, OH: Atlas Books.

Brown, L. (1993). (Ed.). *The new shorter Oxford English Dictionary.* New York, NY: Oxford Clarendon Press.

Bruhn, J. G. (2001). Being good and doing good: The culture of professionalism in the health professions. *Health Care Manager, 19*(4), 47–58.

Bryant-Lukosius, D., DiCensio, A., Browne, G., & Pinelli, J. (2004). Advanced practice nursing roles: Development, implementation and evaluation. *Nursing and Healthcare Management and Policy, 48*(5), 519–529.

Carr-Saunders, A. M., & Wilson, P. A. (1933). *The professions.* Oxford, England: Clarendon.

Ceci, C. (2004). Nursing, knowledge and power: A case analysis. *Social Science and Medicine, 59,* 1879–1889.

Chiang-Hanisko, L., Ross., R., Boonyanurak., P., Ozawa, M., & Chiang., L. (2008). Pathways to progress in nursing: Understanding career patterns in Japan, Taiwan, and Thailand. *The Online Journal of Issues in Nursing, 13*(3), Manuscript 4. doi: 10.3912/OJIN. Vol13No03Man04

Coburn, J. (1987). "I See and Am Silent." A Short History of Nursing in Ontario, 1850–1930. In D. Coburn, C. D'Arcy, G. Torrance, & P. New (Eds.), *Health and Canadian society* (2nd ed.). Markham, Ontario: Fitzhenry and Whiteside.

Cody, W. K. (2006). *Philosophical and theoretical perspectives for advanced practice nursing.* (4th ed.). Sudbury, MA: Jones and Bartlett.

Cronenwett, L., Dracup, K., Grey, M., McCauley, L., Meleis, A., & Salmon, M. (2011). The Doctor of Nursing Practice: A national workforce perspective. *Nursing Outlook, 59,* 9–17.

Curtin, L. (2001). Guest editorial: The ICN Code of Ethics for Nurses: Shared values in a troubled world. *ICN International Nursing Review, 48*(1), 1–2.

Dewey, J. (1980). *The quest for certainty: A study of the relation of action knowledge and action.* New York, NY: Perigree Books. (Original work published in 1929.)

Dierckx de Casterlé, B., Izumi, S., Godfrey, N. S., & Denhaerynck, K. (2008). Nurses' responses to ethical dilemmas in nursing practice: Meta-analysis. *Journal of Advanced Nursing, 63*(6), 540–549.

Dodd, S. J., Jansson, B. S., Brown-Saltzman, M. S., & Wunch, K. (2004). Expanding nurses' participation in ethics: An empirical examination of ethical activism and ethical assertiveness. *Nursing Ethics, 11*(1), 15–27.

Donaldson, S. K., & Crowley, D. M. (1978). The discipline of nursing. *Nursing Outlook, 26*(2), 113–120.

Doris, J. M., & The Moral Psychology Research Group. (2010). *The moral psychology handbook.* New York, NY: Oxford University Press.

Dougherty, C. J. (1990). The costs of commercial medicine. *Theoretical Medicine, 11,* 275–286.

Dougherty, C. J. (1992). The excesses of individualism. For meaningful healthcare reform, the United States needs a renewed sense of community. *Health Progress Journal, 73*(1), 22–28.

Dracup, K., Cronenwett, L., Meleis, A. I., & Benner, P. E. (2005). Reflections on the doctorate of nursing practice. *Nursing Outlook, 53,* 177–182.

Duffy, M. E., & Currier, S. (1999). *Ethics and human rights in nursing practice: A survey of New England nurses. Unpublished report of the survey.* Principal investigators: Sara Fry, Henry Luce Professor of Nursing Ethics, Boston College, Chestnut Hill; & Joan Riley, Director, Department of Nursing Emmanuel College, Boston, MA.

Fawcett, J., & Malinski, V. M. (1999). On the requirements for a metaparadigm: An invitation to dialogue. In J. W. Kenney (Ed.), *Philosophical and theoretical perspectives for advanced nursing practice* (2nd ed., pp. 111–116). Sudbury, MA: Jones and Bartlett.

Fawcett, J., Newman, D. M. L., & McAllister, M. (2004). Advanced practice nursing and conceptual models of nursing. *Nursing Science Quarterly, 17*(2), 135–138.

FEPI. (2012). *Code of Ethics and Conduct for European Nurses.* Brussels, Belgium: Author. Retrieved from http://www.fepi.org/userfiles/file/FEPI_Code_of_Ethics_and_Conducts_170908 .pdf

Fineberg, H. V. (2012). A successful and sustainable healthcare system: How to get there from here? *New England Journal of Medicine, 366*(11), 1020–1027.

Flaming, D. (2004). Nursing theories as nursing ontologies. *Nursing Philosophy, 5*(3), 224–229.

Flexner, A. (1915). Is social work a profession? *Proceedings of the National Conference of Charities and Correction, 581,* 584–588, 590. Retrieved from http://darkwing.uoregon .edu/~adoption/archive/FlexnerISWAP.htm

Fowler, M. (1997). Nursing's ethics. In A. J. Davis, M. A. Aroskar, J. Liaschenko, & T. S. Drought (Eds.), *Ethical dilemmas and nursing practice* (4th ed.). Stamford, CT: Appleton & Lange.

Fry, S. T. (1995). Nursing ethics. In W. T. Reich (Ed.), *Encyclopedia of bioethics* (Rev. ed., Vol. 2, pp. 1822–1827). New York, NY: Simon & Schuster Macmillan.

Fry, S. T. (2002). Guest editorial: Defining nurses' ethical practices in the 21st century. *International Nursing Review, 49,* 1–3.

Fry, S. T., & Grace, P. J. (2007). Ethical dimensions of nursing and health care. In J. L. Creasia & B. Parker (Eds.), *Conceptual foundations: The bridge to professional practice* (4th ed.). Philadelphia, PA: Mosby, Elsevier.

Gilligan, C. (1982). *In a different voice: Psychological theory and women's development.* Cambridge, MA: Harvard University Press.

Grace, P. J. (1998). *A philosophical analysis of the concept "advocacy": Implications for professional–patient relationships.* Unpublished doctoral dissertation, University of Tennessee: Knoxville, TN. Retrieved from http://proquest.umi.com. Publication Number AAT9923287, Proquest Document ID No. 734421751.

Grace, P. J. (2001). Professional advocacy: Widening the scope of accountability. *Nursing Philosophy, 2*(2), 151–162.

Grace, P. J. (2004a). Ethics in the clinical encounter. In S. K. Chase (Ed.), *Clinical judgment and communication in nurse practitioner practice* (pp. 295–332). Philadelphia, PA: F. A. Davis.

Grace, P. J. (2004b). Philosophical considerations in nurse practitioner practice. In S. K. Chase (Ed.), *Clinical judgment and communication in nurse practitioner practice* (pp. 279–294). Philadelphia, PA: F. A. Davis.

Grace, P. J. (2005). Ethical issues relevant to health promotion. In C. Edelman & C. L. Mandle (Eds.), *Health promotion throughout the lifespan* (6th ed., pp. 100–125). St. Louis, MO: Elsevier/Mosby.

Grace, P. J. (2006). Philosophies, models, and theories: Moral obligations. In M. R. Alligood & A. Marriner-Tomey (Eds.), *Nursing theory: Utilization and application* (3rd ed., pp. 67–85). St. Louis, MO: Elsevier/Mosby.

Gross, M. L. (2010). Teaching military medical ethics: Another look at dual loyalty and triage. Cambridge *Quarterly of Healthcare Ethics, 19,* 458–464.

Group, T. M., & Roberts, J. I. (2001). *Nursing, physician control and the medical monopoly.* Bloomington, IN: Indiana University Press.

Hagedorn, S., & Quinn, A. A. (2004). Theory-based nurse practitioner practice: Caring in action. *Topics in Advanced Practice Nursing, 4*(4).

Hardingham, L. (2004). Integrity and moral residue: Nurses as participants in a moral community. *Nursing Philosophy, 5,* 127–134.

Helft, P. R., Chamness, A., Terry, C., & Uhrich, M. (2011). Oncology nurses' attitudes toward prognosis-related communication: A pilot mailed survey of oncology nursing society members. *Oncology Nursing Forum, 38*(4), 468–474.

Henderson, V. A. (1991). *The nature of nursing.* New York, NY: National League for Nursing.

International Council of Nurses. (2012). *Code of ethics for nurses.* Geneva, Switzerland: Author. Retrieved from http://www.icn.ch/icncode.pdf

Kelly, B. (1998). Preserving moral integrity: A follow-up study with new graduate nurses. *Journal of Advanced Nursing, 25*(8), 1134–1145.

Kepler, M. O. (1981). *Medical stewardship: Fulfilling the Hippocratic legacy.* Westport, CT: Greenwood Press.

Mechanic, D. (1998). The functions and limitations of trust in the provision of medical care. *Journal of Health Politics, Policy and Law, 23,* 661–686.

Milton, C. (2005). Scholarship in nursing: Ethics of a practice doctorate. *Nursing Science Quarterly, 18*(2), 113–116.

Nagel, T. (1970). *The possibility of altruism.* Oxford, England: Clarendon.

National Association of Social Workers. (1999). Code of ethics. Retrieved from http://www
.socialworkers.org/pubs/code/code.asp

Nelson, H. L. (1992). Against caring. *Journal of Clinical Ethics, 3,* 8–15.

Newman, M. A., Sime, A. M., & Corcoran-Perry, S. A. (1991). The focus of the discipline of
nursing. *Advances in Nursing Science, 14*(1), 1–6.

Newton, L. H. (1988). Lawgiving for professional life: Reflections on the place of the professional code. In A. Flores (Ed.), *Professional ideals* (pp. 47–56). Belmont, CA: Wadsworth.

Nightingale, F. (1946). *Notes on nursing: What it is and what it is not.* Philadelphia, PA: Lippincott.
(Original work published in 1859.)

Packard, S. A., & Polifroni, E. C. (1992). The nature of scientific truth. *Nursing Science Quarterly,
5*(4), 158–163.

Paley, J. (2012). Book review: The moral psychology handbook. (Edited by John Doris and
the Moral Psychology Research Group. Oxford University Press.) *Nursing Philosophy, 13,*
18–22.

Pavlish, C., Brown-Saltzman, K., Hersh, M., Shirk, M., & Rounkle, A. (2011). Nursing priorities, actions, and regrets for ethical situations in clinical practice. *Journal of Nursing
Scholarship, 43*(4), 385–395.

Pelau, H. E. (1952). *Interpersonal relations in nursing.* New York, NY: G. P. Putnam's Sons.

Reid, T. R. (2009). *The healing of America: A global quest for better, cheaper, and fairer health care.*
New York, NY: Penguin.

Relman, A. S. (2007). Medical professionalism in a commercialized health care market.
Cleveland Clinic Journal of Medicine, 75 (Suppl. 6), S33–S36.

Rest, J. (1983). The major components of morality. In P. Mussen (Ed.), *Manual of child psychology* (Vol. Cognitive Development). New York, NY: Wiley.

Rest, J. R. (1982). A psychologist looks at the teaching of ethics. *Hastings Center Report, 12*(1),
29–36.

Rogers, M. E. (1970). *An introduction to the theoretical basis of nursing.* Philadelphia, PA: F. A.
Davis.

Sasso, L., Steviano, A., Jurado, M. G., & Rocco, G. (2008). Code of Ethics and Conduct for
European Nurses. *Nursing Ethics, 15*(6), 821–836.

Sellman, D. (2005). Towards an understanding of nursing as a response to vulnerability.
Nursing Philosophy, 6(1), 2–10.

Silva, M. C., & Ludwick, R. (2006, March 20). Is the Doctor of Nursing Practice ethical?
Online Journal of Issues in Nursing. Retrieved from http://www.nursingworld.org
/MainMenuCategories/ANAMarketplace/ANAPeriodicals/OJIN/Columns/Ethics
/DNPEthical.aspx

Sullivan, W. M. (1999). What is left of professionalism after managed care? *Hastings Center
Report, 29*(2), 7–13.

Tschudin, V. (2006). How nursing ethics as a subject changes: An analysis of the first 11 years
of publication of the *Journal of Nursing Ethics. Nursing Ethics, 13*(1), 66–82.

Varcoe, C., Doane, G., Pauly, B., Rodney, P., Storch, J. L., Mahoney, K., . . . Starzomski, R.
(2004). Ethical practice in nursing: Working the in-betweens. *Nursing Philosophy, 45*(3),
316–325.

Weston, A. (2011). *A practical companion to ethics* (4th ed.). New York, NY: Oxford.

Whitney, S. N., Ethier, A. M., Fruge, E., Berg, S., McCullough, L. B., & Hockenbury, M. (2006). Decision making in pediatric oncology: Who should take the lead? The decisional priority in pediatric oncology model. *Journal of Clinical Oncology, 24*(1), 160–165.

Williams, J. R. (2009). Dual loyalties: How to resolve ethical conflict. *South African Journal of Bioethics and Law, 2*(1), 8–11.

Willis, D. B., Grace, P. J., & Roy, C. (2008). A central unifying focus for the discipline: Facilitating humanization, meaning, choice, quality of life and healing in living and dying. *Advances in Nursing Science, 31*(1), E28–E40.

Windt, P. Y. (1989). Introductory essay. In P. Y. Windt, P. C. Appleby, M. P. Battin, L. P. Francis, & B. M. Landesman (Eds.), *Ethical issues in the professions* (pp. 1–24). Englewood Cliffs, NJ: Prentice Hall.

Wuest, J. (2006). Professionalism and the evolution of nursing as a discipline: A feminist perspective. In W. K. Cody (Ed.), *Philosophical and theoretical perspectives for advanced nursing practice* (4th ed., pp. 85–98). Sudbury, MA: Jones and Bartlett.

Professional Responsibility, Social Justice, Human Rights, and Injustice

Pamela J. Grace

*Where justice is denied, where poverty is enforced, where ignorance prevails,
and where any one class is made to feel that society is an organized conspiracy to
oppress, rob and degrade them, neither persons nor property will be safe.*
— FREDERICK DOUGLASS, 1886

*As long as justice and injustice have not terminated their ever renewing fight for
ascendancy in the affairs of mankind, human beings must be willing, when need is,
to do battle for the one against the other.*
— JOHN STUART MILL, "The Contest in America," 1862

Introduction

This chapter explores the responsibilities of advanced practice nurses (APNs)
for recognizing and addressing injustices that affect the health of persons.
The APN's ethical responsibilities include "the prevention of illness, the
alleviation of suffering, and the protection, promotion, and restoration
of health" (American Nurses Association [ANA], 2001, preface). These are
simply stated yet complex obligations. Fulfilling these goals may mean that
APNs have to look for the antecedents of a patient's or population's problems in the value structure or politics of the larger community and that
APNs take remedial actions either on their own or collaboratively with concerned others. Two important assumptions of professional nursing practice
are (1) that each patient is equally worthy of attention and (2) the concerns
of patients often cannot be effectively addressed without understanding
the environment in which they live their daily lives. However, it can be very
difficult to balance the needs of individuals within the APN's care with the
needs of other patients or the larger population of patients. It is also difficult

to know what social justice demands of nurses without understanding how ideas of social justice, including individual human rights, developed and why. This chapter first explores the nature of problems associated with asserting that attending to social justice is an obligation of the nurse. Second, solutions and strategies for nurse actions alone or in concert with others are proposed. Finally, underlying assumptions about the relationship of societal conditions and health are explored and illustrated with cases. The following provides a brief overview of these aspects of social justice and APN practice that are developed in more detail within the body of the chapter.

The Concept of Social Justice

Problems with the Concept of Social Justice

Both the International Council of Nurses (ICN) and the ANA posit that nurses should be concerned with addressing social justice issues that affect their populations, but neither entity defines social justice or what social justice demands of nurses. Various definitions and theories of social justice have been proposed, but all are subject to criticisms that they are inadequate to structure just societies for various reasons. Buettner-Schmidt and Lobo (2012) completed a concept analysis of social justice for the purpose of nursing work and settings. They drew on a broad array of related literature from different disciplines. Their definition captures many essential characteristics of the concept as it is generally, if somewhat vaguely, understood. No resulting framework for action is proposed, although the authors do note that one is needed to guide nursing actions. Grace and Willis (2012) propose a framework for remedying injustices in health care that draws on the ideas of Powers and Faden (2006). Their framework may not be applicable to all nursing situations, but it does provide a starting point, and modifications can be made in concert with ethical decision-making tools to address other situations.

Although it remains unclear what a good theory of social justice would look like, there is growing agreement among disparate cultures that justice demands, at a minimum, that each individual be treated as equally worthy of moral concern. This basically means that no individual can be treated as an object or the possession of another. The United Nations' (UN's) Universal Declaration of Human Rights affirms that ". . . recognition of the inherent dignity and of the equal and inalienable rights of all members of the human family is the foundation of freedom, justice and peace in the world"

(UN, 2012/1948). The UN consists of at least 192 member countries from all continents, cultures, and geographic regions, demonstrating that regardless of cultural ideology there is global recognition that respect for individuals is a worthy ideal. However, in balancing the needs of each person within the society against the needs of fellow citizens, some constraints on permissible individual actions are necessary. For example, a person cannot be free to cause another person serious harm. Additionally, balancing is needed in relation to the distribution of benefits and harms that occur as inevitable consequences of communal living. Societal values, nature, and powerful human interests all play a role in the distribution of individual benefits and harms; for this reason some inequities are difficult to avoid and the project of trying to remedy inequities is complex.

Many commentators have proposed that a just society should maintain a just healthcare system; support for this proposition is given later. However, a large body of literature critiques the U.S. healthcare system as being systematically unjust (Mechanic, 2006). The healthcare systems of many other countries, although not as inherently unjust, may well disadvantage or fail to appropriately serve the needs of certain populations. Even within a relatively just healthcare system that is accessible to all—that is, where all are able to get help with the resources needed for the protection or improvement of their health (within the boundaries determined by the society's political process)—nurses may face problems mediating between the needs of a particular patient and the needs of a patient population. Thus, gaining an understanding of the nuances associated with human rights and justice is important for all nurses, but especially APNs, who can be considered the profession's leaders, regardless of country of practice.

The general ideas behind social justice are that within a society everyone has a right to benefit from the collective skills and resources of its members and that any associated burdens should be fairly shared. Claims can be made against a society (via its political institutions) to ensure this right. However, the actualization of this ideal has proven problematic philosophically and politically, as explained in more detail shortly.

Social Justice Solutions

What does ambiguity about the concept of social justice and its warrants mean for APNs who encounter injustices then? Do they just throw up their hands, asking "If the philosophers and politicians can't agree on what a good theory of social justice is or how social institutions ought to be arranged to maximize fairness, then, how can we be expected to address injustices?" The answer is that there are actions that nurses can take (and as a profession have historically taken) to address particular injustices. APNs need not focus on this larger question of how societal institutions should be arranged and/or financed to ensure fairness (e.g., government, the legal system, education, health care, etc.), although they do need to understand the complexities of it. APNs have responsibilities to address injustices that affect their populations of concern. These responsibilities may include political action to influence inadequate local or national policies—indeed they may be the only observers of certain sorts of injustices (as discussed shortly). Problematic policies are those that negatively influence health or mistake the actual source of a problem. Additionally, there may be a lack of policies aimed at anticipating future health problems. In this context political action means activities—informed by nursing knowledge and clinical judgment (see **Table 1**)—undertaken by the nurse, often in collaboration with others and with the purpose of influencing necessary changes in policy at the institutional, local, or societal levels. At no time has it been more crucial for APNs to grasp the importance of this responsibility than now. Many countries are developing APN roles because of otherwise unmet health needs of populations (Ketefian, Redman, Hanucharurnku, Masterson, & Neves, 2001; Pulcini, Jelic, Gul, & Loke, 2010). As disciplinary leaders, APNs have crucial collaborative and integrative roles to play in addressing justice issues for their patients. The next chapter explores APN leadership responsibilities in more detail. The latter part of the chapter provides examples of different types of problems stemming from societal injustices and the nature of healthcare systems more broadly. APN responsibilities for addressing these problems at a multitude of different levels are delineated, and strategies are proposed for effective action, including, where necessary, political activism on behalf of the population served.

Social Justice Assumptions

Societies have formed both historically and contemporarily because no one individual is capable of providing for all of his or her own personal needs. Contemporary societies ostensibly exist to facilitate the lives of the individuals within them. Arguably, and as discussed shortly, not all societies deliberately intend to provide for the freedom or well-being of all persons who fall under their canopy. Historically, many societies have had a free class

■ Table 1 Clinical Judgment in Nursing

Clinical judgment in nursing is the nonlinear process of using knowledge, reasoning, tacit (experiential) skills, and interpersonal skills to determine—within the limits of available information—probable best actions given the inevitable existence of uncertainty about the possession of adequate knowledge and outcome of actions.

Components	Categories
Knowledge	Knowledge base of nursing: ■ Nature of the discipline ■ Purposes and goals ■ Nature of persons and environment ■ Characteristics of good practitioners ■ Scope and limits of practice Knowledge derived from other disciplines: philosophical (including ethical theory), physical, social, psychological, spiritual, biological Knowledge related to the situation: ■ Primary subject/who is involved ■ Subject's understanding of the situation, values, beliefs, and context ■ Goals
Experience	Previous experiences: ■ Personal ■ Professional
Characteristics and skills	Perceptual: ■ Grasp the nature and complexity of issues ■ Identify needed/potential resources ■ Envision resolution ■ Reflect on practice; engage in self-reflection ■ Be creative, articulate Relational: ■ Interpersonal ■ Collaborative ■ Mediation Motivation: ■ Professional responsibility ■ Emotional engagement

and an enslaved or indentured class. Nevertheless, contemporary democratic societies globally have as a guiding principle the idea that all citizens are equal under the law. As the UN Declaration of Human Rights, Article 7 reads, "[a]ll are equal before the law and are entitled without any discrimination to equal protection of the law. All are entitled to equal protection against any discrimination in violation of this Declaration and against any incitement to such discrimination" (2012/1948). That is, everyone is subject to the same freedoms and the same restrictions upon those freedoms that are needed for a fair distribution of the burdens and benefits of societal living. This is a starting place for justice and a helpful foundation for nurses in understanding their dual obligations to individuals and society.

The Historical Development of Ideas of Social Justice

The Social Contract: Hobbes

The mechanisms of many contemporary societies are rooted in some form of the idea of a social contract. This "is the view that persons' moral and/or political obligations are dependent upon a contract or agreement between them to form society" (Friend, 2006). Although traces of social contract theorizing are visible as far back as the time of the ancient Greeks, contemporary theorizing about the structure of a good society arguably begins with the writings and thoughts of Thomas Hobbes (1588–1679). Hobbes is well known in philosophical and other circles, both for his assertion that a social contract is necessary for an orderly and mutually beneficial society and for grounding this assertion in a graphic description of what life would be like for human beings without such a contract.

Like all philosophers, Hobbes' theorizing was influenced by his context. He lived in the turbulent times of the English civil war, a war fought between Royalists (supporters of the monarch) and Oliver Cromwell's supporters, who wanted parliamentary rule. His theory is based on a rather pessimistic view of human nature that does not take into account the possibility of human capacity for altruistic actions (action that is either not primarily or not wholly self-interested). Hobbes felt that an overall ruler, such as a monarch, was necessary to impose order. However, he did not believe that royalty derived its power directly from a supreme being. That is, he did not believe in the divine right of kings. Individuals comprising the potential society would elect a leader they felt could provide the most impartial leadership.

Once elected, the ruler would be entrusted with maintaining social order and permitted to do what was necessary for that end.

Hobbes's particular view of the social contract has been criticized on many levels. Most contemporary critics do not find his characterization of human beings accurate, nor do they agree with the structure he proposes. Nevertheless, his graphic description of life in a state of nature captures some of humanity's worst fears about how human life could be in the absence of some sort of societal structure and how these fears are exemplified currently by the terrible conditions that exist in certain parts of the world, where no identifiable or coherent social infrastructure seems to exist (for example, Haiti, Libya, Afghanistan, Iraq, and Sudan). Some have argued that even within so-called civilized societies, the conditions of certain marginalized groups of people are not so terribly far from Hobbes's conception of life without a social contract (Iceland, 2006; Papadimos, 2006; Rank, 2005).

The Social Contract After Hobbes

As noted, the structures and functioning of many modern societies are based on some conception of a social contract. Ideas about human nature and the social contract, however, have gone through several evolutions since the time of Hobbes. Contemporarily, many scholarly writers in bioethics and justice use John Rawls's (1971) ideas, detailed in *A Theory of Justice* (and explained in more detail in Chapter 1), to explore and/or critique the notion that justice is a particular view of fairness in the distribution of the benefits and burdens of living within a socially contracted society (a distributive justice theory). There are two important principles that emerged from his theorizing: (1) the *principle of equal liberty*, whereby each person has an equal right to the most extensive liberties compatible with similar liberties for all, and (2) the *difference principle*, which states that social and economic inequalities should be arranged so that they are both to the greatest benefit of the least advantaged persons and attached to offices and positions open to all under conditions of equality of opportunity (Rawls, 1971, p. 60).

As discussed, criticisms of these sorts of distributive justice theories derived from ideas of a social contract are varied. Feminists worry that the voices of women, the weak, and the vulnerable are muffled or muted by more powerful societal members, and thus their concerns are left out of the contract (metaphorically speaking). Additionally, the person at the center of the contract is generally conceived to be a self-sufficient, rational individual who is able to reason objectively. However, contemporary philosophers, feminists, and others have pointed out that in fact humans live in a web of relationships that inevitably are influential in complex ways that are not fully understood; therefore, the ideal of a rational person who can be divorced both from emotions and his or her relationships with others for the purposes of objective decision making is a myth. In view of this problem, the existence of a stable, just society is not possible. A more reasonable perspective is that there is an ongoing struggle to achieve justice within society. This struggle entails, among other things, a concerted effort to bring out and magnify the perspectives of the disempowered by those who are in a position to recognize the nature and origins of perceived injustices. It includes efforts to rein in the influence of the powerful or redirect such influences toward a just cause.

One other conception of justice that is sometimes used as a basis for discussions related to the allocation of scarce resources concerns the view that people should receive benefits in proportion to the contributions they have made or according to what they deserve (Pojman, 1999). Whether a person is considered deserving of special consideration or not depends on societal, community, or religious values, and these will be discernible from the supporting rationale. The problem for healthcare providers in relying on a conception of justice based on merit is that their knowledge base includes theoretical and empirical evidence that those who are privileged by supportive backgrounds and environments are often those who will appear more meritorious. It is easier to be meritorious if a person is not caught up in the struggle of merely surviving from day to day, for instance.

Powers and Faden on Social Justice in Public and Health Policy

Recently, Powers and Faden (2006) proposed a theory of justice that does not focus on trying to discover the best ways to distribute goods. Instead of focusing on discovering which conception of justice is correct—which they think is something of a futile quest—they wanted to focus on discovering "[w]hich inequalities matter most" (p. 3) and what is necessary for living a minimally decent life. For this, they concentrated on what they argue are essential dimensions of human living. A life missing, or "seriously deficient," in any one dimension will also have problems in all of the other dimensions because they are interrelated. These dimensions, they assert, are universally shared—people across cultures need a minimal level of each in order to have a meaningful quality of life, and they are not hierarchical. The essential aspects are roughly stated:

- Health—a common sense perspective of physical and psychological well-being or flourishing
- A sense of personal security—not living in constant fear and vigilance
- The ability to reason (theoretical as well as practical reasoning) — allows understanding of the world, helping individuals "make logical connections and detect logical errors . . . allowing [them] to navigate both the natural and the social world." (p. 20)
- Respect—self-respect, as well as respect for and from others
- Attachment—being able to form trusting relationships with others
- Self-determination—a person's ability to make his or her own choices, act on them, and be accountable for them

Powers and Faden were especially concerned with the effects of missing or inadequate dimensions in the lives of children, because effects on children tend to be pervasive and long term. Danny Willis's work exploring the experience of healing from childhood abuse exemplifies their point (currently prepublication). His study, which included only men who perceived themselves as healing subsequent to abuse, revealed that for most the healing process took decades. For many the main dimension affected could probably be pinpointed as a loss of sense of personal security—they reported persistent problems with physical and psychological health, inability to make and retain relationships, poor self-respect, and problems with reasoning and consequently self-determination (Grace & Willis, 2012). For the present purposes, then, Powers and Faden's (2006) ideas about social justice are helpful in many situations (although probably not all) that APNs face. Their main purpose was to determine "which inequities matter most" (p. 3). The next section provides a very abbreviated and simplified account of the evolution of contemporary democratic societies and the relationships of individuals to the societies in which they are members by virtue of location or abode. The purpose of this section is to highlight the nature and source of tensions that exist between individuals and society and, thus, implications for advanced practice in negotiating the levels of professional responsibility that exist.

Individuals and Society: Tensions

There are, of course, many different types of societies. The idea of a social contract is implied in some societies and not in others. Not all societies either historically or currently have held respect for individuals as a crucial value. In many societies, the interests of the group, or some other value, are considered by the society's rulers or traditions to be more important than respect for the individual. And, as noted earlier, even when consideration for the equal moral worth of each person is valued, some individuals are more powerful than others and thus more capable of ensuring that they are accorded respect.

The sinking of the Titanic provides a striking example of this point. The Titanic was a new type of oceangoing ship, touted as being indestructible. However, after a catastrophic encounter with an iceberg, many of the lower-class passengers traveling in steerage class were trapped below deck by gates meant to separate the classes. This meant that they could not easily reach the lifeboats (of which there were too few to accommodate everyone) as the ship was sinking. It was obvious that the lower classes were not treated as equally worthy of moral concern as the upper classes—their very lives were obviously deemed less important than those who had paid more for their passage. Although that event took place almost a century ago, disparities based on class and race continue.

For the purposes of this chapter, though, and because this text is written primarily for APNs in contemporary democratic societies such as the United States, the discussion assumes the existence of a society that (1) takes itself to be democratic, (2) values each citizen as being of equal consideration in the distribution of the benefits and burdens of community living, and (3) has developed implicit and explicit (moral and legal) rules for the conduct of its daily business. Another way of saying this is that within the society each citizen is considered the equal of any other citizen in influencing policy. Ideally all have a say in determining what goods and services are important and what restrictions on personal freedoms are necessary to achieve the desired ends. These assumptions, which represent values espoused in the Constitution of the United States of America and in the constitutional documents of many other countries, allow for critique of contemporary healthcare arrangements or policies that unfairly disadvantage people.

Democratic Societies, Cooperation, and Legal Protection

Democratic societies are to a certain extent cooperative, meaning that such things as goods and services are gained that would not otherwise be accessible to individuals, and such things as materials, time, labor, and money are given in exchange for needed goods and services. Cooperation permits efficiency in the production of goods and the delivery of services, but it also means that the actions of individuals within society necessarily have an impact on the lives of others with whom they interact or, even more broadly, on others in society. The impact may be positive in that mutual benefit occurs or negative in that someone's freedom is restricted or the expected or contracted service is not provided.

Tensions between the needs, desires, and freedom of individuals and what is perceived to be the good of the larger society are inevitable and often lead to political unrest. Not surprisingly, it is frequently those who are the most powerful or who have the most resources, natural and/or material, whose interests prevail. For societies to be successful in balancing individual interests with the interests of the larger group, effective rules and guidelines are needed to deal with inevitable tensions. These rules or guidelines are necessarily influenced by philosophical analysis and empirical evidence about problems, their antecedents, and promising remedies. Each democratic society, supposedly, develops its own system of justice based on the values of the society. "The provision of goods, when these are deemed by the society as vital for the well-being of individuals in the society . . . are safeguarded" (Grace, 1998, p. 98) by a system of laws. "The legislative system [of the society] determines in what manner, and to what extent, people will be legally protected from having their rights to these crucial goods violated" (Grace, 1998, p. 99). These, then, are the legal rights that a person within a society can claim as his or her due. Legal rights, however, are only one type of right. Moral rights also exist. The basis for moral rights may be the same as or different from those of legal rights depending on the underlying value systems of the society, that is, what sorts of belief systems are accorded legitimacy within the system and which values are deemed important enough to protect via formal sanctions.

Moral Rights

General Moral Rights

In addition to legal rights that are conceived within the society (and in democratic societies with the input of citizens) and for which impingements warrant formal sanctions of some kind, other conceptions of rights exist. So-called moral rights, Feinberg (1973) asserts, "exist prior to, or independently of, any legal or institutional rules" (p. 84). Moral rights may or may not be protected by laws. But what does the term *moral rights* mean? How do these rights differ from legal rights? As usual, in philosophy there is a variety of answers that can be given to these questions—as many answers as the different perspectives or theories that exist. Some of the important aspects of moral rights are sketched in the following paragraphs.

The idea that an individual has certain moral rights is centered on conceptions that some human goods are critically important and should be protected, preserved, or promoted. What is held to make these goods important may differ with varying religious and cultural beliefs, but there is a subset of goods that is universally important because without them people would not survive. These can be called *critical human goods*. The actions of protecting, preserving, or promoting critical human goods imply interactions taken by others on behalf of the subject. An evaluation of the proposed or actual actions is made on the basis of whether the action can or does actually serve its purpose. Moreover, some actions may be forbidden if they are likely to cause more harm than good.

In moral philosophy, the appraisal of actions usually falls into one of three categories. The action by the agent is required (obligatory), permissible (neutral), or forbidden. Although here the discussion is about action framed in positive terms, refraining from acting when action is needed to prevent harm or further a person's good is also subject to moral appraisal. The moral status of actions is generally linked to values espoused within a society—such as freedom of speech and equality of opportunity. These values may be based on a variety of moral theories (deontology, utilitarianism, virtue, and so on) or on a belief in divine rules. For example, say that a patient (an individual within a society) is conceived of as having a right to make his or her own decisions by virtue of societal values; no provider may interfere with that decision, all things being equal (in the absence of some reason to suppose that the person is incapable of acting independently). Admission to the hospital does not remove that right. This may seem rather obvious, but it is not always honored, and patient rights were frequently not respected historically. Physicians were often considered to know what was best for a patient whether or not the physician had a sense of the patient's own values. Moral rights are not always subject to legal enforcement, although they may be.

Although it is beyond the scope of this chapter to engage in, or even present, some of the many philosophical debates related to rights and obligations, it is perhaps helpful to note one differentiation that is sometimes made between a positive moral right—where a claim may be made against someone or some institution for assistance or for the provision of goods and services (often requires more government regulations)—and negative moral rights—or the right to be left alone and to be free from the interference of others or from the state (often implies limits on government interference or regulations). To make a claim that an individual has a right to health care is a positive right in this sense. Positive rights mean that a claim may be made against some entity to ensure a right—in this case the government of an individual's society. Claims about a right to health care are often made on the basis of human rights. Human rights are one type of important or critical moral right that are said to belong to humans regardless of the values held by their particular society. The belief that health care is a human right has implications for healthcare providers. The implications stem from the supposition that human beings all have the right to at least a minimally good life (Nickel, 2005; Powers & Faden, 2006).

Human Rights

HUMAN RIGHTS AS A CATEGORY OF MORAL RIGHTS: HISTORY

Human rights are a specific type of moral right that is no less important in healthcare settings than in wider contexts. But what are they? Where do they come from? And what is their force? In developed countries human rights are as natural as having legs or lungs: their existence is not questioned, and people believe that these rights are theirs to claim. People object to murder and torture whenever they occur and consider these acts violations of human rights. To take away a person's life puts an end to all of that person's potential future choices, aspirations, and actions. It ends their humanity.

Modern ideas about human rights trace their origins as far back as the Magna Carta of 11th-century England. Under pressure from his noblemen, King John was swayed to institute what was essentially a contract between the king and his subjects. It limited the power of the state to control its populace and delineated what individuals could lay claim to in the courts (British Bill of Rights, 1994). In essence, it served as the foundation for contemporary rules of law. This was an important development because prior to the Magna Carta the citizens of many societies were subject to the whims and desires of their leaders, often kings. Individual freedom was limited by the dictates of these rulers. The Magna Carta was pivotal for certain political changes but did not extend to all subjects, only to those who already had some power.

It was several centuries later during the Enlightenment when the issues of moral rights and human rights were taken seriously. The Enlightenment represents a period in American and European philosophy when the use of reasoning or analytic thought became valued as the main route to knowledge and was viewed as an essentially and uniquely human characteristic. Locke (1690/2003), for example, claimed that rights naturally flowed from the nature of humans as free and rational beings. Kant's ideas about the innate dignity of human beings served as his justification for the existence of human rights. According to Kant (1785/1967), human beings by virtue of their capacity for rational thought and for making moral rules are, and thus should be allowed to be, self-governing. For this reason, they should never be used purely as a means of serving someone else's advantage. Kant had a complicated argument for this but basically proposed that it is irrational to use an individual purely or primarily as a means to someone else's advantage. For example, if a person assented to this, that person would essentially be saying, "Everyone can treat anyone else as a means to an end" (this is Kant's Categorical Imperative roughly stated). But people would not want to be treated purely as a means to someone else's end; thus, it is irrational to treat someone else as a means to one's own end.

Moral rights, then, include such things as being free to make one's own choices and being free from the interference of the state in personal affairs. Human rights are a more fundamental category of rights. Whereas particular moral rights are based in theories of moral philosophy and may or may not hold depending on the values of a society, human rights are asserted to apply to every human simply by virtue of their humanity. Therefore, human rights apply to everyone regardless of the society to which they belong. Some human rights are considered to be inalienable, that is, they cannot be given away by the person. A classic example of an inalienable right is the right to be free. This means that a person cannot agree to be enslaved even if this would benefit his or her family in some way because it is the nature of humans to be free. It is important to note that there is no agreement about exactly what is the set of rights that are called human rights, although certain rights are generally agreed to be included.

HUMAN RIGHTS: CONTEMPORARY UNDERSTANDINGS

Following the Enlightenment period, attention to the issue of human rights waned temporarily. However, renewed interest emerged partly as a result of human abuses during World War II (1939–1945) as documented in Chapter 6, *Research Ethics: Advanced Practice Roles and Responsibilities*. This prompted a revisiting of the issue of human rights and attempts to further define what they are and why they should be honored. Fagan (2006) noted that contemporarily, "human rights have been defined as basic moral guarantees that people in all countries and cultures allegedly have simply because they are people." According to Nickel (2005), human rights "are concerned with ensuring the conditions . . . of a minimally good life" (p. 386) and, as noted earlier, Powers and Faden (2006) based their theory on this same premise. Fagan (2006), in his thoughtful discussion of human rights, noted that this idea of a minimally good life "has been enshrined in various declarations and legal conventions issued during the past fifty years, initiated by the Universal Declaration of Human Rights (1948) and perpetuated by, most importantly, the European Convention on Human Rights (1954) and the International Covenant on Civil and Economic Rights (1966)." Conceptions of a minimally good life are necessarily different depending on the society and its resources.

The idea behind an assertion that all human beings have rights simply by virtue of being human derives from the "philosophical claim: that there exists a rationally identifiable moral order, an order whose legitimacy precedes contingent social and historical conditions and applies to all human beings everywhere and at all times" (Fagan, 2006). This can be stated a little differently by saying either each human is equally worthy of moral consideration (viewed as important in his or her own right) or no one is. If no one is to be accorded moral consideration, then any person at any time might find their interests discarded on someone else's whim. Indeed, using Rawls's ideas about people in the original position deliberating behind "a veil of ignorance" (Rawls, 1971), it is imaginable that no one would feel secure about abolishing human rights for fear his or her position in society and assets might make them particularly vulnerable to the absence of such rights.

Human rights, however, are not bound to a particular society but are taken to apply across societal and national borders and political contexts. The declarations cited earlier allude to human rights as supporting such goods as a basic standard of living that includes education, provisions for health care, and protection from the effects of destitution. They prohibit torture, slavery, and exploitation. Unfortunately, the interpretation of these rights and how they should be applied in actual situations is a more difficult undertaking than asserting that they exist—as is enforcing them. Currently, in moral philosophy and bioethics circles there is debate about whether human rights imply the right to a certain basic level of health care that is consistent with the status of healthcare knowledge and societal resources.

Complicating things further is the absence of a definition of health that everyone can agree upon.

Is There a Right to Health Care?

This question has been raised by many scholars in the United States and elsewhere. It is an important problem to explore in this text because nurses assert, via the policies and position statements of their professional bodies (ANA, 2003; ICN, 2012) and the writings of scholars, that they exist to attend to the health needs of individuals and society in a nondiscriminatory manner (Ballou, 2000; Gaylord & Grace, 1995; Grace, 1998, 2001; Raphael, 1997; Spenceley, Reutter, & Allen, 2006). Thus, clarity about the influence of all of the following on health is important: universal human rights and their demands on societies, societal values implied (what people would tell you) versus actual (how societal institutions are set up), a person's social and/or economic standing, and the nature and accessibility of healthcare services. These factors are fundamental for understanding what actions are required to meet the health needs of an APN's population (where the definition of health depends both upon the patient's conception of this and insights from nursing knowledge development and the APN's specialty knowledge base).

Nurses, as Curtin (1979) and many other commentators have pointed out, are often the ones who "attend patients when distress is immediate . . . for sustained periods of time" (p. 4) and thus have the opportunity to experience patients in all of their humanity, including the struggle of the poor and otherwise disadvantaged for survival in an inequitable environment. Certain living conditions have been shown to contribute to or exacerbate health problems perhaps even more than a lack of access alone, although often persons living in substandard conditions also lack easy or adequate access to healthcare services. Thus, there are inextricable links among living conditions, social standing, economic status, and health (Danziger & Haveman, 2001; Iceland, 2006; Powers & Faden, 2006; Rank, 2005). For this reason, even if it can be agreed that there is a right to a basic level of health care, this will not ensure good health because even more fundamental justice problems arise within society that also require attention, such as needs for adequate nutrition, housing, and security, as discussed shortly.

Human Rights Arguments for Justice in Health Care

Before discussing professional advocacy for individual and societal health— which means comprehending the effects of poverty, socioeconomic standing, and abuse and neglect on persons' lives and their functioning and flourishing—it is important to gain an understanding of the relationship between human rights and rights to health care. Dernier (2005) notes when it is asserted that a right to health care exists, several related claims are essentially being made. A right to health care means that everyone encompassed by the society (regardless of status and perhaps even including so-called "illegal" immigrants), by virtue of being human, is entitled to a certain level of access to health care and society has a collective responsibility to ensure this. It is a strong societal obligation. This obligation should be reflected in policy debates, and failure to meet this obligation can be said to constitute an injustice.

As a profession, nursing takes the stance that providing basic healthcare services, including those that facilitate the prevention of illness, and the promotion and preservation of health for all members of society are a moral responsibility and should be treated as a human right (ICN, 2007). This is a starting place. A further question that is beyond the scope of this text to explore in detail is to ask, "What are the scope and limits of this right?" Buchanan (1984) noted in the 1980s that there was a growing belief in the idea that "the right to a decent minimum of health care" exists; indeed this is the title of his book. However, d'Oronzio (2001), along with many other philosophers, ethicists, healthcare professionals, and citizens, is concerned that viewing a basic minimum of health care as a human right is not compatible with the current U.S. healthcare financing arrangements. Although efforts to change the U.S. healthcare delivery system are in process, certain professional healthcare groups, notably the ANA (2008), have affirmed their belief that there is a right to health care and that this means the system must change. "The ANA endorses a single payer system as a way to integrate services and facilitate accessibility. ANA believes that health care is a basic human right . . . Thus, ANA reaffirms its support for a restructured health care system that assures universal access to a standard package of essential health care services for all citizens and residents" (ANA, 2008, p. 2).

The following section explores the scope and limits of an APN's responsibilities to patients and society. Role responsibilities are described as both narrow and broad. An argument is presented for understanding responsibilities in three areas: to individual patients, to influence societal conditions that affect groups of patients in terms of access to care or other influences on health, and to overcome obstacles to good care caused by the environment of practice.

Advanced Practice Nursing and Professional Advocacy

Professional Advocacy: A Broad Conception of Role Responsibilities

The term *advocacy* is commonly used in nursing circles as an ideal of practice. However, efforts are ongoing to define what this means in nursing contexts (Bu & Jezewski, 2007; Chafey, Rhea, Shannon, & Spencer, 1998; Grace, 1998, 2001; Mallik, 1997; Snowball, 1996; Spenceley et al., 2006). Consequently, the boundaries of nursing responsibilities related to advocacy are often not fully understood and shift depending on the definition of advocacy assumed. The term has various meanings to various people. I know this to be true both from available literature and from informal surveys of the many graduate and undergraduate students I have encountered over the years. Some say advocacy means defending patients' rights (Abrams, 1978; Curtin, 1982; Gadow, 1990; Jezewski, 1993; Miller, Mansen, & Lee, 1983; Pagana, 1987; Shirley, 2007; Zussman, 1982); some say it means ensuring that patients get their immediate needs met; still others might say that it is a role-related responsibility of nursing, meaning that any action taken by the nurse while acting in the role of a nurse is advocacy. Indeed, all of these definitions appear in the nursing and allied literature (ANA, 2001; Annas, 1974/1990; Bernal, 1992; Chafey et al., 1998; Gaylord & Grace, 1995; Grace, 2001; Hewitt, 2002; MacDonald, 2007; Mallik, 1997; O'Connor & Kelly, 2005; Snowball, 1996; Spenceley et al., 2006).

Elsewhere, I have examined the concept of advocacy in great detail (Grace, 1998, 2001); indeed, it was the topic of my doctoral dissertation. A colleague and I were initially stimulated to explore this topic by an article that appeared in the *Hastings Center Report* in 1992 by non-nurse ethicist Ellen Bernal. In the article, she chastised nursing for taking the stance that nurses are patient advocates. She argued that nursing uses advocacy to advance its autonomy as a discipline and thus improve its professional status. On closer reading, we realized she was using an interpretation of advocacy as meaning only a defense of patient rights and were moved to explore in more depth what nursing means by advocacy (Gaylord & Grace, 1995). This problem of ambiguity of meaning and thus expectations of the nurse became the impetus for a whole program of study related to professional responsibility.

Perhaps the most interesting insight gained during this investigation of advocacy concerned the roots of the term in legal settings. Advocacy as a practice ideal has its origins in the field of law. In law, it means the verbal act of arguing for a person's cause against the cause of an adversary. Lawyers, while advocating, have responsibilities only for that client (or group of clients) and the client's cause. If there are system injustices, these are dealt with outside of the immediate lawyer–client situation.

Nurses, however, do not have such limited responsibilities. In advocating for one patient to have his or her needs met, nurses may well cause disadvantage to another. For example, a primary care nurse practitioner (NP) in a busy clinic is told by one of her patients that she is being physically abused by her boyfriend. This is an urgent matter and the patient needs time and attention. But the nurse is in a practice with two physicians, who in response to economic pressures have limited the time allocated for nurse visits. The NP is the sole available provider this afternoon, and she has three other patients who are also waiting to be seen. She must make a decision that will affect somebody's care. An immediate decision must be made that balances the risk to the other patients against the likely benefit to the abused patient of spending more time with her. The NP has simultaneous responsibilities to more than one patient; thus, advocating for one to receive extra attention may well disadvantage others. Thus, her responsibilities cannot end with the immediate decision and ensuing action. The problem of inadequate visit time is recurring and results in part from a misunderstanding about the APN role, deliberate or inadvertent, on the part of the collaborating/supervising physicians.

Therefore, a different way of looking at the advocacy role of the APN is to view it as any action taken to further professional goals (ultimately related to promoting patient good). This permits nurses to see that their advocacy actions may be directed at different levels. "Professional advocacy, then, may be conceived both as actions taken to further nursing's purposes on behalf of individual patients and actions taken to expose and redress underlying problems that are inherent in the larger contexts of institutions, policymaking, and the health care delivery system" (Grace, 2001, p. 161). Many so-called advocacy situations "have their fundamental roots in such things as national health policy decisions, economic conflicts of interests, miscommunication, institutional barriers or a host of other grounds" (Grace, 2001, p. 152).

To provide some coherent structure to the exploration of advocacy viewed as professional responsibility to further nursing goals (responsibilities of the nursing role), the next section is divided into three parts. The first part describes advocacy viewed as the APN's professional responsibilities to individual patients encountered in practice settings. Second, advocacy is viewed as a responsibility to address the environment in which the APN practices. Finally, the APN's role in influencing social policy is explored. However, this is an artificial categorization because in many cases all three levels of responsibility coexist. When the APN is faced with a tension between trying to provide what is needed for a particular patient and the needs of others within the practice, clinical judgment is needed to prioritize action. Clinical judgment in this sense is synonymous with ethical or moral reasoning (see Table 1).

CASE STUDY: AN EXAMPLE OF COMMON ISSUES

This case appeared in the *Louisville Courier-Journal* (Coomes, 2007). It exemplifies the various levels of advocacy needed to ensure good care for this patient. Although this case might be considered peculiar to the United States, a review of associated international literature highlights similarities between Ms. Henley's situation and those in poverty in other countries. Research data from The Commonwealth Fund (2007) found that although the United States lags behind on many healthcare benchmarks, "experiences in all countries (Australia, Canada, Germany, The Netherlands, New Zealand, United Kingdom, United States) indicate the need for more integrated, patient-centered care 'systems.'" The object of the article was to point out that three simple things are all that is needed to improve health for many people. "They should stop smoking, eat better and exercise more" (Coombes, 2007). However, as the reporter noted, "Lack of access to health care providers, healthy foods and safe places to exercise can be roadblocks to healthier lives for those in rural areas and the poor across the state." Ms. Henley is just one example of a pervasive problem in healthcare settings. Healthcare providers know from empirical evidence what strategies are needed for health promotion or maintenance, but more than this is needed to keep people healthy. We need to know what the roadblocks are and help them negotiate these.

Additionally, Ms. Henley's predicament is familiar, one to which many nurses at all levels of practice can relate. "Portia Henley, a 50-year-old [African American] grandmother from Louisville [is] unable to keep a steady job. She has diabetes and struggles to pay for the better food and special drugs her condition requires; asthma inhibits her ability to exercise. 'I'm fighting a real battle,' said Henley. 'It's hard to stay on the straight and narrow in terms of what you eat when you don't have the income to handle the price of medicine, the price of going to doctors and the price of keeping a roof over your head, plus the cost of buying food for this one specific health problem.'"

Professional Advocacy for Individual Patients

THE NURSE–PATIENT RELATIONSHIP

The essence of nursing care is the individual nurse–patient relationship. This is a fiduciary relationship based on trust. Whether patients do or do not actually trust their nurses, in the sense of knowing who their nurses are and having confidence in their abilities, nevertheless, they are forced to trust that nurses have their patients' best interests in mind, know what they are doing, understand the limits of their knowledge and skills, and will steer patients in the right direction or put patients in touch with needed resources when they have reached the limits of their expertise. For this reason, transparency of purpose and affiliation is important. In some cases, especially in advanced practice settings, nursing's work is not directly aimed at patient benefit. Some examples are performing pre-employment wellness screenings or serving in the role of research nurse coordinator. In such cases, APNs have responsibilities to reveal their purpose and any existing conflicts of interest, to address misunderstandings, and to direct the involved person to a source of help as needed.

However, mostly the APN's role is to further patient good related to individual persons' actual or potential health needs. To further this good APNs use clinical judgment to determine appropriate actions. A definition of clinical judgment that was synthesized from extant literature in nursing, medicine, and the cognitive sciences appears in Table   1. Clinical judgment is needed to identify patients' needs, anticipate future needs, and facilitate care that is most likely to meet these needs. Because the goals of care involve understanding what is best for the patient whose life is necessarily contextual and nuanced, nurses need to engage with a patient (and with family members when this is indicated) to discover a patient's beliefs, values, and preferences so that the nurse's actions are tailored to that person's needs. Additionally, because nurses too are human and have their own beliefs, values, and biases, they must be careful to understand what these biases are and how such prejudices (prejudgments about the nature or attributes of a person) are likely to affect their clinical judgment in particular situations.

BIASES

Ms. Henley's case serves as an example of a possible bias (Doris & The Moral Psychology Research Group, 2010) that providers may exhibit related to poverty. Many people do not have a good understanding of the nature of poverty and its antecedents. Coryn (2002), in his literature review, noted that there are three distinct categories of attitudes people have related to poverty: these are "individualistic/internal, structural/external, and fatalistic." In the United States, the predominant attitude of the middle class is individualistic/internal, meaning the poor person is blamed for possessing a character flaw such as laziness or lack of ambition that has led to his or her present condition. Perhaps not surprisingly, among the poor themselves the predominant attitude is structural/external, meaning they attribute poverty to external circumstances (Coryn, 2002). Because most healthcare professionals are middle class, a bias against the poor can be anticipated (Crandall, 1990).

One way to avoid the effects of bias that arise from inexperience or ignorance is to try to understand what a person's life is like. What are the person's daily experiences and struggles like? Other biases or prejudices may exist because of negative past experiences with someone. For example, a nurse whose parent suffered from alcohol abuse may have a negative attitude toward patients she views as alcoholic. Advocacy, viewed as professional responsibility to further the goals of the profession for good care, obligates nurses to understand who patients are, what is needed for their care, and what obstacles exist to getting them the care they need.

IDENTIFYING AND ADDRESSING OBSTACLES

Obstacles to providing what the APN determines to be necessary for the good of an individual patient may take many shapes and forms. **Table** 2 lays out the different levels at which obstacles may present and provides a synopsis of common problems. Strategies to address obstacles are presented shortly. The specialty chapters of this text provide strategies that are particular and pertinent to that specialty, but issues of poverty and disadvantages of various sorts are commonly encountered across settings. For Ms. Henley there are many obstacles to achieving optimal health even within the limits of her complex issues. Because some of these issues arise as a result of social inequities, addressing these requires influencing social policies, as addressed shortly.

In caring for Ms. Henley at the nurse–patient relationship level, the immediate concern is assisting with her current problems. Professional advocacy at this level means using an approach that is based in nursing's

■ Table 2 Categories of Obstacles to Ethical Nursing/Health Care

Category	Obstacles

Individual patient	1. Patient not viewed as unique:
	  ■ Standardized patient care
	  ■ Provider lacks understanding of the influence of important contextual details
	  ■ Patient "labeled" by others
	2. Prejudgment of patient (bias/prejudice)
	3. Patient or family's need for knowledge not fully addressed (related to #2)
	4. Interpersonal conflict:
	  ■ Provider–patient
	  ■ Patient–family
	  ■ Provider–provider
	5. Poor communication:
	  ■ Provider–patient/family
	  ■ Provider–provider
	6. Power imbalances—coercion/silencing
	7. Inadequate time—resources to evaluate and address needs (also a practice environment problem)
	8. Patient's moral agency diminished (does not see self as having meaningful choices (Blacksher, 2002)

Practice environment	1. Lack of primary focus on patient good:
	  ■ Economic conflicts of interest
	  ■ Practice philosophy is to meet economic goals
	2. Autonomous practice constrained:
	  ■ Senior colleagues
	  ■ Institutional mission
	  ■ Managed care mandates
	3. Unsupportive environment

Social injustices	1. Unjust aspects of the healthcare system:
	  ■ Access
	  ■ Financing
	  ■ Priorities
	  ■ Failure to attend to the real origins of certain health problems

(continues)

Category	Obstacles
	2. Socioeconomic disparities:
	■ Education
	■ Poverty
	■ Discrimination
	3. Lasting effects of violence, abuse, neglect
	4. Profit motive or business emphasis
	5. Fragmented services

philosophy of care and goals of practice. Although priority goals are to meet her immediate needs, it is still necessary to have an idea of who Ms. Henley is as a person. In the absence of a life-threatening emergency that would require immediate measures, it is not possible to adequately help meet her health needs if the nurse does not know more about her. The nurse needs to know, for example, how her maladies are affecting her, what she views as the priority issue, what she knows about her physical conditions, what resources are available to her, and what are her priorities. Advocacy at the level of nurse–patient relationship, then, means professional responsibility to ensure good patient care. This entails understanding what good actions are likely to be for this patient, working with her to determine what are good avenues of action from her point of view, and recognizing and accounting for potential and actual obstacles to good action.

Advocacy viewed as professional role responsibilities for good care presents the same obligations regardless of setting and is based in nursing's philosophy of care and disciplinary goals. Thus, Ms. Henley could have presented for care at any number of different specialty practices—primary care adult health, family practice, women's health primary care, emergency room, as a preanesthesia workup, in a diabetes or asthma clinic, and so on. The time required to address all of her issues may be different in different settings because some aspects of her care may well be beyond the knowledge and skills of the clinician, who will then need to refer Ms. Henley to others for care of those aspects. Nevertheless, the APN's responsibilities include evaluating the quality and appropriateness of the referral made.

Advocacy, as described earlier, can be seen as an onerous and unrealistic responsibility given current environments of practice with their inevitable time constraints and pressures. This view is not uncommon and may be true in many settings. Nevertheless, the APN's role responsibilities include understanding and influencing the context of care so that nursing goals can be met. In those situations where the APN finds intractable differences between his or her philosophy of care and those of her practice colleagues, it is the nurse's responsibility to consider whether a different type of setting might be more fitting.

Nurses see firsthand the effects of unaddressed or poorly addressed problems upon their population of patients. They may be the first or only ones to understand both what those effects are and what changes are needed. Therefore, nurses' responsibilities do not end when the presenting patient's priority needs are met, especially when it is recognized that the practice environment may actually be working against nursing goals of providing care for the patient as a person.

Professional Advocacy and Practice Environments

The varied environments in which APNs work and care for patients also give rise to problems that can interfere with optimal care for a given patient (see Table 2). Role responsibilities exist so that nurses can understand how a particular setting and its values are impinging on ethical patient care. The problem may involve a particular patient or may be seen as recurrent. In the case of Ms. Henley, a practice focus of constricted time slots or on managing only the acute presentation would lead to fragmented care, is at odds with nursing goals that include anticipation and prevention of future problems, and would affect many of the patients within the practice. As another example, in correctional settings the facility's goal of prisoner behavior control may interfere with a nursing emphasis on providing for an individual prisoner's well-being. In yet other settings, unit, institutional, or practice policies, conventions, or expediencies may raise barriers to good patient care. Like other healthcare providers in primary care settings especially, constraints related to financing arrangements, reimbursement issues, and managed care practices pose some of the most troubling, difficult, and time-consuming problems for NPs (Creel & Robinson, 2010; Johnson, 2005; Ulrich et al., 2006; Ulrich & Soeken, 2005).

Professional Advocacy and Social Injustices

At the broadest level, APNs in concert with other nurses, physicians, and allied health professionals have a collective interest in addressing social injustice. This is because the goals of almost all healthcare professions have to do with improving the health of individuals. Improving the health of individuals often requires addressing injustice that is deeply rooted in a society. It is not expected that most APNs will be capable of single-handedly tackling an issue; however, their knowledge and experiences place them in the ideal situation to join with colleagues or collaborate with other professionals to inform policy debates.

Nurses, both because they provide direct care and have a perspective and approach that permits hearing patients' health and illness stories within the contexts of patients' daily lives, may be the first or only ones to recognize existing and developing patterns of injustice or disparity. Nurses, along with other healthcare providers, see firsthand the end results of poor access to health care or poor health maintenance. Thus, viewing advocacy as a broader responsibility to further professional goals at both the individual and societal level highlights the range of knowledge, skills, and actions that may be needed. In addition to the fact that taking a broad view of nursing responsibilities is needed for meeting nursing goals, positive action at a level different from the immediate situation is also a way of mitigating the moral distress or unease felt when APNs are unable to provide the care needed for a particular patient because of environmental or other obstacles (Arthur, 1995; Corley, 1995; Corley, Minick, Elswick, & Jacobs, 2005; Erlen & Sereika, 1997; Fowler, 1989).

HEALTH DISPARITIES AND POVERTY

Although health disparities are by no means the only nursing care issues that require professional advocacy at the societal level, the issue of poverty internationally and its pervasive influence on health provides an important exemplar and argument for APNs to take seriously their ethical responsibilities to advocate for health policy changes. Poverty affects people in a variety of ways that are not always easily discernible but that have been well documented in the literature and supported by empirical studies (Danziger & Haveman, 2001; Iceland, 2006; Rank, 2005). Patients like Portia Henley, for whom daily life is an ongoing struggle to make ends meet, may delay seeking care until their problems are out of control. They may have inadequate insurance, transportation difficulties, lack of family support, be the primary caretaker for others whose needs they put first, or have any number of other obstacles to getting the assistance they need. As a diabetes clinical nurse specialist (CNS) or APN, my immediate goal would be to assess Ms. Henley's priority needs for knowledge, self-care, nursing, and other necessary therapeutics, which would include understanding her values and priorities. Next steps would be to help her obtain the resources and supports she needs to achieve a level of health that she desires and that is realistic in the context of her life. Finally, what is really needed is an exploration of the environmental and economic conditions that resulted in her current status.

The next section briefly presents some ideas for influencing change in the broader healthcare environment. Nursing has a rich history of activism to improve health care, starting with the efforts of Florence Nightingale (1820–1910). Nightingale used evidence and influence to change the way wounded soldiers were treated during the Crimean War, and she used her knowledge, skills, and influence to ensure that a patient's environment would be conducive to his or her healing.

Professional Advocacy: Influential Strategies

APNs are uniquely positioned to research and articulate the likely consequences of problematic practices to those in charge of policy decisions, whether this is at the institutional, local, and/or societal levels. The current healthcare climate necessitates the political action of nurses individually, collectively, and in collaboration with others and is exceptionally open to the input of nurses because "physicians have lost much of their influence and control to corporate medicine in recent years" (Mechanic & Reinhard, 2002, p. 7). Although not all nurses can, as Malone (2005) notes, "become policy experts . . . in addition to providing direct patient care . . . all nurses can assess, identify, and articulate for [or on behalf of] patients" on certain problematic issues and "provide information to patients on options for impacting policy; and work to effect policy change through professional and advocacy organizations" (p. 136).

Nurses can (and should) include in their nursing assessments possible "policy factors that may have preventive, etiological, or therapeutic significance" (Malone, 2005, p. 136). This may sound complicated but is actually elementary. For example, it means asking why certain poor patients with diabetes are not managing their diet and medicines well. Is the reason that they are unaware of resources (the system is not allowing for adequate patient education), cannot afford the medicines (health insurance problems), have access problems, or some other issue? One effective strategy is for an APN to join forces with other nurses, physicians, and allied professionals whose concerns mirror their own. As a group they can publicize the problem, provide convincing rationale, and outline probable consequences.

Individual patient narratives as exemplars of a larger problem can be very powerful. Blacksher (2002), a philosopher, documented the life of her mother (only on reading the acknowledgments does the reader discover that Sally is her mother). Sally was born into extreme and unremitting poverty. She had no opportunities to develop a sense of self. She was periodically abused by others—beaten by her mother and then her husband. This affected her health, development of a sense of self as worthwhile, and ability to rise above. Blacksher's vivid portrayal is of a woman who was "stuck." She was unable to develop and exercise moral agency, that is, to choose actions that would benefit either herself and others. In fact, she did not see herself as having choices. "Chronic socioeconomic deprivation can create environments that undermine the development of self and capacities constitutive to moral agency—i.e., the capacity for self-determination and crafting a life of one's own" (pp. 455–456). What nursing can do in such cases on an individual level is to provide a "key" to unlock a person's potential and facilitate the development of a sense of self as worthwhile. Nursing actions include treating patients with respect, providing resources and referral, and empowering—this is a process. But it is also important to examine the particular aspects of the environment that served to perpetuate the patient's situation. In Sally's case, years of neglect from health care and social systems alike had an impact.

Providing a submission to the op-ed page of a newspaper or a letter to the editor often gets public attention and raises questions for discussion in a more public forum. Membership in relevant institutional or local committees is another good strategy and can serve as an important forum for educating other committee members about nursing concerns. For example, acute care CNSs or NPs can provide a valuable voice for patients when they sit on hospital ethics committees and patient care committees.

APNs can be instrumental in educating and providing information for grassroots patient organizations. They should recognize that the information they have about patient situations is valuable and can be articulated in a variety of arenas and forums to inform needed changes. For example, family nurse practitioner (FNP) students joined with their mentors and a specialty organization to change the practice of one managed care company related to antihistamine prescriptions. The formulary allowed only diphenhydramine for seasonal allergy treatments, but this was making many of the children drowsy. A letter-writing and publicity campaign managed to change the practice and make better options available to these children. Another example of effective nursing political activity was given by Murphy, Canales, Norton, and DeFilippis (2005) and is related to improved pain control. "Through regulatory policy advocated for by nurses and many others in the political arena, optimal pain control is now part of standard practice" (p. 22). Nurses are urged to join with colleagues and/or collaborate with allied professionals to publicize a problem. This can also be done via letters to the editor of local papers, or by emailing, calling, or writing to local or state representatives.

Conclusion

Professional advocacy is synonymous with the idea that all nursing actions have ethical implications. This is because all nursing actions have the ultimate purpose of furthering the goals of nursing related to patient well-being. The goals of nursing involve providing health and well-being for individuals who are inextricably a part of the larger society in which they reside. Consequently, patients are susceptible to inequities occurring as a result of societal arrangements. Good patient care often requires attention to the underlying circumstances that have given rise to the need for nursing's services, including poverty and other disparities that leave patients especially vulnerable to their healthcare needs.

Summary

This chapter provides an essential background for understanding the breadth of APN responsibilities to attend to the health needs of both individuals and society. An argument is provided for the importance of balancing the needs of individuals with societal needs related to health and health care. To fulfill professional goals, APNs need to engage with individual patients, taking into account their patients' unique needs and addressing obstacles that prevent meeting these needs. Additionally, APNs may need to engage in political activity at a variety of levels, either singly or in collaboration with others.

Discussion Questions

1. All nurses have patients or types of patients who we find ourselves avoiding. This is human nature. The person reminds us of someone in the past, perhaps, who treated us badly or at whose hands we suffered, the person may just be difficult to please, or their problems may seem intractable, as in the case of Blacksher's mother, Sally. Other intractable problems might be a person with an addiction whose problem seems overwhelming or who exhibits drug-seeking behavior. In the United States there are a set of patients, often homeless, who are labeled "frequent flyers" because of their repeated visits to the emergency department. In light of the discussion of advocacy, explore ways in which you might make a connection with a difficult patient. What are a nurse's responsibilities related to different levels of advocacy?

   To what extent do you see such problems as ones of human rights, moral rights, and social justice?

2. In your practice or from your nursing experience, identify the common barriers/obstacles that make it difficult for you to give the care that in your clinical judgment is required. How should such problems be addressed?

3. You are one of the two APNs in a group practice. You and your colleague are being pressured to assume the same approach to practice as your physician colleagues and the physician's assistant. Your colleagues are receptive to your input and you have a collegial relationship. How would you explain to them that your nursing perspective requires a different approach?

4. What does it mean to be self-reflective? How does one know when you have been genuinely self-reflective (versus justifying your values)?

5. Do you think that everyone should have access to the same basic level of health care? What would this include?

References

Abrams, N. (1978). A contrary view of the nurse as patient advocate. *Nursing Forum, 17,* 258–267.

American Nurses Association. (2001). *Code of ethics for nurses with interpretive statements.* Washington, DC: Author.

American Nurses Association. (2003). *Social policy statement*. Washington, DC: Author.

American Nurses Association. (2008). *Health system reform agenda*. Retrieved from http://ana.nursingworld.org/MainMenuCategories/HealthcareandPolicyIssues/HealthSystemReform/Agenda.aspx

Annas, G. J. (1974/1990). The patient rights advocate: Can nurses effectively fill the role? In T. Pence & J. Cantrall (Eds.), *Ethics in nursing: An anthology* (pp. 83–86). New York, NY: National League for Nursing Publication.

Arthur, E. (1995). Coping with moral distress. *Minnesota Nursing Accent, 67*(3), 5.

Ballou, K. A. (2000). A historical-philosophical analysis of the professional nurse obligation to participate in sociopolitical activities. *Policy, Politics, & Nursing Practice, 1*(3), 172–184.

Bernal, E. W. (1992). The nurse as patient advocate. *Hastings Center Report, 22*(4), 18–23.

Blacksher, E. (2002). On being poor and feeling poor: Low socio-economic status and the moral self. *Theoretical medicine and bioethics, 23*(6), 455–470.

British Bill of Rights. (1994). *The Magna Carta*. Retrieved from http://www.hrweb.org/legal/otherdoc.html

Bu, X., & Jezewski, M. A. (2007). Developing a mid-range theory of advocacy through concept analysis. *Journal of Advanced Nursing, 57*(1), 101–110.

Buchanan, A. (1984). The right to a decent minimum of health care. *Philosophy and Public Affairs, 13*(1), 55–78.

Buettner-Schmitt, K., & Lobo, M. L. (2012). Social justice: A concept analysis. *Journal of Advanced Nursing, 68*(4), 948–958.

Chafey, K., Rhea, M., Shannon, A. M., & Spencer, S. (1998). Characterizations of advocacy by practicing nurses. *Journal of Professional Nursing, 14*(1), 43–52.

Commonwealth Fund. (2007). International health policy survey in several countries. Retrieved from http://www.commonwealthfund.org/Surveys/2007/2007-International-Health-Policy-Survey-in-Seven-Countries.aspx

Coomes, M. (2007, May 11). Kentucky's health: Critical condition. *Louisville Courier-Journal*. Retrieved from http://www.courier-journal.com/apps/pbcs.dll/article?AID=/20051214/NEWS01/512140410&template=printart

Corley, M. C. (1995). Moral distress of critical care nurses. *American Journal of Critical Care, 4*, 280–285.

Corley, M. C., Minick, P., Elswick, R. K., & Jacobs, M. S. O. (2005). Nurse moral distress and ethical work environment. *Nursing Ethics, 12*(4), 381–390.

Coryn, C. (2002). Antecedents of attitudes towards the poor. Unpublished paper. Retrieved from http://www.iusb.edu/~journal/2002/coryn/coryn.html

Crandall, L. A. (1990). Advocacy of just health policies as professional duty: Cultural biases and ethical responsibility. *Business and Professional Ethics Journal, 9*(3&4), 41–53.

Creel, E. L., & Robinson, J. C. (2010). Ethics in independent nurse consulting: Strategies for avoiding ethical quicksand. *Nursing Ethics, 17*(6), 769–776.

Curtin, L. (1979). The nurse as advocate: A philosophical foundation for nursing. *Advances in Nursing Science, 1*(3), 1–10.

Curtin, L. L. (1982). What are human rights? In L. L. Curtin & M. J. Flaherty (Eds.), *Nursing ethics: Theories and pragmatics* (pp. 3–16). Bowie, MD: Brady Communications.

Danziger, S. H., & Haveman, R. H. (2001). *Understanding poverty*. Cambridge, MA: Harvard University Press.

Dernier, Y. (2005). On personal responsibility and the human right to healthcare. *Cambridge Quarterly of Healthcare Ethics, 14,* 224–234.

d'Oronzio, J. C. (2001). A human right to health care access: Returning to the origins of the patients rights movement. *Cambridge Quarterly of Healthcare Ethics, 10,* 285–298.

Doris, J. M., & The Moral Psychology Research Group. (2010). *The moral psychology handbook*. New York, NY: Oxford University Press.

Douglass, F. (1982). U.S. abolitionist. In J. W. Blassingame (Ed.), *The Frederick Douglass Papers*. New Haven, CT: Yale University Press. Original speech April 1886, Washington, DC.

Erlen, J. A., & Sereika, S. M. (1997). Critical care nurses, ethical decision-making and stress. *Journal of Advanced Nursing, 26,* 953–961.

Fagan, A. (2006). Human rights. *The Internet encyclopedia of philosophy*. Retrieved from http://www.iep.utm.edu/hum-rts/

Feinberg, J. (1973). *Social philosophy*. Englewood Cliffs, NJ: Prentice Hall.

Fowler, M. D. M. (1989). Moral distress and the shortage of critical care nurses. *Heart and Lung, 18,* 314–315.

Friend, C. (2006). Social contract theory. *The Internet encyclopedia of philosophy*. Retrieved from http://www.iep.utm.edu/s/soc-cont.htm

Gadow, S. (1990). Existential advocacy: Philosophical foundations of nursing. In T. Pence & J. Cantrall (Eds.), *Ethics in nursing: An anthology* (pp. 40–51). New York, NY: National League for Nursing. Reprinted from *Nursing Images and Ideals*, 1980, pp. 79–101.

Gaylord, N., & Grace, P. (1995). Nursing advocacy: An ethic of practice. *Nursing Ethics, 2*(1), 11–18.

Grace, P. J. (1998). *A philosophical analysis of the concept "advocacy": Implications for professional–patient relationships*. Unpublished Dissertation. University of Tennessee, Knoxville. Retrieved from http://proquest.umi.com. Publication No. AAT9923287, Proquest Document ID No. 734421751.

Grace, P. J. (2001). Professional advocacy: Widening the scope of accountability. *Nursing Philosophy, 2*(2), 151–162.

Grace, P. J., & Willis, D. G. (2012). Social justice and professional responsibilities: An analysis in support of disciplinary goals. *Nursing Outlook, 60,* 198–207.

Hewitt, J. (2002). A critical review of the arguments debating the role of the nurse advocate. *Journal of Advanced Nursing, 37*(5), 439–445.

Hobbes, T. (1967/1651). Leviathon. In A. I. Melden (Ed.), *Ethical theories: A book of readings* (2nd ed., pp. 218–231). Englewood Cliffs, NJ: Prentice Hall. Original work published in 1651.

Iceland, J. (2006). *Poverty in America* (2nd ed.). Berkeley, CA: University of California.

International Council of Nurses. (2007). ICN Position statement: Nursing and development. Geneva, Switzerland: Author. Retrieved from http://www.icn.ch/publications/position-statements/

International Council of Nurses. (2012). Code of ethics for nurses. Geneva, Switzerland: Author. Retrieved from http://www.icn.ch/about-icn/code-of-ethics-for-nurses/

Jezewski, M. A. (1993). Culture brokering as a model for advocacy. *Nursing and Health Care, 14,* 78–85.

Johnson, R. (2005). Shifting patterns of practice: Nurse practitioners in a managed care environment. *Research and Theory for Nursing Practice, 19*(4), 323–340.

Kant, I. (1967). Foundations of the metaphysics of morals. In A. I. Melden (Ed.), *Ethical theories: A book of readings* (pp. 317–366). Englewood Cliffs, NJ: Prentice Hall. Original work published in 1785.

Ketefian, S., Redman, R. W., Hanucharurnku, S., Masterson, A., & Neves, E. P. (2001). The development of advanced practice roles. Implications in the international nursing community. *International Nursing Review, 48,* 152–163.

Locke, J. (2003). *Two treatises of government and a letter concerning toleration.* I. Shapiro (Ed.). Binghamton, NY: Vail-Ballou Press. Original work published in 1690.

MacDonald, H. (2007). Relational ethics and advocacy in nursing: Literature review. *Journal of Advanced Nursing, 57*(2), 119–126.

Mallik, M. (1997). Advocacy in nursing—a review of the literature. *Journal of Advanced Nursing, 25,* 130–138.

Malone, R. E. (2005). Assessing the policy environment. *Policy, Politics, & Nursing Practice, 6*(2), 135–143.

Mechanic, D. (2006). *The truth about health care: Why reform is not working in America.* Piscataway, NJ: Rutgers University Press.

Mechanic, D., & Reinhard, S. C. (2002). Contributions of nurses to health policy: Challenges and opportunities. *Nursing and Health Policy Review, 1*(1), 7–15.

Mill, J. S. (1862). The contest in America. *Harper's New Monthly Magazine, 24*(143), 683–684.

Miller, B. K., Mansen, T. J., & Lee, H. (1983). Patient advocacy: Do nurses have the power and authority to act as patient advocates? *Nursing Leadership, 6*(6), 56–60.

Murphy, N., Canales, M. K., Norton, S. A., & DeFilippis, J. (2005). Striving for congruence: The interconnection between values, practice, and political action. *Politics, Policy, & Nursing Practice, 6*(1), 20–29.

Nickel, J. (2005). Poverty and rights. *Philosophical Quarterly, 55,* 385–402.

O'Connor, T., & Kelly, B. (2005). Bridging the gap: A study of general nurses' perceptions of patient advocacy in Ireland. *Nursing Ethics, 12*(5), 53–67.

Pagana, K. D. (1987). Let's stop calling ourselves "patient advocates." *Nursing, 17,* 51.

Papadimos, T. J. (2006). Charles Dickens hard times and the academic health center: A tale of the urban working poor and the violation of a covert covenant, an American perspective. *Online Journal of Health Ethics, 1*(2), 71–72.

Pojman, L. (1999). Merit: Why do we value it? *Journal of Social Philosophy, 30*(1), 83–102.

Powers, M., & Faden, R. (2006). *Social justice.* New York, NY: Oxford University Press.

Pulcini, J., Jelic, M., Gul, R., & Loke, A. Y. (2010). An international survey on advanced practice nursing education, practice, and regulation. *Journal of Nursing Scholarship, 42*(1), 31–39.

Rank, M. R. (2005). *One nation underprivileged: Why American poverty affects us all.* New York, NY: Oxford University Press.

Raphael, A. R. (1997). Advocacy oral history: A research methodology for social activism in nursing. *Advances in Nursing Science, 20*(2), 32–43.

Rawls, J. (1971). *A theory of justice.* Cambridge, MA: Belknap/Harvard University Press.

Shirley, J. L. (2007). The limits of autonomy in nursing's moral discourse. *Advances in Nursing Science, 30*(1), 14–25.

Snowball, J. (1996). Asking nurses about advocating for patients: Reactive and proactive accounts. *Journal of Advanced Nursing, 24,* 67–75.

Spenceley, S. N., Reutter, L., & Allen, M. N. (2006). The road less traveled: Nursing advocacy at the policy level. *Policy, Politics, & Nursing Practice, 7*(3), 180–194.

Ulrich, C. M., Danis, M., Ratcliffe, S. J., Garrett-Mayer, E., Koziol, D., Soeken, K. L., & Grady, C. (2006). Ethical conflict in nurse practitioners and physician assistants in managed care. *Nursing Research, 55*(6), 391–401.

Ulrich, C., & Soeken, K. L. (2005). A path analytic model of ethical conflict in practice and autonomy in a sample of nurse practitioners. *Nursing Ethics, 12*(3), 305–316.

United Nations. (2012). The universal declaration of human rights. Retrieved from http://www.un.org/en/documents/udhr/index.shtml

Zussman, J. (1982). Want some good advice? Think twice about being a patient advocate. *Nursing Life, 2*(6), 46–50.

To Engage or Not Engage: Choices Confronting Nurses and Other Health Professionals

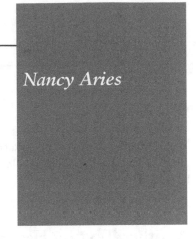

Nancy Aries

OVERVIEW

Healthcare professionals of the 21st century must understand how the government, together with providers, consumers, and insurers, interacts in the health policy process. This chapter provides a comprehensive overview of the essential elements that drive and shape health policy in America. By understanding the politics of policy making and program implementation, health professionals will be better prepared to advocate for a healthcare system that best meets the population's needs.

OBJECTIVES

- To understand the formal definition of health policy
- To understand the policy-making process, which includes the following:
  - Describing the ways competing concepts of federalism create the structure within which policy is determined
  - Explaining the role of the market and the government in the framing of health policy
  - Identifying the competing interests that shape health policy and the ways these competing interests determine policy outcomes
  - Recognizing the role that implementation plays in the policy process
- To describe the opportunities and constraints that health professionals and their patients face as a result of policy decisions
- To recognize different ways that healthcare advocates can impact policy and programmatic decisions

KEY TERMS

- Advocacy
- Federalism
- Government programs: Taxation, provision or purchase of services, regulation
- Implementation

- Policy: Social policy, health policy
- Policy-making process
- The role of markets and government
- Stakeholders and interest groups

Another Text on Health Policy and Politics: Why?

Numerous text books are available that describe the healthcare delivery system in the United States or step back to explain how politics and policy making influence the organization of care delivery. Why are we putting another text on the market that purports to address many of the same questions? Our answer is both simple and complex.

Simply put, we believe that many of these books fail to address the reality of health care as experienced by nurses and other health professionals. Many of the students and practitioners with whom we work are totally absorbed in the day-to-day demands of their jobs. They work hard just to keep up with the needs of patients and their families, health colleagues, physicians, and administrators. Many describe themselves as running up a down escalator that speeds up every time they think that they might make some forward progress. One consequence of this consuming daily struggle is that there is no time or intellectual space to step back and reflect on the larger institutional, social, political, and economic forces that shape their professions and their industry.

The more complex answer is that students often recognize that the hospitals, community-based agencies, and other health facilities that employ them are under severe pressure to cut costs and that they, as front-line workers, bear the brunt of these cost-cutting measures when their organizations are understaffed and the demand for productivity is increasing. If they are going to act to improve this situation, they need to know exactly how the dots that define health policy connect to the dots that define care and treatment. This book is intended to provide an understanding of policy that is rooted in the perspectives of nursing and other health professionals but at the same time helps make students conversant with the politics and economics that generate the rules of the game under which they work with such skill and dedication.

In this book, we want to put the opportunities and constraints that confront our professions in a larger perspective. By developing a more nuanced understanding of the ways policy shapes the organization of the healthcare system, we hope to provide those working in healthcare delivery with the tools that they need to influence these decisions. One book cannot change how we conduct our professional lives, but it can change how we understand our options. This book demonstrates that we have options other than hoping to get by or finding positions where we do not experience the pain of those whose care is compromised. To take no action is to allow decisions to be made by others. Engagement in the policy world can be an effective way to overcome a sense of helplessness about the current state of the healthcare system. By more fully understanding the healthcare system and the levers for change, it becomes possible to influence more actively the direction that the system takes.

This plea for engagement is shaped by our own experiences of the healthcare system. There has not been a time in recent history when the problems of healthcare costs, access, and quality were not serious concerns. In the early 1970s, we achieved greater access to care after the implementation of Medicare and Medicaid, but healthcare costs began to escalate. Access was expanded, but no one was sure how it could be sustained. In the mid 1980s, healthcare expenditures topped 10% of gross domestic product (GDP), and the concept of managed care gained salience as a way to control costs while maintaining quality. Cost control, but not necessarily quality improvement, was achieved, whereas access declined as the number of uninsured increased. In the early 1990s, President Clinton's healthcare reform proposal reached Congress. Through a complicated system labeled managed competition, the plan was purported to increase access, control costs, and improve quality. The bill was defeated. Healthcare costs stayed flat through most of the 1990s, as managed care became the predominant insurance model; however, access became more restricted, and there were growing concerns regarding quality of care.

We cannot continue on our present course. Healthcare expenditures reached $2.3 trillion in 2008, or 16% of GDP. That amounted to $7,681 per person. The health share of the GDP is projected to reach 19.5% by 2017 (National Health Expenditure Data Fact Sheet, 2008). The number of uninsured Americans was nearly 47 million, or 16% of the population in 2005, the latest government data available (DeNavas-Walt et al., 2007). This is an increase of almost nine million people since 2000. The United States probably has one of the most sophisticated healthcare systems—yet it ranked twenty-sixth internationally for mortality of children under 5 years of age (State of the World's Mothers, 2007).

Although it is critical that we describe the ways that health policy has shaped the healthcare system, it is equally important to understand that policy making is an interactive process. In some instances, government dictates the response of providers. In other cases, providers dictate the response of government. Then there is the business sector, insurance companies, public health organizations, professional associations, and advocacy groups. Each one is trying to be heard and push the system to become more responsive in its needs and the needs of its constituents. In this book, we want you to recognize that as health professionals you can play a similar role in this process. You are in a position to advocate for your professions and for the patients that you serve. Your voice can and should be heard. The combination of describing the health system and explaining how complex policy processes shape it and the ways you can become instrumental in that process distinguishes this book.

In order to provide the context for understanding the policy and the policy-making process, this chapter addresses the following issues. In the first section, we define policy and consider how it shapes our experience of the healthcare system. When we are successful in our jobs, it is often because of policies. When we fail, it is often the case that policies have created an environment in which it is difficult to operate. Policy, as will be explained, can have many meanings. In this book, the term policy is used to refer to government programs. The second section highlights the different ways that government policy and programs intervene in the organization and delivery of health services in order to assure greater social equity in the distribution of goods and services. This involves understanding the competing concepts of federalism and the ways that it impacts the development of government programs. After this framework is established, we can consider the actual programmatic tools available to government to achieve its goals. The choice of tools is determined by the balance established between the market and the government in overseeing the organization of healthcare delivery.[1] Although we have a mixed system, each presents a different set of opportunities and constraints for policy makers. Next, we examine the actual process by which government policy is made. This involves understanding which groups have a stake in the development of government programs, how their interests get expressed in the political process, and whose interests are ultimately reflected in the government programs. This chapter does not explain the legislative process. That is better left to a civics text. Rather, it explains how interest groups influence that process in order to achieve what they perceive to be a more favorable outcome. Policy making, however, does not stop with the passage of legislation. Implementation is equally important, although sometimes overlooked. Implementation is also an opportunity to influence how policy is realized on a day-to-day basis. The final section of the chapter brings this discussion back to the nurses and other health professionals for whom this text is written. We reconsider why a better understanding of policy not only impacts our work and the experiences of those seeking health care but also provides a framework for better understanding how to become more effective players within the field.

Health Policy Defined

Policy in the broadest sense is the manifestation of ideology or belief systems about how the world should work (Rushefsky, 2008). For example, as a nation, we have watched our beliefs about foreign relations shift from being highly isolationist to becoming the protector of democratic values. We have strong beliefs about the value of rugged individualism, which is manifest in rags-to-riches stories. One way our beliefs are manifest is in government actions. This means we should be able to analyze government actions in terms of the ways that they are reflective of dominant social values or ideology. The ideological justification for the Iraq War put forward by President Bush was our nation's responsibility to promote democracy. Similarly, the passage of welfare reform in the 1990s can be rooted in a social value of financial independence.

Public policy, the term used to describe government actions, is typically divided into three areas: foreign policy, economic policy, and social policy (Lowi & Ginsberg, 1998). The objective of foreign policy is to defend national sovereignty. Economic policy is designed to promote and regulate markets. Although foreign and economic policy seeks to improve the overall well-being of society by promoting the political and economic well-being of American society, typically policies in these areas do not have equal impact on all sectors of society. Some groups may

---

[1]The terms "market" and "government" are short-hand expressions to describe the two alternative ways in which society conducts its business. "Market" means reliance on generally voluntary exchanges between private parties. Sometimes these exchanges are mandated and regulated by government, as is the case with mandatory liability insurance to own a motor vehicle. "Government" means reliance on the direct provision of a service by government employees, as is the case with Veterans Affairs hospitals. It is not uncommon to use a combination of markets and government, as is the case with Medicare and Medicaid, where government makes payments to private providers to care for individuals who the government is seeking to service.

benefit, whereas others might find themselves suffering undue consequences. The North American Free Trade Agreement benefited the economy overall, but many persons who held manufacturing jobs found themselves unemployed as production moved from the United States to countries with lower production costs. Social policy often becomes the means by which the unintended consequences of policies that seek to better the overall condition of American society are addressed. Government actions become the means by which we ensure the provision of the basic necessities: food, shelter, health care, and education (Midgley & Livermore, 2008). Social policy is redistributive by its very nature. Its goal is to achieve greater social equity.

Health policy can be located within the larger realm of social policy. Because policy generally is rooted in social values and ideologies, our discussion of health policy begins with the recognition of the values and ideology that are reflected in the organization of the healthcare system. The historic course of American health policy is best described in terms of our shifting beliefs about how access to care is provided. Sometimes we have stridently pursued health care as a right for all. Sometimes we have treated it as a privilege (Knowles, 1977). In fact, these competing values (i.e., a right versus a privilege) are simultaneously and continually at work in the outcomes of our health policy. Therefore, to understand health policy requires that we delve further into explaining how values can shape a complex set of actions.

The American approach to health insurance provides a good illustration of this duality. On one hand, we have a health insurance program that covers practically all Americans over the age of 65 years. One argument underscoring the creation of Medicare was that the older population had worked for the benefit of society and should

not risk poverty in old age because of high healthcare costs. For those over 65 years of age, health care was deemed a right. The opposite holds true for the working-age population and their dependents. No universal health insurance program is available to Americans under 65 years of age. Either they can obtain health insurance as a benefit of employment, or they can purchase health insurance out of pocket. Health insurance, however, is costly. The average premium in 2007 was $2,613 for an individual health insurance policy. For those who cannot afford to purchase insurance, there is an array of safety net programs that provide marginal care and have been unable to address the needs of the rising number of uninsured (Center for Policy and Research, 2007). How did this situation come to pass? To get the answer, we need to understand how policy in this area evolved. We begin by understanding the nature of our federal system of policy making.

The Framework for Public Policy Making

Federalism

In order to understand the process of policy formation in the United States, it is necessary to grasp the meaning of federalism in the American context (Bovbjerg et al., 2003). American federalism is a system of governance in which the exercise of sovereign power is split between the 50 states and the national government. Hence, the federal government is limited in its actions in several important ways. First, there is the dual nature of our system of state and federal governance. When the nation was founded, the states ceded certain responsibilities to the federal government but retained others for themselves. In addition, within the federal government, there is a separation of powers among the legislative, executive, and judicial branches. This further constrains the power of the national government by dividing the government against itself. Finally, the Constitution limits government by protecting individual rights that cannot be denied except by extraordinary procedures.

According to the framers of the Constitution, the central government has express powers to levy taxes, declare war, and oversee interstate commerce. All power not expressly delegated to the federal government falls under the jurisdiction of the states. This system of dual federalism provides the context in which the patchwork quilt pattern of health policy exists. Although there is a strong national government, the states were initially more important than the national government in virtually all policies governing the lives of Americans, such as economic regulation, public health, and education. When President Pierce vetoed a law setting aside millions of acres of federal land to benefit the mentally ill, he argued that mental health was a state, not a federal, responsibility (Rothman, 1971).

Despite the fact that social policy relating to individual welfare is a state responsibility, there has been a constant expansion of federal power in this area since the Civil War. By the 1930s, scholars saw such a radical departure in the conduct of federalism that the New Deal has been characterized as a shift from a system of dual federalism to a system of cooperative federalism (Kernell & Jacobson, 2006). This shift was brought on by the severe social hardship of the Great Depression. During this period, the ability of states to protect the well-being of their citizens was diminished, as states had limited ability to raise funds through taxation or deficit financing; therefore, the states turned to the federal government, which initiated and funded many social programs. Using grants-in-aid programs, Congress appropriated money to state and local governments with the condition that

the money be spent for particular purposes as defined by Congress. The Maternal and Child Health program, which was created under Title V of the Social Security Act in 1933, is an example of such a grants-in-aid program. This program sought to improve the health of low-income mothers and children. From a policy perspective, cooperative federalism is important because Congress began to set national goals and influence state activity in the realm of social programs.

Federal power increased through the 1960s as opposition grew to the variability in the ways that states implemented social programs. The federal government assumed a larger role in terms of shaping and funding social welfare programs by imposing national standards on the states through regulations and unfunded man-

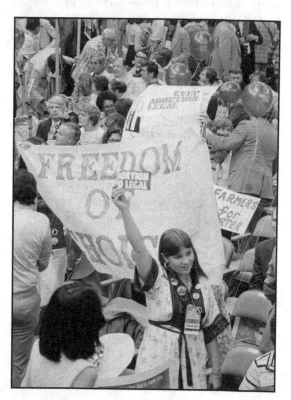

dates (Conlan, 2006). Typically, the costs of regulatory compliance were not funded by the federal government. Hence, these were labeled as unfunded mandates. States needed to comply with the regulations or risk penalty such as the withholding of grant money. Federal regulatory authority was further advanced by the social movements of the 1960s. Civil rights advocates demanded greater regulation of federal programs in their efforts to achieve racial and social equity. One response of the federal government was to create categorical programs that made program funding directly available to community-based providers (Davis & Schoen, 1978). This meant federal funding bypassed the state governments entirely. The community health centers that were funded by the Office of Economic Opportunity provide an example of a categorically funded program. In this instance, the federal government bypassed the sovereign powers of the state governments and contracted directly with the healthcare providers for specified services.

In the late twentieth century, there was one more shift in the relationship between the federal government and the states. Starting with President Nixon but affirmed during Reagan's presidency, there has been a push to return authority to the states. Called the new federalism, it involves devolution of authority to the states to define social welfare programs that are funded by the federal government (Anton, 1997). The expressed intention is to permit the states to accommodate their diversity better. This is not possible when the federal government attempts to impose a "one size fits all" approach to social programs. The use of block grants is the mechanism by which greater discretion has been given to the states to shape programs to meet their specific needs. The block grants essentially combine funding from several grant-in-aid programs and allowed states to determine how the money will be spent to achieve broad social goals.

The very nature of federalism is that it results in an inherently fragmented system of governance (Steinmo & Watts, 1995). Nowhere is this clearer than in the arenas of social policy and health policy. Laws addressing similar needs are being passed at the federal, state, and local levels. As a result, there is no uniformity in health policy and related health programs. One of the consequences is the fragmentation and duplication of services caused by the different programs that address a particular need. Examples of gaps in services, duplication of services because of the nonalignment of program requirements, are easily recognized by persons serving older persons. An individual seeking long-term care is confronted with myriad programs. These include the Medicare and Medicaid programs as well as social service programs developed under Title XX of the Social Security Act and the Older Americans Act. Individuals must navigate this maze to determine their eligibility for services or providers must try to integrate the various funding streams in order to make available coordinated and comprehensive services for consumers. Although insurance regulation is a seemingly obscure problem, it has negatively impacted the nation's ability to develop a system of national health insurance. States have regulatory authority over insurance, including health insurance, but the Employment Retirement Income Security Act of 1975 supersedes state laws relating to benefit plans. This means businesses that self-insure for employee health as part of their benefits program are exempt from state insurance regulations. The significance of this dual regulatory system is that neither the states nor the federal government can easily mandate employers to offer health benefits because neither governing body has regulatory authority over all businesses in a particular area (Mariner, 1996).

Markets versus Government

Although individual well-being is a state responsibility, we do not depend on the government to provide for our basic needs. We acquire most goods and services, including health care, through the market. Our decisions and choices are influenced by the signals we get from sellers in terms of the prices at which they offer products. An obvious example is the ways in which the cost of gasoline is shifting consumer preferences away from large, fuel-inefficient automobiles toward smaller, fuel-efficient cars. Less obvious, perhaps, but more important are the ways in which the market responds to broader shifts in society. Consider how the housing market is responding to the reality of an aging population. As the population ages, the number of persons looking for housing alternatives that offer service options not readily available in single-family or multiunit dwellings is growing. Companies such as Marriott are entering the senior housing market in response to this demand. These are cases in which consumers influence producers. There are also cases in which business tries to influence consumer behavior. The direct marketing of pharmaceuticals to consumers through television and print advertising is intended to influence consumer perceptions about possible remedies for their health conditions.

A fundamental problem with the market is that it cannot respond adequately to social needs and preferences that cannot be expressed in terms of price. In a market, one only has a "right" to purchase the goods and services that one can afford. Those who cannot afford their desired goods and services are not entitled to them. What if, however, the service is essential to an individual's welfare or the welfare of a society? In these cases, the market is an inadequate distributive mechanism because competition puts those with fewer resources at a disadvantage in terms of accessing health services. Most Americans less than 65 years of age rely on health insurance as the means by which they can afford and therefore access health services; however, a growing number of small businesses have limited their benefit packages, no longer offer health insurance to family members, or have dropped their health insurance plans altogether (Reschovsky et al., 2006). To buy individual insurance policies is extremely expensive, which means the number of uninsured Americans is rising. As this case demonstrates, the market is limited in its ability to assure distributive justice. The market assumes an exchange among equals, but such an exchange is not possible in a society with unequal distribution of income (Arrow, 1963).

The government intervenes in these situations (Lowi & Ginsberg, 1998). The government's role derives from this fundamental tension between the economic organization of the production and the distribution of goods and services. Although the market pulls in the direction of economic inequality, political beliefs demand counterbalance in terms of the distribution of rights and opportunities. The government becomes the arena to address the needs of those persons who cannot provide for themselves through the exchange of goods and services in the market (Arrow, 1974). Through its policies and programs, government mediates the interests of the market and interests that have no expression in the market. It is the mechanism by which a society seeks to achieve greater equality. Its policies and programs are redistributive. By looking at who benefits and who is overlooked, one can see a broader theme about whether we are advancing social justice or reinforcing social inequality.

This tension between the role of the markets and government can be seen in the history of government programs such as Medicare. Medicare is a universal entitlement, which means that a defined population is eligible for care regardless of ability to pay. With few exceptions, a package of health services is available to persons over the age of 65 years. Such programs tend to be more expensive because of their all-inclusive nature, but they also tend to have broader political support because all persons can ultimately expect to benefit from the program (Brown & Sparer, 2003). Medicare benefits have come to be seen as a right, but the right is being questioned as the cost of Medicare continues to increase. In light of what is perceived to be the government's failure to organize care efficiently, proposals seek to balance the market and government as providers of this important benefit (Steuerle & Bovbjerg, 2008). Many alternatives to the existing Medicare program have been proposed, including making Medicare a premium support program rather than a defined set of benefits. This means that individuals would receive a predetermined sum to purchase a basic health plan. The amount might vary by age, gender, or geographic location. Those persons desiring more comprehensive coverage would have to pay an additional out-of-pocket charge.

Alternatively programs may be more selective in the population being served. Medicaid is an example of a selective program, in that it has need-based criteria for eligibility (Brown & Sparer, 2003). Medicaid creates a safety net for those who cannot afford to access health services through the market. Such programs are less expensive because they serve a subset of the population. The benefits are often more redistributive or in the case of Medicaid more comprehensive than the benefits of a universal program such as Medicare. Such selective programs tend to have less political support because they typically serve needy populations whose claim for services is considered questionable and because they often provide a level of service that is greater than can be accessed in the market by persons who are slightly above the cutoff. As a result, they are an easier target for

cutbacks because their benefits are not available to the general population.

Governmental Intervention

The government has several tools at its disposal to intervene when the market cannot adequately address a problem (Stone, 2002). Among these are taxation, service provision, and regulation. Most often we think about taxation as the means by which government raises money in order to support its spending. Medicare Part A is financed by payroll taxes to which employers and employees contribute. Taxation, however, can also be used as a way to influence behavior. Many states place a high tax on the sale of cigarettes in order to influence personal choices about cigarette use (DeCicca et al., 2008). Higher cigarette taxes have resulted in lower rates of consumption. The revenues raised in this way can be either targeted for programs to support the desired behavioral change or contribute to the state's general revenues.

Another tool is the use of government revenues to support service provision. In some cases, the government is the actual provider of services. Public hospitals are locally financed institutions that were organized to serve persons who could not afford care. The Veterans Administration is a comprehensive healthcare system provided by the federal government to the men and women who have medical problems related to their injuries after discharge from the service. Both are "socialized" medicine in that the programs are managed and provided by government agencies. Alternatively, the government can purchase services from the private market. Medicaid is an example of such a program. Medicaid enrollees seek services from providers who have contracted with the state government to provide services. These providers bill the government for their services and are reimbursed for the medical care they provide. Such spending is designed to increase access of persons with limited resources to the market. The government can also be a producer and a purchaser of services. This is the case with biomedical research. The National Institutes of Health has a large biomedical research complex that supports numerous researchers. In addition, the National Institutes of Health fund independent researchers at universities and research laboratories across the country.

The purchase of service may also take an indirect form whereby the government subsidizes specific sellers to encourage their participation in markets that might not be competitive based on price. For example, medical education is an extremely costly endeavor (Koenig et al., 2003). Hospitals that train physicians cannot compete on price with nonteaching hospitals given the additional costs incurred for resident and faculty salaries and the additional resources used for each patient seen by a resident. As a result, Medicare funds physician training by funding the salaries of residents and subsidizing the hospitals where residents are trained. Another example is the orphan drug program (Grabowski, 2005). The government subsidizes pharmaceutical companies to develop and produce drugs that are used by a very small number of persons and therefore are unprofitable to develop and produce. Through these types of programs, the government offsets what might be the high cost of services or encourages program expansion in specific areas.

A third programmatic tool is government regulation of the market. Regulations are legal restrictions that aim to produce outcomes that otherwise might not occur. Examples of regulation include the licensure of physicians and other health professionals (Grumbach, 2002). These regulations were adapted in the early twentieth century as a way to protect the public from practitioners who were not deemed qualified to provide care. Through a series of educational and practice requirements and an examination, states regulate who can and cannot provide medical and healthcare services. Another example of government regulation is state-mandated nursing staff to patient ratios for hospital-based care (Conway et al., 2008). These regulations are designed to protect patients by maintaining a minimum number of nurses in a department at any time. These regulations are intended to prevent hospitals from cutting corners financially by understaffing a unit.

The Policy-Making Process

Interest Groups

Federalism creates the structure within which social policy is made. Federalism, however, does not explain what will be the content of a particular program and how programs are changed over time. The substance is determined by those individuals and groups that have interests in the field, and change occurs as the power of these groups to influence outcomes rises and falls (Smith, 1993). The healthcare field is comprised of many players who can be found inside and outside of government. There are physicians, nurses, hospital administrators, insurance companies, and on and on. They represent multiple interests, and each one is trying to influence the direction of government policy. The challenge for policy analysts is to understand how these interests are organized and which ones have the most influence and why.

Because health and health care are fundamental to each of our well-being, it is a sphere of activity that garners everyone's interest even if in passing. Although it is possible to speak generally about the public's interest in health care, there are multiple pressure groups that represent discrete interests in the health sector and that want to influence the outcome (Kernell

& Jacobson, 2006). These groups are generally known and identifiable. They typically work on their own behalf when issues are quite specific. They form coalitions when the issues are more general. These groups must be examined more closely as they shape the content of health policy making.

Figure 1 provides a schema for understanding which groups are part of the healthcare field and how their interests can be understood in relation to each other and the field as a whole. Healthcare providers are most central to the dis-

cussion of health policy. They are surrounded by persons who use the healthcare system and by three groups that support the operation of the system: payers, the medical supply industry, and knowledge producers. Although there are stronger and weaker ties between each of these groups, their actions have impacts that reverberate throughout the field.

Healthcare providers can broadly be categorized in two groups: clinicians and the organizations where they work. On the clinical side, one can speak about physicians, nurses, and other

Figure 1 Health policy field.

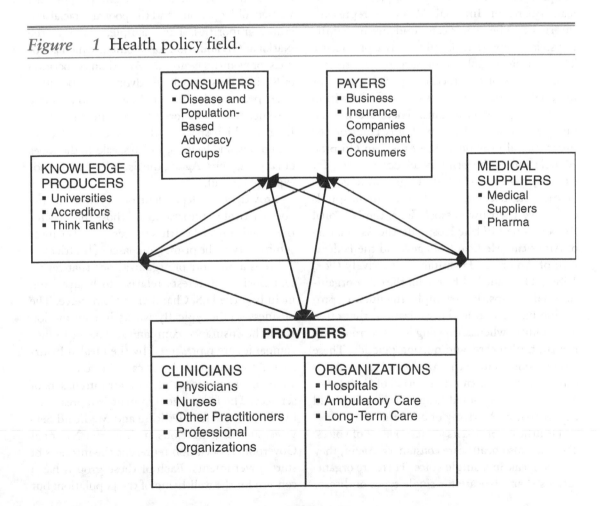

advanced practice providers. On the institutional side, there are hospitals, long-term care organizations, and ambulatory care organizations. Although it is possible to identify broad categories of interest, none of these groups speak with a single voice. Physicians as a group are represented by the American Medical Association (AMA); however, on specific policies, the AMA may avoid the issue because the specialists' point of view differs from the interests of primary care physicians. As a result, there are many physician organizations representing unique sets of interests. For example, the American Board of Internal Medicine represents internists. The American Academy of Family Physicians represents family practice physicians. The American College of Surgeons represents practitioners of this medical specialty, and the list goes on. Such divisions can be found within other groups of clinicians. There are myriad nursing groups. The same holds true for the institutional providers. The American Hospital Association is the primary advocacy group for the hospital industry, but public hospitals, academic health centers, and for-profit hospitals each have their own associations: the National Association of Public Hospitals, the Association of American Medical Colleges, and the Federation of American Hospitals, respectively (Fox, 1986). The same holds true for the other organizational groups. For example, the nursing profession has several lead organizations that often work jointly when addressing issues surrounding health, health care, and nursing practice. These associations include the American Nurses Association, the American Association of Colleges of Nursing, the National League of Nursing, and the American Academy of Nursing.

Healthcare providers are just one set of voices. There are also healthcare consumers. Again, they do not speak in a single voice. There are organizations that advocate for single types of disease such as the American Cancer Association, the American Lung Association, and the National Mental Health Association. This list is also long, with organizations representing persons with specific diseases such as Parkinson's, lupus, arthritis, and autism. In some cases, their concerns are specific to advancing the treatment of the specific illness, and in other cases, their agendas more broadly relate to better financing of a discrete set of services. In addition to disease-specific groups, there are population-based groups that speak on behalf of their membership's need for health services. The largest groups represent women, older persons, and the poor and racial and ethnic minorities. For example, there is the National Organization for Women, which advocates for women's health; the American Association of Retired Persons, which advocates on behalf of older persons; the National Association for the Advancement of Colored People and the Urban League, which speak to the interests of African Americans; and La Raza, which speaks to the issues of Latino groups. Again, the list is long and is not explained in full.

Providers are dependent on revenue to survive. Critical to the system are those that pay for the provision of health services. The business community is the prime purchaser of health care. There is a plethora of organizations that represent business interests relative to health care, including the U.S. Chamber of Commerce. The business sector typically works in conjunction with the insurance companies. The insurance companies are represented by the Health Insurance Association of America. The federal and state governments are also major purchasers of services. The federal government is represented by the Centers for Medicare and Medicaid Services, and organizations such as the National Governors Association represent the interests of state governments. Each of these groups has a concern for the well-being of the population, but each one also has a stake in how health services are financed and reimbursed.

Closely aligned to the clinical providers is what is termed as knowledge producers. The most obvious are the universities and biomedical research organizations. These groups are concerned with advancing the knowledge that underpins medical care and establishing and maintaining standards for medical practice. One of the most central organizations is the American Association of Medical Colleges. Beyond the university, there are think tanks that are concerned with the production and dissemination of knowledge and the associations such as the Institute of Medicine, the PEW Commission, and the Commonwealth Fund, as well as the Joint Commission on the Accreditation of Healthcare Organizations that are concerned with maintaining the standards of medical practice through accreditation, examinations, and licensing.

The last group to consider is the medical supply industry. This sector is assuming a larger role in health policy decisions as technology plays a greater role in the provision of health care. The fastest growing part of this sector is the pharmaceutical industry, which is represented by the Pharmaceutical Research and Manufacturers of America. The growing set of suppliers of medical devises such as stents and medical equipment such as imaging machines should be taken into account also. The American healthcare system is known for its technological know-how. This means that these interests must be considered when decisions are made that impact their use.

Interest Group Power and Influence

Although all groups aim to influence the policy-making process, the power of these groups is not equal. On any given issue, one must understand the constant give and take between the many interests described previously and within the framework of power. It is the interplay between these groups that shape policy (Smith, 1993). Historically, physicians were the dominant group shaping health policy (Morone, 1995). The power of the AMA was legendary, particularly when discussing the possibility of national health insurance. Power was ceded to the medical profession at the turn of the last century (Freidson, 1970; Starr, 1982). Physicians had a claim to technical expertise that justified their control over the organization and delivery of medical services. Second, their professional authority was extended to state-supported control over the healthcare field. Physicians determined the regulation of medicine through state licensing procedures. Finally, physicians actively sought to control health politics. They historically advocated against programs such as national health insurance that were perceived to undermine their authority by increasing the role of the state to regulate the provision of health services. Later they began to advocate for programs that enhanced physician authority such as the Peer Review Organizations (Starr, 1982).

Although nurses and other healthcare providers are a larger group in terms of actual numbers, it is physicians who set the terms of the debate historically. Their expertise was the basis for their having authority over nursing practice (Gordon, 2005). Although nurses have autonomy over their professional scope of practice, they take their directions from doctors for all matters related to direct patient care. Physicians' knowledge base is oriented toward cure, and the healthcare system is directed toward that end (Glouberman & Mintzberg, 2001). Nursing practice is oriented toward care. This function, however, is often secondary in the ways that we organize the healthcare delivery, although there has been a constant call for its centrality to achieving health (Gawande, 2007).

In addition to physicians, the other centers of power until the 1980s were the hospitals and the academic medical centers in particular (Tierney, 1987). The advancement of both groups augmented the work of physicians. Their growing strength can be seen post–World War II when increased pressure was put on the federal government to provide support for health care. The federal government could not intervene directly and support the provision of health services because such proposals were aggressively opposed by physicians as being precursors to socialized medicine. Physicians acceded to government funding of hospital construction and biomedical research spending, which enhanced their ability to practice medicine (Stevens, 1971). The Hill-Burton Act of 1946 made money available to rebuild and expand the deteriorating hospital infrastructure. The federal government also dramatically increased its support for the National Institutes for Health that became the vehicle for funding biomedical research at the universities where doctors trained (Daniels, 1971).

The balance of power between these groups is not constant. A shift began to occur in the 1980s because of a convergence of several factors. Most important was the increasing cost of care. Healthcare expenditures rose from 5.1% of the GDP in 1960 to 9.1% by 1980 (National Health Expenditure Data, 2008). With the country in an economic downturn, the rising healthcare costs put pressure on payer groups to find a solution to the problem. Second, the government was fast becoming one of the largest payers of health services with the growth of the Medicare and Medicaid programs. A third trend was the growing corporatization of the healthcare field (Relman, 1980; Starr, 1982). The growth of for-profit facilities and multifacility corporations were seen as shifting institutional goals away from public benefit toward more narrow concerns for financial profitability. Finally, technology and demographic trends pointed to ever-increasing costs caused by the rate of medical innovation and the aging of the population that would require increased services (Bodenheimer, 2005; Marmor, 2001).

The growing complexity of the healthcare system led to its transformation from what was termed a physician-dominated system to a finance-driven system (Starr, 1982). When the issue was recast as one of constraining costs, professional expertise was no longer the critical skill needed to resolve the problem. Doctors' ability to influence and direct the organization and delivery of care began to give way to the administrators of the system, including third-party payers. These groups were in a better position to control the cost of care by creating the appropriate financial incentives to influence physician practice patterns. By the 1990s, authority over health policy was becoming firmly rooted in the organizations that paid for health services. This includes big business, the insurance companies that are represented by the Health Insurance Association of America, and increasingly the federal and state governments.

The challenge to physician dominance was not limited to the financial sector of the industry. Patients were also advocating for greater autonomy and sovereignty over the decisions that affect their health (Schneider, 1998). They wanted to demystify the role of physicians and enable patients to become active participants in their own care. Patients' loss of trust in the medical profession became manifest in many ways (Mechanic, 1996). Among these was the use of the courts for recourse to care that they found negligent. The number of malpractice suits began rising in the 1980s, which led to a crisis of sorts related to the cost and availability of malpractice insurance (Studdert et al., 2004). What started with protest groups outside of the healthcare system became a legitimate concern within the medical field. In 2003, several physician groups spearheaded by the American Board of Internal Medicine issued a statement on medical professionalism that reaffirmed the importance of the patient/physician relationship being defined by integrity, respect, and compassion (American Board of Internal Medicine, 1994).

Finally, other healthcare practitioners began to challenge physician authority. The healthcare labor force has historically been described as a pyramid with physicians at the apex directing all related medical practice. As the provision of care becomes increasingly complex, alternative practitioners have begun to seek professional status and the right to independent practice. Research demonstrates that they provided care comparable to or of higher quality than their physician counterparts (Cromwell, 1999; Maule, 1994). These practitioners are capable of providing quality care at a lower cost. Thus, they offer a cost effective alternative to physicians. Professional associations of groups such as physical therapists and nurse practitioners are lobbying on a state-by-state basis to change licensing laws so that these clinicians can practice independently and receive direct reimbursement for their services. Such laws create an alternative center of authority.

Agenda Setting and Policy Adoption

Although there are numerous policy advocates with numerous policy alternatives, not all of their ideas can be acted on. Some ideas have a greater chance to succeed than others (Bachrach & Baratz, 1962; Smith, 2002). Why do some ideas take precedence over others in shaping policy? The objective conditions, or what we might term the actual problem, are always a necessary foundation for a social policy idea to succeed, but

not a sufficient one. The first step is for an idea to become part of the public agenda. National health insurance is an interesting case study because it has moved on and off the public agenda since the early twentieth century but has never been affirmed as policy despite the fact that there is an actual problem (Cairl & Imershein, 1977; Skocpol, 1995; Steinmo & Watts, 1995). It was last considered in 1993 when Clinton's healthcare proposal was defeated in Congress. Once again, national health insurance has been put on the agenda with the election of Barack Obama as president, but the uncertainty in the economy makes action highly uncertain.

Numerous factors can elevate the status of an issue to the extent that it might be acted on by the government (Peterson, 1993). In some instances, there are triggering events such as Hurricane Katrina. Many public health issues that had been ignored before the hurricane, such as emergency preparedness, were suddenly perceived as needing immediate action (Fee & Brown, 2002). In other instances, interest groups have used the courts to further their policy change agenda. The series of law suits brought against the tobacco companies in the 1990s led these companies to seek a compromise with the government that would provide liability protection in exchange for greater regulation (Pertschuk, 2001). Interest groups found an effective way to use the courts to get their issues on the agenda. Such groups have many tools available to them. They can meet with legislators. They can meet with corporate executives. They can also organize conferences to inform policy makers and the public about a particular issue. Political action is another means to build consensus about the need for action. Whether on the mall or at corporate headquarters, demonstrations are intended to be a show of support for a set of issues and thus pressure legislatures to act. Persons in political power can also put issues on the public agenda. The President sets the agenda each year when he gives the State of the Union address. Legislators also advance particular interests. Harrison Wofford's special Senate run in 1991 for U.S. Senator from Pennsylvania was framed by a single issue, national health insurance. His upset victory was a major impetus for President Clinton to advance healthcare reform as one of his first legislative initiatives following his 1992 election victory.

Although the tactics used by different groups to elevate their issues are important, the fact remains that some groups find themselves struggling to be heard, whereas others have greater access to policy makers and their proposals have greater credibility. This was the case with AIDS during the 1980s (Shilts, 1987). The policies and programs that are most reflective of the strongest interests in the healthcare field have greatest chance of being taken under consideration (Schnattschneider, 1960). These are the groups that hold the most power within society generally and the healthcare field specifically. The healthcare field has been characterized as being comprised of five broad groups of actors, and within each broad group, some players are more powerful than others. Physicians have typically

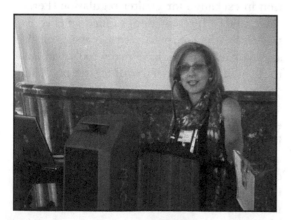

dominated nurses in policy debates. Recently, nurses and other health professionals have found themselves with greater authority and they are leading several of the policy discussions. It is notable that the Obama administration appointed a nurse, Mary Wakefield, to oversee the Health Resources and Services Administration. The business community carries more weight than consumer advocacy groups in regard to policies related to health insurance. The interests of the academic medical centers often outweigh those of community hospitals. These groups' strength is reflected in their ability to organize, the cohesion of their members, their funding, their expertise on the issue, and their legal status (Howlett & Ramesh, 2003).

The culmination of the policy-making process is the adaptation of policy via the legislative process. Elected officials decide the broad outlines of policy when they enact laws. Legislators do not act in isolation. There are many centers of power both inside and outside of government that try to influence the process. As a result, legislators usually seek a middle ground that is responsive to these competing interests (Smith, 2002). When looking for this middle ground, two of the most important issues for having a policy alternative recognized in law are its technical feasibility and its acceptability among different political constituencies (Kingdon, 1995; Tierney, 1987). Legislators are often looking for programs that are small and limited in scope because implementation is not as difficult to achieve and the programs are more likely to succeed. As proposed programs becomes more complex and impact a greater number of groups, developing legislation that is acceptable to all of the parties involved becomes more difficult (Morone, 1995). In these cases, legislators are looking for proposals around which they can build public support. Such proposals have often been termed "safe." This means legislators are seeking to adjust existing programs rather than proposing fundamental change to the status quo (Bachrach & Baratz, 1962).

There are moments of exceptionalism when programs disrupt existing social relations that define the organization and delivery of services. The passage of Medicare and Medicaid in 1965 is the most notable example in the healthcare field. These programs sought to redistribute control over access to healthcare resources (Ball, 1995), but even such major pieces of legislation are rooted in past programs and shaped in response to existing political interests (Vladeck, 1999). Medicare succeeded in making health insurance available to persons over 65 years of age, but the legislation must also be understood as an extension of the existing healthcare system. The hospitals supported Part A because its charges would be determined retrospectively based on actual costs. This meant that hospitals would see a growth in revenue from persons who previously had difficulty paying for hospital care. Physicians and the AMA supported Part B because it was voluntary and did not create a broader precedent for the government provision of care. Along with Medicaid, Congress preserved the principle of a safety net as opposed to the principle of health care as a right. The insurance companies supported Medicare because they would be responsible for claims administration. Also, there was bipartisan support in Congress. For Democrats, Medicare was a social insurance program that provided universal coverage for persons over 65 years of age for hospitalization, a high-cost health service. The Republicans ultimately supported the legislation because it maintained a program of voluntary insurance for physicians' services and therefore did not set a precedent for the socialization of the healthcare system (Marmor, 1973).

Implementation

Although often ignored, policy implementation is a continuation of the politics of policy creation in the administrative arena and cannot be divorced from the policy-making process. Legislation provides the broadest possible outline of a program. The specificity of the law determines the flexibility that the administration has in its implementation (Lowi, 1979). Congress can attempt to be specific in its formulation of programs in order to control the actions of a possibly hostile administration, or Congress can choose to leave the details of implementation to the administering agency. There are advantages and disadvantages to both choices. A bill in which details are clearly specified may encounter difficulty in Congress because groups may oppose the particulars as opposed to the overarching program. Clinton's health insurance plan was a victim to this approach (Brady & Buckley, 1995). A consensus can be more easily built around a law with broad, overarching goals, but few details. In this case, decisions about implementation are left to the administering agencies.

Program implementation is the responsibility of the executive branch and its administrative agencies. At the federal level, the Department of Health and Human Services has responsibility for realizing the legislation's goals through the administration of programs created by Congress (Pressman & Wildavsky, 1973). Implementation can be difficult because the abstract agreements made during the legislative process often fall apart if underlying conflicts have not been resolved. This makes the administrative leadership and organizational capacity of administrative agencies even more important. How an agency chooses to implement the program can have tremendous influence on its outcome (Jacobson & Wasserman, 1999; Morone, 1995; Pressman & Wildavsky, 1973). The leadership of the agency must be in accord with the program's goals so that it does not languish, and the personnel must also have program expertise to implement the program effectively. The State Children's Health Insurance Program, commonly referred to as SCHIP, is a case in point. As power over program implementation devolved back to the states in the late 1980s and early 1990s, there was concern about the capacity of the states to implement such a complex health program. The states, however, have developed capacity in these areas over the past decades, as it was their intent to expand children's access to health care (Kinney & Chang, 2004). They had supportive leadership and developed the internal capacity required to operate the program.

As in the case of the legislation process, administrative agencies do not work in a vacuum. Organized interests that are instrumental in mobilizing and building support for policies throughout the legislative process play a comparable role during its implementation. They work with the administrative agencies to insure that implementation meets their interests by monitoring the process (Pressman & Wildavsky, 1973). The agency staff also develops a stake in the programs that they oversee (Peterson, 1993). As they become expert in a given field, they also become influential in the policy-making process. It is not atypical for government employees to work with advocacy groups and Congressional committees to advance their program's interests. Given their expertise in a given field, the situation exists where professionals move between these sectors—sometimes working for the government and sometimes working in the private or nonprofit sectors.

Healthcare professionals and their patients experience the impact of the implementation process on a daily basis. How patients are recruited to programs such as SCHIP and Part D of Medicare is determined by the regulations of these programs. Which companies have contracts to provide Medicare Managed Care programs is also a result of program guidelines. The same is true for the nurse-to-patient ratios specified in the laws of California or the limit on the hours that medical residents can work in New York State hospitals (which came about in response to a patient's death in a city hospital). These are all examples of programs that were developed by federal and/or state legislatures and implemented by federal and state administering agencies. Although their work is seemingly distant, its impact is immediate in terms of access to quality health care.

What Is at Stake for Nurses and Other Health Professionals?

The work of nurses and other health professionals tends to be highly individualized. By interacting with patients, they see the many problems that result from policy decisions made at a distance. They understand how the loss of healthcare insurance can result in patients deferring care much to their detriment. They understand that the pursuit of quality patient care is dependent on their ability to engage and use nursing resources effectively, which will likely become more challenging as the nursing shortage persists and resources become increasingly limited (Draper, Felland, Liebhaber, & Melichar, 2008).

In many cases, these professionals become the patients' advocates, but historically, they have not played a major role in the initial development of the policies that have such a tremendous subsequent impact on the lives of their patients and on their work. Some have attributed this to the heavy workloads. Others have discussed the educational process that socializes nurses to distance themselves from politics. Still others speak about the difficulty nurses have asserting their professional authority when they find themselves up

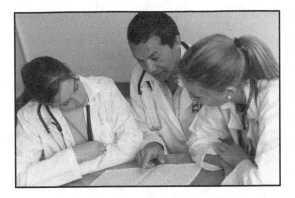

against dominant interests such as physician groups, hospitals, and payers. Regardless of cause, there is now a growing concern that nurses and other health professionals find an even greater voice in the policy-making process (Thomas & While, 2007; Wolf & Greenhouse, 2007).

By understanding the policy-making process and how it has shaped the organization and delivery of health care, it is possible to understand the many ways one can become politically engaged. Since the 1990s, we have looked to the market to bring greater efficiency to the organization and delivery of care. It is the failure of this approach that is reinvigorating interest in the politics of health care. We know that health costs are rising, that the risk of becoming uninsured is increasing, and that the quality can suffer despite

the best efforts of healthcare providers. The critical challenge will be determining how health care should be organized and delivered so as to ensure the best possible health outcomes for the population. With the worsening financial situation of the country, the stresses that ordinary Americans will experience will be evidenced in the healthcare arena through even greater numbers of uninsured and even greater numbers of persons who are delaying or foregoing care. Determining what will be the tradeoffs between access, costs, and quality will impact the situation that nurses and other professionals confront every day. Nurses and other healthcare providers need to become one of the dominant voices in the policy-making and policy-implementation process if we are to have a healthcare system that best meets the needs of the people it serves.

References

American Board of Internal Medicine. (1994). Project professionalism medical professionalism in the new millennium: a physician charter. *Annals of Internal Medicine, 136,* 243–246.

Anton, T. (1997). New federalism and intergovernmental fiscal relationships: The implications for health policy. *Journal of Health Politics Policy and Law, 22*(3), 691–720.

Arrow, K. J. (1963). Uncertainty and the welfare economics of medical care. *The American Economic Review, 5*(5), In *Bulletin of the World Health Organization, 82*(2), 141–149.

Arrow, K. J. (1974). *The limits of organization.* New York: W.W. Norton and Co.

Bachrach, P., & Baratz, M. (1962). Two faces of power. *American Political Science Review, 56,* 4632–4642.

Ball, R. (1995). What Medicare's architects had in mind. *Health Affairs, 14*(4), 62–73.

Bodenheimer, T. (2005). High and rising health care costs. Part 2: Technologic innovation. *Annals of Internal Medicine, 142,* 932–937.

Bovbjerg, R., Wiener, J., & Housman, M. (2003). State and federal roles in health care: Rationales for allocating responsibilities. In J. Holahan, A. Weil, & J. Wiener (Eds.), *Federalism and Health Policy* (vol. 3, pp. 25–51). Washington, DC: The Urban Institute Press.

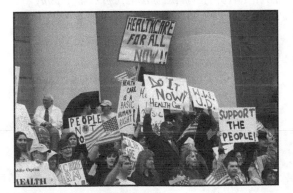

Brady, D. W., & Buckley, K. M. (1995). Health care reform in the 103d Congress: A predictable failure. *Journal of Health Politics Policy and Law, 20,* 447–454.

Brown, L. D., & Sparer, M. S. (2003). Poor program's progress: The unanticipated politics of Medicaid policy. *Health Affairs, 22*(1), 31–44.

Cairl, R., & Imershein, A. (1977). National health insurance policy in the United States: A case of non-decision-making. *International Journal of Health Services,* 7(2), 167–178.

Center for Policy and Research. (2007). *Individual Health Insurance 2006–2007: A Comprehensive Survey of Premiums, Availability, and Benefits.* Retrieved July 1, 2008, from http://www.ahipresearch.org/pdfs/Individual_Market_Survey_December_2007.pdf

Conlan, T. (2006). From cooperative to opportunistic federalism: Reflections on the half-century anniversary of the commission on intergovernmental relations. *Public Administration Review, 66,* 663–676.

Conway, P. H., Tamara Konetzka, R., Zhu, J., Volpp, K. G., & Sochalski, J. (2008). Nurse staffing ratios: Trends and policy implications for hospitalists and the safety net. *Journal of Hospital Medicine, 3*(3), 193–199.

Cromwell, J. (1999). Barriers to achieving a cost-effective workforce mix: Lessons from anesthesiology. *Journal of Health Politics Policy and Law, 24,* 1331–1361.

Daniels, G. H. (1971). *Science in American society: A social history.* New York: Alfred Knopf.

Davis, K., & Schoen, C. (1978). *Health and the war on poverty: A ten year appraisal.* Washington, DC: Brookings Institution.

DeCicca, P., Kenkel, D., Mathios, A., Shin, Y. J., & Lim, J. Y. (2008). Youth smoking, cigarette prices, and anti-smoking sentiment. *Health Economics, 17,* 733–749.

DeNavas-Walt, C., Proctor, B., & Smith, J. (2007). U.S. Census Bureau, *Current population reports, P60-233, Income, Poverty, and Health Insurance Coverage in the United States: 2006.* Retrieved September 26, 2008, from http://www.census.gov/prod/2007pubs/p60-233.pdf

Draper, D., Felland, L., Liebhaber, A., & Melichar, L. (2008). The role of nurses in hospital quality improvement. *Center for Studying Health System Change, 3,* 1–8.

Fee, E., & Brown, T. M. (2002). The unfulfilled promise of public health: Déjà vu all over again. *Health Affairs, 21*(6), 31–43.

Fox, D. (1986). The consequences of consensus: American health policy in the twentieth century. *The Milbank Quarterly, 64,* 176–199.

Freidson, E. (1970). *Profession of medicine: A study of the sociology of applied knowledge.* New York: Dodd, Mead.

Gawande, A. (2007). *Better: A surgeon's notes on performance.* New York: Picador.

Glouberman, S., & Mintzberg, H. (2001). Managing the care of health and the cure of disease: Part I: Differentiation. *Health Care Management Review, 26*(1), 56–69.

Gordon, S. (2005). *Nursing against the odds: How health care cost cutting, media stereotypes, and medical hubris undermine nurses and patient care (the culture and politics of health care work).* Ithaca, NY: Cornell University Press.

Grabowski, H. (2005). Encouraging the development of new vaccines. *Health Affairs, 24*(3), 697–700.

Grumbach, K. (2002). Fighting hand to hand over physician workforce policy: The invisible hand of the market meets the heavy hand of government planning. *Health Affairs, 32*(5), 13–27.

Howlett, M., & Ramesh, M. (2003). *Studying public policy: Policy cycles and policy subsystems.* Toronto, ON: Oxford University Press.

Jacobson, P., & Wasserman, J. (1999, June). The implementation and enforcement of tobacco control laws: Policy implications for activists and the industry. *Journal of Health Politics Policy and Law, 24,* 567–598.

Kernell, S., & Jacobson, G. C. (2006). *The logic of American politics* (3rd ed.). Washington, DC: CQ Press.

Kingdon, J. W. (1995). *Agendas, alternatives, and public policies.* New York: Harper Collins College Publishers.

Kinney, G., & Chang, D. I. (2004). The state children's health insurance program: Successes, shortcomings, and challenges. *Health Affairs, 23*(5), 51–62.

Knowles, J. H. (1977). The responsibility of the individual. In J. H. Knowles (Ed.), *Doing better and feeling worse: Health in the United States.* Cambridge: American Academy of Arts and Sciences.

Koenig, L., Dobson, A., Silver, H., Jonathan, M., Siegel, J. M., Blumenthal, D., & Weissman, J. S. (2003). Estimating the mission-related costs of teaching hospitals. *Health Affairs, 22*(6), 112–122.

Lowi, T. (1979). *The end of liberalism: ideology, policy, and the crisis of public authority* (2nd ed.). New York: Norton.

Lowi, T., & Ginsberg, B. (1998). *American government* (5th ed.). New York: Norton and Co.

Mariner, W. (1996). State regulation of managed care and the employee retirement income security act. *New England Journal of Medicine, 335,* 1986–1990.

Marmor, T. (1973). *The politics of Medicare.* Chicago: Aldine Publishing Co.

Marmor, T. (2001). How not to think about Medicare reform. *Journal of Health Politics, Policy and Law, 26*(1), 107–117.

Maule, W. (1994). Screening for colorectal cancer by nurse endoscopists. *New England Journal of Medicine, 330,* 183–186.

Mechanic, D. (1996). Changing medical organization and the erosion of trust. *The Milbank Quarterly, 74*(2), 171–189.

Midgley, J., & Livermore, M. (Eds.). (2008). *The handbook of social policy* (pp. 3–20). Los Angeles: Sage.

Morone, J. (1995). Elusive community: Democracy, deliberation, and the reconstruction of health policy. In M. Landy & M. Levin (Eds.), *The new politics of public policy* (pp. 180–204). Baltimore, MD: Johns Hopkins University Press.

National Health Expenditure Data. Aggregate, per capita amounts, percent distribution, and average annual percent growth, by source of funds: Selected Calendar Years 1960–2006. Retrieved July 14, 2008, from http://www.cms.hhs.gov/NationalHealthExpendData/downloads/tables.pdf

National Health Expenditure Data Fact Sheet. Retrieved September 26, 2008, from http://www.cms.hhs.gov/NationalHealthExpendData/25_NHE_Fact_Sheet.asp#TopOfPage

Pertschuk, M. (2001). *Smoke in their eyes: Lessons in movement leadership from the tobacco wars.* Nashville, TN: Vanderbilt University Press.

Peterson, M. A. (1993). Political Influence in the 1990s: From iron triangles to policy networks. *Journal of Health Politics, Policy and Law, 18,* 395–436.

Pressman, J. L., & Wildavsky, A. (1973). *Implementation.* Berkeley, CA: University of California Press.

Relman, A. S. (1980). The new medical-industrial complex. *New England Journal of Medicine, 303,* 963–970.

Reschovsky, J. D., Strunk, B. C., & Ginsburg, P. (2006). Why employer-sponsored insurance coverage change, 1997–2003. *Health Affairs, 25,* 774–782.

Rothman, D. J. (1971). *The discovery of the asylum: Social order and disorder in the New Republic.* Boston: Little, Brown.

Rushefsky, M. (2008). *Public policy in the United States: At the dawn of the 21st century* (4th ed.). Armonk, NY: M.E. Sharpe.

Schnattschneider, E. E. (1960). *The semisovereign people: A realist's view of democracy in America.* New York: Holt, Rinehart and Winston.

Schneider, C. E. (1998). *The practice of autonomy: Patients, doctors, and medical decisions.* New York: Oxford University Press.

Shilts, R. (1987). *And the band played on: Politics, people and the AIDS epidemic.* New York: St. Martin's Press.

Skocpol, T. (1995). *Boomerang: Clinton's health security effort and the turn against government in US politics.* New York: W.W. Norton.

Smith, M. (1993). *Pressure, power and policy: State autonomy and policy networks in Britain and the United States.* Pittsburgh, PA: University of Pittsburgh Press.

Smith, D. G. (2002). *Entitlement politics: Medicare and Medicaid 1995–2001.* New York: Aldine de Gruyter.

Starr, P. (1982). *The social transformation of American medicine.* New York: Basic Books.

State of the World's Mothers. (2007). *Saving the lives of children under 5.* Retrieved September 26, 2008, from http://www.savethechildren.org.au/australia/publications/mothers_report/mothers_report.html#findings

Steinmo, S., & Watts, J. (1995). It's the institutions, stupid! Why comprehensive national health insurance always fails in America. *Journal of Health Politics, Policy and Law, 20,* 329–372.

Steuerle, C. E., & Bovbjerg, R. R. (2008). Health and budget reform as handmaidens. *Health Affairs, 27,* 633–644.

Stevens, R. (1971). *American medicine in the public interest.* New Haven, CT: Yale University Press.

Stone, D. (2002). *Policy paradox: The art of political decision making.* New York: Norton.

Studdert, D. M., Mello, M. M., & Brenna, T. A. (2004). Medical malpractice. *New England Journal of Medicine, 350,* 283–292.

Thomas, P., & While, A. (2007). Should nurses be leaders of integrated health care? *Journal of Nursing Management, 15,* 643–648.

Tierney, J. (1987). Organized interests in health politics and policy-making. *Medical Care Review, 44*(1), 89–118.

Vladeck, B. (1999). The political economy of Medicare. *Health Affairs, 18*(1), 22–36.

Wolf, G. A., & Greenhouse, P. K. (2007). Blueprint for design: Creating models that direct change. *Journal of Nursing Administration, 37,* 9381–9387.

Photo Credits

Public Health Policy: Promotion, Prevention, and Protection

Mary Mincer Hansen and Mary Jones

OVERVIEW

Public health touches everyone's life every day. Healthy children are better learners. Healthy workers are more productive. Healthy countries are more prosperous and peaceful. Doctor Margaret Chan (2008a), Director of the World Health Organization (WHO), eloquently states that "health care is a critical contributor to social cohesion. Social cohesion is the best protection against social unrest . . . (and) healthy human capital is the foundation of economic productivity." Her point is further explicated by a statement from WHO (2008b): "The prevention of illness and the promotion of health through the delivery of efficient and effective public health services lie at the core of society's ability to create a virtuous circle of better health, more productive citizens and affordable health care." Public health has impacted the history of the United States in many ways. One of the more notable contributions being that the average life span of Americans was increased by 25 years because of public health initiatives during the last century (Centers for Disease Control and Prevention [CDC], 1999). Given its undisputed contribution to our nation and the world, it is stunning to realize that the United States annually spends more than $1.7 trillion in health care but less than 4 cents of every dollar is spent on prevention and public health (Lambrew, 2007). This resource disparity is directly related to the lack of a strong public health voice in health policy development and advocacy.

This chapter defines public health in the context of its history and service components. Service delivery in the areas of health prevention, promotion, and protection is delineated. Factors transforming global and national public health service delivery, including a focus on wellness, chronic and infectious diseases, environmental assets and threats, health inequity, and emergency preparedness are discussed. An analysis of the priority issues of accreditation, globalization, media, economics, and workforce that are shaping the future of public health is presented. This chapter concludes with a discussion of the skills and strategies integral for public health advocacy and policy formulation.

Historical Underpinnings of Public Health

Precisely defining public health is difficult. From its origins in ancient times to the mid 19th century when the first formal governmental health departments were established in the United States and into the 21st century, public health has evolved over a number of landmark eras in history. Table 1 provides an overview of these eras, the paradigms associated with each era, analytical approaches, and actions used during that time and initiatives that continue to be a critical part of public health practice (Awofeso, 2004).

The earliest landmark era in public health dates from ancient times to the 1830s. This era began with health protection that addressed disease prevention by enforcing regulation of human behavior through social structures. For example, this included enforcement of spiritual practices or customs imposed by ruling elites. Quarantine and some environmental protection laws were used. The next era was sanitation control, which surfaced in the 1840s through the 1870s, and addressed unsanitary environmental conditions that would cause disease. Community approaches were used through implementation of minimum standards for sewage, drainage, and refuse disposal, leading the way for potable water and early sanitation programs. This landmark time was the foundation from which the public health legal framework and disease surveillance and epidemiology methodology evolved.

Contagion control or the germ theory marked the next landmark era in public health history, dating from 1880 to the 1930s. The central theme of this era was the "demonstration of infectious origins of disease," which focused on the presence of disease-causing microorganisms, their hosts, and modes of transmission. These discoveries led to vaccinations, improved water filtration, and more standardized disease outbreak control strategies. Evidence-based public health practice came to light during this time. From the 1940s through the 1960s, the preventative medicine era emerged, focusing on the prevention and cure of diseases in high-risk populations. These included the treatment of communicable diseases and interventions directed at disease vectors. This moved public health program planning toward high-risk population groups and created an environment for gaining a better understanding of the pathogenesis of communicable and noncommunicable diseases.

Primary health care was the priority in the 1970s and 1980s, giving rise to a focus on the community. This meant that effective health care was geared toward the community, for the community, and by the community. Although preventative health care was at the forefront, emphasis was also placed on equity, accessibility, and the social determinants of health such as poverty and education. This led to a more global approach to public health and closer linkages between health promotion and disease prevention. Multicultural health emerged, healthy city initiatives grew, and community participation in public health surfaced. Early in the 1990s the era of health promotion and advocacy for health became the focus. This created supportive environments for impacting optimal health at the

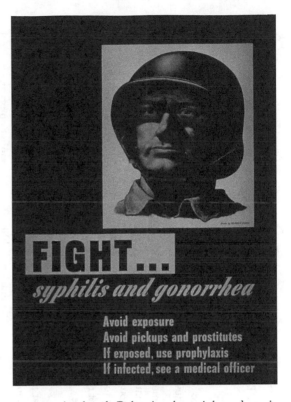

community level. Behavioral, social, and environmental changes could be made as a result of education, economic, and political actions. This assisted individuals and the community in strengthening actions toward optimal health (Awofeso, 2004).

The 21st century ushered in another era in public health. In the first few years of this century, the terrorist attacks on the United States in 2001 and subsequent anthrax-laden letters sent through the U.S. Postal Service, Severe Acute Respiratory Syndrome (SARS) in 2003, and the threat of another pandemic demonstrated how the world is changing in terms of vulnerability to public health threats. Concerns about the United States public health system's preparedness for epidemics and disasters have been elevated. According to a WHO (2007a) report, SARS confirmed fears generated by the bioterrorism threat that a

Table 1 Six Eras in the Evolution of Public Health

Public Health Era	Dominant Paradigm	Analytic Approaches	Action Frameworks	Legacies Incorporated into Contemporary Public Health
1. Health Protection (antiquity–1830s)	Diseases may be prevented by enforced regulation of human behavior, mediated through societies' social structures.	Interpretation/promulgation of religious and cultural rules that are thought by the ruling elites to protect the health of the individual and the community	Enforcement of spiritual practices, community taboos, customs, and quarantine	Quarantine of illegal migrants; enforcement of some environmental protection laws; aspects of spirituality in prevention and coping with disease; some occupational and transport safety laws
2. Miasma Control (1840s–1870s)	Addressing unsanitary environmental conditions may prevent diseases.	Demonstration that poor health and epidemics resulted directly from unsanitary physical and social environments	Centralized action to improve environmental sanitation; public health legislation relating to minimum standards for drainage, sewage, and refuse disposal	Aspects of Healthy Cities initiatives; potable water and sanitation programs; legal framework for implementing public health activities; foundations of modern epidemiology and surveillance
3. Contagion Control (1880s–1930s)	Germ Theory is a positivist approach to demonstration of infectious origins of diseases.	Demonstration of the presence of disease-causing microorganisms in infected media, their isolation, and experimental transmission	Interruption of disease transmission through improved water filtration processes, vaccination, standardized disease outbreak control measures	Evidence-based public health practice; ethical vaccination practices; foundations for international cooperation in health; foundations for modern chemotherapy
4. Preventive Medicine (1940s–1960s)	Improvements in public health through focus on	Definition of, and interventions aimed at, main avenues for disease	Environmental interventions directed at disease vectors	Focus on "high-risk groups" in the planning and implementation of public health such

the prevention and cure of diseases in "high-risk groups"	transmission. Medical dominance, with focus on treatment of communicable diseases and primary care of "special populations" (e.g., pregnant women and factory workers)	identification and use of "useful" microbes; enhanced medical care for "high-risk groups"; foundations of modern clinical pathology	as mosquitoes; programs; improved understanding of the pathogenesis of communicable and noncommunicable diseases
5. Primary Health Care (1970s–1980s)	Health for All: effective health care geared toward the community, for the community, and by the community	Largely preventive health care approach, underpinned by emphasis on equity, community participation, accessibility of services, and social determinants of health	Emphasis on global cooperation and peace; adapting health services to countries and communities; links between health care and socioeconomic development; intersectoral cooperation in health promotion and disease prevention; equity in health care	Concepts underpinning multicultural health and Healthy Cities initiatives, health inequalities, and community participation in health promotion activities
6. Health Promotion (1990s–present)	Advocacy for health; enabling individuals and communities to attain optimal health	Individuals and communities may be assisted by educational, economic, and political actions to increase control over, and improve, their health through attitudinal, behavioral, social, and environmental changes	Encapsulated by the key action areas of the Ottawa Charter: build healthy public policy; create supportive environments; strengthen community action; develop personal skills; and reorient health services	Encapsulated by the key action areas of the Ottawa Charter: build healthy public policy; create supportive environments; strengthen community action; develop personal skills; and reorient health services

Source: Table 1 from Awofeso, N. (2004). What's new about the new public health? *Am J Public Health, 94*(5), 705–709. Used with permission of the author.

new or unfamiliar pathogen would have profound national and international implications for global public health security.

Organization of Public Health Services

Public health cannot be completely defined without a discussion of its infrastructure. One of the earliest designers of governmental public health infrastructure can be traced back to Lemuel Shattuck (1850) in his *Report of the Sanitary Commission of Massachusetts*. From the time the report was written, several decades had passed before state and local public health agencies began to form. By 1900, health departments existed in nearly all states, and the first county-based health department was formed in 1911 (Turnock & Barnes, 2006). As state and local public health agencies began to form, serving different population sizes and addressing diverse health issues, the structure, governance, and statutory frameworks of these agencies varied depending on health needs.

Governmental public health is intrinsically a network of local, state, and federal agencies that are collectively responsible for health promotion and protection and disease prevention. These agencies provide basic community services, including collecting vital statistics, prevention services, and the promotion of health education and healthy life styles. In addition, these services include ensuring clean drinking water, sanitation, and prevention and control of diseases. The focus of traditional public health practice occurs at the community level and is aimed at the population. The practice must allow for flexibility in order to deal with specific community health needs, which vary from jurisdiction to jurisdiction (Institute of Medicine [IOM], 1988).

Public health is primarily the responsibility of the state. Although primary responsibility belongs to the state, a majority of public health services are provided at the local level. Thousands of local, state, and federal agencies participate in public health practice and are governed independently by varying degrees of authority. The U.S. public health agencies are products of federalism—a system of government in which power is distributed between a central authority and the constituent units. The agencies are regulated by the orders of boards at the local level, governors at the state level, and primarily secretaries at the federal level.

Governance of public health practice is driven by administrative and bureaucratic realities, meaning that programs are influenced and shaped by their political context. It is a culmination of science and politics coming together in the public arena and being influenced by political forces. The translation of turning plans into action requires a great deal of perseverance and negotiating skill. If successful, it comes with varying degrees of support in terms of funding and infrastructure. As political alliances rise and fall, so does public health. In essence, public health is not defined by what the profession is capable of doing; instead, it is driven by the decisions made by a political system within a jurisdiction (IOM, 1988).

The shaping of public health occurs as a result of the health problems needing to be addressed in a particular community and by the political system within which it functions. It is at that local level that an understanding of how programs should function and what resources are necessary to address particular health needs are realized. It is at the state level that resource acquisition, coordination, and evaluation occur. It is at the federal level that coordination of national public health initiatives takes place, state and local governmental public health is supported, and a national vision is articulated. This vision is captured by the IOM's definition of the public health system (1988): "A complex network of individuals and organizations that, when working together, can represent 'what we as society do collectively to assure the conditions in which people can be healthy.'"

Service Delivery

Based on the 1988 IOM report the *Essential Public Health Services*, ideas about service delivery were developed in 1994 (see Table 2). This broad framework is used across the nation by public health leaders to articulate what public health does. Based on this framework, basic service delivery includes preventing epidemics and the spread of disease, protecting against environmental hazards, preventing injuries, promoting healthy behaviors, and addressing public health emergencies.

Preventing epidemics and the spread of disease encompasses surveillance and investigation to determine the etiology, virulence, and communicability of actual and potential sources of disease. Based on these data, public health practitioners design, implement, and evaluate control strategies to prevent, reduce, or eliminate infectious disease. The SARS epidemic in 2003 confirmed the need to ensure that the nation's public health system has the capacity to prevent, detect, respond to, and manage outbreaks of infectious disease.

Protecting against environmental hazards involves assessing both the natural and built environments to determine health risk factors. Programs and activities focus on mitigating the effects of harmful substances and structures that endanger individuals and populations. This involves monitoring environmental risk factors and enforcing regulation. Examples of activities include ensuring food safety, conducting housing inspections, and monitoring air and water quality. More recently, environmental health includes exploring links between community design and public health. This expanded role is geared toward protecting against and preventing injury and disease by improving where we live, work, shop, and play (Heishman & Dannenberg, 2008).

Preventing injuries encompasses activities that facilitate the prevention, reduction, or elimination of intentional or unintentional injuries. This involves studying how, when, and why injuries occur; designing new strategies to prevent injuries; and educating the public about evidence-based prevention strategies. The goal is to keep people safe from injury and violence with a reduction in disabilities, death, and medical expenses across all life stages (CDC, 2006a).

Services that promote healthy behaviors include activities that prevent and reduce illness and disease. These activities support and incentivize individuals and communities to develop healthy behaviors. The result is increased wellness and quality of life with a decrease in chronic disease, premature mortality, and disease burden.

Addressing public health emergencies includes activities to prepare the public health system to respond to public health threats, emergencies, and disasters and to assist in the recovery process. In order to address these threats, the public health system must have adequate capacity and capability to reduce morbidity and mortality from infectious diseases either naturally occurring or intentionally introduced. Coordination of prevention and response activities, along with strong linkages among multiple partners, is integral in public health preparedness.

Throughout history, the context of public health practice has been transformed a number of times and continues to be transformed today given the demographic change in age and diversity of the population, globalization, the explosion in technology, and national security. Each period of transformation is the result of changing health threats to our nation that either add new responsibilities to public health or change

Table 2 TEN ESSENTIAL PUBLIC HEALTH SERVICES

1. Monitor health status to identify community health problems.

2. Diagnose and investigate health problems and health hazards in the community.

3. Inform, educate, and empower people about health issues.

4. Mobilize community partnerships to identify and solve health problems.

5. Develop policies and plans that support individual and community health efforts.

6. Enforce laws and regulations that protect health and ensure safety.

7. Link people to needed personal health services and assure the provision of health care when unavailable.

8. Assure a competent public health and personal healthcare workforce.

9. Evaluate effectiveness, accessibility, and quality of personal and population-based health services.

10. Research for new insights and innovative solutions to health problems.

Source: Centers for Disease Control and Prevention, 1994.

its focus in order to ensure optimal health for the population. One of the earliest public health actions (quarantine) in protecting health is still used, and many of the legacies left by each public health era continue today. Thus, precisely defining public health remains problematic; however, three key themes continue to surface and have survived the test of time toward defining public health: promotion, prevention, and protection. These themes are the cornerstones of public health and public health practice.

Factors Transforming Global and National Public Health Service Delivery

Public health is a complex mosaic of programs that focus on the interconnected roles of protecting and promoting health and preventing illness in populations. This complexity has been amplified by rapidly changing factors that are transforming public health practice and service delivery: a focus on wellness, increased incidence of chronic disease, actual and potential emergence, re-emergence of lethal infectious diseases, population-focused programs to address health inequities, the increased role of public health in assisting with disasters, and the myriad environmental factors influencing health.

Wellness and Chronic Disease

Wellness is optimal health for individuals and groups. Wellness focuses on realizing maximum potential of the individual physically, psychologically, spiritually, and socioeconomically. When wellness is realized, it creates the additional benefit of healthy individuals being able to participate fully in their roles as members of families and the community (Smith et al., 2006).

The major threats to achieving wellness for the United States at the beginning of the 21st century are chronic and preventable diseases, which account for the majority of mortality, morbidity, and healthcare costs. Cardiovascular disease, cancer, chronic obstructive pulmonary disease, and diabetes account for two thirds of all deaths in the United States (CDC, 2004). More than half of all Americans live with one or more chronic disease (DeVol et al., 2007).

Risk factors that the majority of chronic diseases have in common include excess caloric intake, physical inactivity, and tobacco use. These are lifestyle choices, and therefore, the chronic diseases attributable to them are considered preventable by risk factor modification (Office of the Surgeon General, 2001). The need for risk factor modification is amplified further by the fact that our country has the highest rate of preventable disease of the industrialized nations (Nolte & McKee, 2008).

Approximately 24% of Americans were obese in 2005 compared with 15% in 1995 (CDC, 2006b). The implications of this statistic are staggering. One study postulates that a 20-year-old obese man could experience a 17% reduction in life expectancy (Fontaine et al., 2003). Our children's life spans may be shorter than their parents for the first time in a hundred years (Olshansky et al., 2005). In addition, obese children are at risk for a range of physical and mental problems that may negatively impact school performance (Dietz, 1998).

Obesity contributes to 75% of hypertension cases (American Obesity Association, 2008). Statistics show that approximately 90% of middle-aged Americans will develop hypertension, with almost 70% of these individuals failing to achieve adequate blood pressure control (American Heart Association, 2003).

One of the most prevalent chronic diseases related to obesity is diabetes. More than 20 million American adults have type 2 diabetes. An additional 54 million are prediabetic, and 2 million of those are adolescents (Cowie et al., 2009). Approximately 20% of cancer in women and 15%

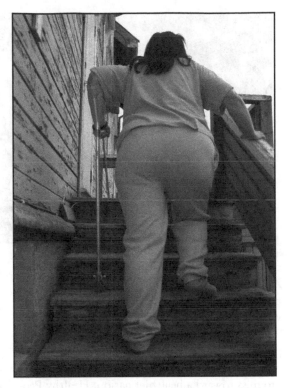

of cancer in men can be attributed to obesity (CDC, 2004). These statistics emphasize the health impact on the population created by the obesity epidemic and the important role of public health.

Another health behavior that contributes to chronic disease is tobacco use, use which is the cause of nearly 5 million deaths per year (WHO, 2008c). It is the leading preventable cause of death in the United States. Smoking and second-hand smoke kill approximately 440,000 people in the United States annually (Armour et al., 2005). It is one of the major risk factors for coronary heart disease. This is significant because coronary heart disease is the leading cause of death in the United States (CDC, 1993).

The U.S. public health system has attempted to deal with the epidemic of chronic and preventable diseases by using a national consensus process

ONE WEAPON THAT KILLS FROM BOTH ENDS.

SECONDHAND SMOKE KILLS.

CALIFORNIA DEPARTMENT OF PUBLIC HEALTH

PAID FOR BY THE TOBACCO TAX INITIATIVE

to develop an agenda for improving the health of Americans and promoting wellness. Through this process, a document entitled *Healthy People 2010* was created. The two goals of Healthy People 2010 are (1) to increase life expectancy and improve quality of life and (2) to eliminate health inequities (Keppel et al., 2007). In order to measure progress toward a healthier nation, Healthy People 2010 has identified 10 leading health indicators that will be used to monitor progress in improving the health of our nation: physical activity, overweight and obesity, tobacco use, substance abuse, responsible sexual behavior, mental health, injury and violence, environmental quality, immunization, and access to care. A complete copy of the Healthy People 2010 plan can be found at http://www.healthypeople.gov.

This discussion has documented that chronic diseases are among the most preventable health problems facing our nation. Evidence-based interventions for risk-factor modification can prevent or delay much of the burden while mitigating the devastating consequences. This is accomplished by implementing public health initiatives that promote both healthy behavior choices and community policies and practices that create a culture of wellness (CDC, 2004).

Infectious Disease

The public health system came into existence as the first line of defense against infectious disease. Investment in this system waned with the advent of effective pharmaceuticals and the belief that we had conquered infectious disease as a threat to human health; however, over the past 40 years, 39 new infectious diseases have been discovered, among which are some that drug therapy has been unable to cure. The most deadly of these include HIV/AIDS, Ebola, and SARS (The Millennium Project, 2009). Another disease that has become a serious threat to health is hepatitis C. An estimated 4.1 million Americans have been infected, with 3.2 million suffering chronically (CDC, 2005).

A further complication of infectious diseases is that illnesses previously identified and responsive to medical therapy such as tuberculosis have mutated and developed drug resistance, making them harder to treat. Drug resistance makes the infection less responsive to current therapies and more difficult to treat (WHO, 2007a). Influenza is another disease that has proven to be difficult to both treat and prevent. The United States public health surveillance systems find that seasonal flu results in 200,000 hospitalizations and kills an average of 36,000 Americans yearly (CDC, 2008a).

One of the most deadly and debilitating diseases worldwide has been HIV/AIDS, with 33 million people living with HIV and approximately 7,500 new infections occurring daily. In the United States, an estimated 1.1 million people are infected with HIV. Of serious concern is the projection that approximately one in five persons living with HIV in the United States is unaware that he or she is infected and may be unknowingly transmitting the virus to others (CDC, 2008b).

Our rapidly changing world has led to challenges in implementing public health strategies to contain infectious disease spread. For example, "Airlines now carry more than 2 billion passengers a year, making it possible for any [infectious] diseases they may have to pass from one country to another in a matter of hours" (WHO, 2007a). Globalization will contribute to the rapid spread of the next influenza pandemic. A severe pandemic is projected to "result in 90 million Americans becoming sick, 2.2 million deaths, and the second worst U.S. economic recession since World War II" (Trust for America's Health [TFAH], 2007, p. 6).

Another challenge has been the recent phenomenon of some people refusing immunizations. Six years after the original 2000 target date for the worldwide eradication of polio, the disease persists in countries where the virus is endemic, and new outbreaks are occurring in previously polio-free areas. Public health workers are finding that socioeconomic factors are hindering attainment of complete global obliteration. An example is the suspension of polio vaccination programs in Nigeria in 2003 and 2004 because of a rumor that the vaccine would cause infertility and infection with HIV (Pallansch & Sandhu, 2006).

Environmental

Our environment is both friend and foe. The National Academy of Sciences estimates that 25% of developmental diseases, such as cerebral palsy, autism, and mental retardation, are caused by environmental factors acting alone or together with genetic risk factors. The WHO (2006) estimates that 13 million deaths annually are due to preventable environmental causes.

The WHO sounded a warning on the dangers of ignoring environmental hazards in their recent report on global public health security. The report stated that an inadequate investment in public health, resulting from a false sense of security that vector diseases were eradicated, led to control programs being discontinued and a reduction in training and employment of specialists in the 1980s. The result being that within the following 20 years many important vector-borne diseases, including dengue hemorrhagic fever and malaria, emerged into new areas or re-emerged in areas where the diseases were previously controlled (WHO, 2007b).

Indoor and outdoor air pollution is estimated to be responsible for nearly 5% of the global burden of disease. Childhood asthma in the United States has more than doubled over the last 2 decades, and this rise has been linked to indoor and outdoor air quality. The WHO estimates that about 40% of lower respiratory infections occurring in developing countries are related to environmental conditions. In addition, poor air quality is related to the incidence and severity of heart and lung diseases, allergies, and several types of cancers (National Center for Environmental Health: Office of Global Health).

Environmental factors contribute to higher incidence of chronic disease. Research shows that over 50% of American adults do not get enough physical activity to provide health benefits. There has been a marked decline in children walking or biking to school, 13% today compared with 66% in 1974. This can be directly related to the fact that the United States has the lowest prevalence of walking and biking among developed countries. Research also demonstrates that living in sprawling counties like the United States contributes to individuals walking less, weighing more, and having a higher prevalence of hypertension than those living in compact counties.

The environment can also be a positive force for health. The design and development of communities can promote physical activity and act as a public health intervention to promote wellness. One example of doing this is the concept of healthy places. Healthy Places, also known as Smart Growth or New Urbanism, builds physical activity into daily life by creating walk-able, mixed-use communities. Healthy Places takes into account multiple factors that impact health including transportation, land use planning, housing, school siting, public safety, and access to goods and services. The goals of Healthy Places are as follows (Association of State and Territorial Health Officials [ASTHO], 2006):

- Create safe and walk-able communities
- Create a range of housing opportunities and choices
- Provide a variety of transportation choices
- Develop mixed land uses
- Preserve green space

This discussion has demonstrated that our environment is both an asset and a threat. Improving our environment whether it is in the home, workplace, or community is integral to a healthy future for all citizens of the world.

Inequity

Public health is viewed as a safety net for those individuals without access to health care, the majority of whom are from low-income and minority groups having higher exposure to health threats such as violence and environmental hazards. The combination of these factors contributes to decreased health outcomes and increased strain on the safety net (TFAH, 2008a).

Consequences of inequities are illuminated by the following statistical examples. Rates of death from heart disease for black adults were 29% higher than their white counterparts in 2000. Similarly, death rates from stroke were 40% higher (Office of Minority Health & Health Disparities, 2008). Black males are more than twice as likely to die of prostate cancer (Pfizer Facts). Another alarming statistic is that black, American Indian, and Puerto Rican infants have higher death rates than white infants (Office of Minority Health & Health Disparities, 2004).

It is not only ethnic inequity that leads to poor health. Individuals in lower income levels have fewer opportunities to access health care and make healthy choices. There is limited access to nutritious, affordable foods in low-income areas because of fewer and smaller grocery stores in the community. Individuals in these areas often pay more for fresh fruits and vegetables if they are even available for purchase (TFAH, 2008a). This is also an important environmental issue because there is a correlation between the presence of grocery stores and lower rates of obesity, with higher rates of obesity related to the presence of convenience stores (Morland et al., 2006). A lack of health insurance is also a risk factor for poor health. Thirteen percent of white Americans are uninsured—that figure nearly doubles to 22% among blacks, and nearly triples to 36% among Latinos (Kaiser State Health Facts, 2007).

Emergency Preparedness

Preparedness is a relatively new role for public health. After the September 11, 2001, terrorist attacks, the federal government has invested more than $6 billion to improve public health emergency preparedness (Cohen et al., 2004); however, sustained investment needs to be a priority. Having the system and resources to prepare for and respond to such epidemics as SARS, which infected more than 8,000 people and left 774 dead, is the essence of public health preparedness (TFAH, 2008d).

Our ability to respond effectively to public health emergencies also has economic implications. It is estimated that SARS cost our world 30 to 50 billion dollars in terms of lives lost, quarantines, and lost tourism dollars (Aldrich & Newcomb, 2005).

Public health is a critical partner in emergency response. During 2007, there were 63 federally declared disasters, with health agencies responding to almost all of them (Federal Emergency Management Agency, 2008). At the state level, almost 90% of state public health agencies were involved in a response that required activation of their incident command system or involvement in a statewide multidepartment emergency operations center (ASTHO, 2008a).

The public health system plays a critical role in all types of emergencies. Terrorism, natural disasters, infectious disease, environmental hazards, infrastructure failures, and food-borne outbreaks all require that public health coordinates the protection and provision of health care for large numbers of people (ASTHO, 2008a).

Issues Shaping the Future of Public Health

Accreditation

Many accreditation programs have been developed as a result of internal or external pressure to improve the quality and value of services provided by an industry, whether public or private. In addition, accreditation seeks to strengthen the viability and competitive position of the agency or organization. Today there are a number of accreditation programs that address health and public service organizations, including medical care providers, insurers, education, and public safety to name a few. Within the United States healthcare system, accreditation programs have emerged to provide consumers, employees, and other stakeholders with assurance of complying with a basic set of service delivery standards. Public health agencies, however, "remain one of the few organizational components of the U.S. health and social service system that have yet to develop an accreditation program tailored to their specific scope of activities" (Mays, 2004, p. 4).

In a white paper prepared for the Robert Wood Johnson Foundation (RWJF), several important policy considerations were identified from other service industries that deserve consideration for public health accreditation, including the following (Mays, 2004):

- The potential for promoting improvements in service deliver, operations, and outcomes
- Costs being weighed against the potential benefits to determine feasibility and value
- Costs being distributed and financed equitably to ensure that they do not preclude participation by organizations that could benefit the greatest
- Strong incentives for seeking and maintaining accreditation are essential to the viability and success of the program
- Governance for the accreditation program should include representation from multiple stakeholders engaged in the field of practice
- Accreditation programs, which should be driven by evidence-based practice and focus on performance standards that are linked to service outcomes

A national accreditation program for public health is inevitable. Many momentous initiatives have set the stage for accreditation and modernizing public health and public health practice. Two landmark reports by the IOM—*The Future of Public Health* in 1988, indicating that the governmental public health infrastructure was in disarray, and in 2003 a second report, *The Future of the Public's Health in the 21st Century*, focusing on several broad themes, including population health, determinants of health, strengthening the public health infrastructure, partnerships, accountability, evidenced-based practice, and communication—have been critical in this work. Both reports prompted movement by policy makers, public health agencies, and educational institutions toward greater awareness, investments, and accountability in public health practice.

The 1988 report planted the seed for the development of the IOM's *Essential Public Health Services* (1994) (National Public Health Performance Standards Program) as a method to identify and describe better the activities used to promote health and prevent disease (Table 2). Essential public health services were the precursor to the development of national public health performance standards to improve the quality of public health practice and the performance of the public health system. Another ground breaking activity, *Exploring Accreditation Project*, a partnership coordinated by the ASTHO and the National Association of County and City Health Officials, including the American Public Health Association and the National Association of Local Boards of Health, released final recommendations for a Voluntary National Accreditation Program for State and Local Public Health Departments (CDC, 2008c).

In May of 2007, a national Public Health Accreditation Board was formed through funding support from the CDC and the RWJF. The goal of the voluntary national accreditation program is to improve and protect the health of the public by advancing the quality and performance of state and local public health departments (RWJF, 2006–2007).

Through consensus, a proposed model for a voluntary national accreditation program for state and local health departments has been developed. This model addresses feasibility, cost, structure of the program, and desirability. Feasibility includes existing building blocks of current state programs, a cadre of existing and evolving best practices, and interest of funders and potential applicants. Cost is addressed in the model by applicant fees, governmental support, and private grants. The accreditation program is structured according to national standards, proven evaluation processes, specific financing and incentive plans, and a negotiated governance structure. Desirability encompasses improving quality, performance, accountability, and credibility, as well as recognizing excellence and increasing the visibility of public health (RWJF, 2006–2007).

Several states have developed and implemented accreditation programs while monitoring the ongoing evolution of a national accreditation program. If a national accreditation program is implemented and accomplishes what it is intended to do, the public can be assured that basic public health services are equitably and consistently available regardless of location. Ultimately, however, success will be dependent on sustained policy maker and constituent support and financial commitment.

Accreditation may hold strong potential for improving public health; however, it should not be viewed as a single solution. Meaningful and sustained improvements in public health capacity and service delivery require a systems approach to improvement through workforce education, performance evaluation, quality improvement, professional certification and licensure, system financing, leadership development, and public and policy maker engagement.

Globalization

The amazing advancements in travel and technology have led to international interconnectedness that influences the health of individual citizens in ways never before seen in the history of humankind. The WHO serves as the hub for data and policy in this new world of globalized health problems. According to the WHO, global health is defined by Lee (2003) as the transnational impacts of globalization upon the health of persons that is beyond the control of individual nations.

The WHO delineate major effects of globalization on health as the "inequities caused by patterns of international trade and investment, the effects of global climate change, the vulnerability of refugee populations, the marketing of harmful products by transnational corporations and the transmission of diseases resulting from travel between countries" (Smith et al., 2006, p. 3). Although these threats have global consequences, they must be dealt with simultaneously at the international, national, state, and local level. This requires partnering and priority setting by and among all levels of the public health and healthcare systems (Smith et al., 2006).

Collaboration, however, can be elusive. Without changing human behavior and value systems, sustained change at the global level is unattainable. Global public health strategies require the cooperation of individuals, populations, political leaders, the military, and policy makers working in conjunction with public health professionals to institute sustainable change.

A major issue of globalization is public health security. This refers to the need to protect the world from natural, accidental, or intentional biological, chemical, and radiological agents that threaten human health. A recent WHO report delineates some of the factors controlled by humankind that are contributing to the threats against public health security. These factors include inadequate investment in public health, a false sense of security with a reduction in acute infectious disease outbreaks, policy changes that undermine evidence-based public health interventions such as mandatory immunizations, conflicts that lead to the displacement of individuals to unsanitary and impoverished living conditions, and inadequate animal husbandry and food processing practices that endanger a healthy food supply (WHO, 2007a).

A recent WHO report entitled *A Safer Future: Global Public Health Security in the 21st Century* offers key recommendations to secure the highest level of global public health security. These include cooperation in global surveillance and disease outbreak alert and response, transparency in sharing information and technologies; joint research on samples of disease causing organisms, joint efforts to build a strong public health infrastructure in all countries that includes training, emergency preparedness capacity, and prevention strategies; and improved cross-sector collaboration by governmental agencies within and across (WHO, 2007b).

"Given today's universal vulnerability to these threats, better security calls for global solidarity," said Dr. Margaret Chan, Director-General of WHO. "International public health security is both a collective aspiration and a mutual responsibility. The new watchwords are diplomacy, cooperation, transparency and preparedness" (World Health Organization, 2007b).

A recurring theme in discussions of global health is the importance of strong political advocacy. At the Sixth Global Conference on Health Promotion in Bangkok, this was a major focus. The participants came together and reiterated the need for political advocacy, investment in strategies and infrastructure that address the determinants of health, regulatory interventions, and building health promotion capacity and partnerships. They stressed that these strategies were essential in addressing the challenges posed by globalization (WHO, 2005).

Media

The role of media in public health is pervasive. The Internet, television, radio, newspapers, and magazines are often the most influential sources of information about health. The flow of information has become interactive in that the media presents scientific information and government policies to the public while providing a real-time venue for the public to express their concerns (WHO, 2002). Public health media can be either reactive or proactive. During an acute public health event such as SARS, public health must respond to media-driven requests for information.

According to a study by the Nuffield Trust, the media can either heighten levels of anxiety or provide reassurance at times of acute public health events. Authorities such as governments may use the mass media but can seldom keep control of the information delivered. They have to strike a difficult balance between saying too much and saying too little: One course of action may cause an overreaction; the other may seem complacent (McInnes, 2005).

They also have to be aware that lack of information creates a vacuum that the media will fill. Thus, it behooves public health professionals to respond quickly, conveying competence and control of the situation.

During an acute public health situation, the media can be a valuable public health partner. The use of the web to collect data, communicate findings, and collaboratively plan interventions can facilitate a rapid, comprehensive, and effective response that can reduce morbidity and mortality. Electronic and print media can be used to inform the public about ways they can protect themselves, their family, and their community and mitigate the consequences of the incident. For example, in the case of a food-borne disease outbreak, the public can provide information about the incidence of illness and can be instructed on how to avoid exposure based on the findings of the epidemiological investigation.

The media is also critical to disease prevention and health promotion activities. One example was offered by Lambrew (2007), who recommends a national Wellness Trust and argues that a major component would be electronic infrastructure that includes both an electronic prevention record system similar to the electronic medical record and online options for prevention, control, and community resources (Lambrew, 2007). A second example is the CDC's National Center for Health Marketing. The Center director's inaugural blog entry includes a quote from legendary newsman Daniel Shorr, "If you do not exist in the media, for all practical purposes you do not exist" (Bernhardt, 2006). The CDC now has its own MySpace page, using this electronic social networking tool to dialogue with other health sites. Their presence on Internet social networking sites is based on the belief that this venue has incredible potential to "protect health when accurate and relevant information is shared between trusted peers to support positive and healthy decision-making" (Bernhardt, 2006).

These innovative technologies have also impacted global public health. Internet-based health information is now being accessed by the most socially isolated communities and populations. "Any serious consideration of public health populations must thus be cognizant of the role of the media in both representing and constructing [public health] problems and policies." The reality, however, is that public health often has to fight to make sure that their voice is heard by the media (Bunton & Crawshaw, 2006).

Economics

Economics influences the future of public health in two major ways. Public health has a critical role in controlling and reducing healthcare costs; however, the funding of public health is woefully inadequate, thus jeopardizing its capacity and capability to meet the needs of society as well as reduce healthcare costs.

"The skyrocketing costs of health care threaten to bankrupt American businesses" (TFAH, 2008c, p. 13). It is clear that we must implement public health strategies to promote healthy lifestyles and manage chronic illnesses to reverse this economic crisis.

The most prevalent chronic diseases are costing our country more than $1 trillion every year. Some projections predict that this figure could reach $6 trillion by the middle of this century. Failure to reduce these costs threatens the capacity to provide universal health insurance and adequate health care for a rapidly aging population (DeVol et al., 2007).

Older persons are particularly prone to chronic illness. The Kaiser Family Foundation estimated that 87% of Medicare beneficiaries have at least one chronic illness. Another study concluded that most all of the spending growth in Medicare over the past 15 years was related to caring for individuals with multiple chronic conditions (Thorpe & Howard, 2006).

Affordable, accessible health care is only one aspect of the economic consequences of chronic disease. Other indirect consequences include the financial drain of chronically ill workers utilizing sick days; presenteeism, where workers come to work, but have sub-par productivity; and the loss of productivity of caregivers who must miss work to care for chronically ill family members. The combined cost of these indirect factors was estimated at approximately $1 trillion in 2003.

DeVol et al. (2007) analyzed the economic factors associated with chronic disease-reduction strategies. The researchers found that modest reductions in avoidable factors such as unhealthy behavior, environmental risks, and lack of early detection and innovative treatment would lead to 40 million fewer cases of illness. This translates into a gain of over $1 trillion annually in labor supply and efficiency by 2023. The analysis also compared this best case scenario to one in which costs would be incurred under the status quo and found a 27% reduction in total economic impact. These authors further postulated that this projection was low because it did not take into account the ability to redirect these savings into education and training for future generations.

The exponential increase in the incidence of chronic disease is costing lives, quality of life, and prosperity. It is up to the public health workforce to take the lead in advocating for an increased proportion of healthcare spending to be directed toward the promotion of specific health behaviors that will reduce smoking, obesity, and substance abuse. A reduction in these unhealthy behaviors would yield a significant return on investment (DeVol et al., 2007).

Public health cannot take the lead without adequate capacity. According to the TFAH, there is currently a $20 billion annual deficit in spending on public health (TFAH, 2008b). This deficit prevents public health from adequately fulfilling its core responsibilities of:

- Monitoring health status and health problems
- Enforcing public health laws
- Mobilizing community partnerships
- Developing policy related to individual and community health strategies
- Assuring an adequate and competent public and healthcare workforce

- Linking individuals to health programs
- Evaluating population based health services
- Researching innovative evidenced-based approaches to health promotion and protection and disease prevention

To meet these responsibilities, the TFAH report recommends that the current federal, state, and local public health spending of approximately $35 billion per year ($120 per person) should be increased to $55 to $60 billion annually (approximately $187 per person) (TFAH, 2008b).

Workforce

Adequate funding is only one component of assuring a strong public health system. The workforce in public health is facing critical challenges, namely a steep decline in numbers and resources. These challenges will undermine the ability of a dedicated workforce to protect the public's health. Underserved areas will not have the health services they need. Communities will be ill prepared to deal with disasters, and the public will not have the information needed to protect themselves from an emerging infectious disease, such as pandemic flu or mumps (Perlino, 2006).

The ASTHO (2008b) has compiled some startling statistics that delineate this problem:

- Since 1988, the ratio of public health workers per 100,000 Americans has decreased by 39% while their responsibilities have increased.
- Retirement rates are projected at 56% in some public health agencies by 2012.
- Vacancy rates are up to 25% in some public health agencies.
- In some parts of the country, workforce turnover rates reach 29%.
- The average age of a public health worker in state government is 47 years.

- In 2006, approximately 6,800 individuals graduated from an accredited school of public health. Most took jobs in the private sector.

The most severe shortages are found in the areas of epidemiology, nursing, laboratory science, and environmental health (Perlino, 2006). Nursing is the largest professional group of the public health workforce, with an average age of 49 years. Seventy-eight percent of state public health laboratories report difficulty recruiting and retaining bioterrorism preparedness staff. Additionally, environmental health graduates have dropped 50% since 1998 (ASTHA, 2008b).

Recruiting, training, and retaining the public health workforce is complicated, and there is not one typical career path. The field encompasses a range of specialties. The IOM (2001) points out that public health professionals "receive their education and training in a wide range of disciplines and in diverse academic settings, including schools of public health, medicine, nursing, dentistry, social work, allied health professions, pharmacy, law, public administration, veterinary medicine, engineering, environmental sciences, biology, microbiology, and journalism."

Barriers that have been identified as causative factors to the public health workforce shortage include budget shortfalls, resulting in noncompetitive wages, a lack of an understanding regarding the opportunities of a public health career, and bureaucracy. The ASTHO (2008b) has identified ways to address these barriers:

- Facilitate a broader awareness of the public health workforce crisis
- Advocate for additional resources
- Foster research to address public workforce challenges
- Improve marketing of public health careers

- Forge public–private partnerships to ensure a strong public health workforce

Public Health Advocacy and Policy Formulation

In order to address the myriad of challenges facing public health, it is imperative that health professionals have the knowledge, skills, and competencies required to influence public policy. This will require adopting new approaches to engage the public, communities, business, and policy makers collectively. Success depends on a well-informed public and a valuing of individual, community, and global health. It also requires a culture that views the public health system as an essential component of the well being of the world. This means that policy makers must commit to an increased and sustained investment in public health in order to address effectively the complex health challenges facing this nation in the 21st century (Benjamin, 2006).

The current healthcare system focuses on curing and treating disease and places less value on health promotion and protection and disease prevention. Research has found that prevention is effective in both economic savings and healthy outcomes; however, "a common focus on creating broader access to preventive programs and services continues to fail to get real traction. Because of this, public health advocates now argue that it is time to balance the investment with a greater emphasis on prevention" (Benjamin, 2006, p. 1040).

To transform the paradigm to one in which public health is viewed as the foundation for a vibrant society, health professionals must effectively engage each stakeholder group in policy development, advocacy, and implementation. A strong case must be made regarding the value of public health as a partner in shaping healthy communities and that healthy communities provide tangible benefits for all stakeholders.

A model that can be used by public health professionals to engage partners is megacommunity. The impetus for the development of this model was the authors' experiences in dealing with complex global challenges in the areas of security, economics, health, and safety. These challenges are within public health's sphere of responsibility and influence, having biological, cultural, and geopolitical roots. Because of the complexity of these challenges, "multisector, multilateral, collaborative and innovative solutions" are required (Gerencser et al., 2008, p. 10).

Megacommunity is based on the idea that communities of organizations need to act as vehicles for change. These communities "come together across national, organizational, and sector boundaries to reach goals they cannot achieve alone" (Gerencser et al., 2008, p. 28). The model identifies business, government, and civil society as the three power sectors that must work together to address complex mutual problems. Each sector brings their sphere of influence to the table. The resultant dynamic tension leads to excitement and energy that fosters sustained strategy formulation and leads to transnational solutions necessary in this age of globalization. One caveat the authors have is that sustainable strategy must not compromise future generation's ability to meet their needs. This is consistent with public health's mission to promote and protect the health of the population by enforcing clean air and water regulations and promoting healthy lifestyles to reduce societal economic burden.

Megacommunities may also have a significant effect on globalization. The author's definition of globalization is the interdependence of human activity that is enabled by innovative types of technology, communication, and financial interrelationships. An example of a public health policy that exemplifies this is the preparation for pandemic influenza. Technologies such as real-time disease reporting by healthcare providers to public health and emergency alerting systems are now in place. Multisector and multidisciplinary information sharing regarding issues such as novel infectious diseases and suspicious agents have been developed through a megacommunity approach. Public–private partnerships exist where all three sectors integrate resources and expertise to enhance the response to public health emergencies and disasters (Gerencser et al., 2008).

In order to use megacommunities effectively to influence public health policy, it is necessary to build network capital through negotiated relationships and shared control over processes and goal attainment. Recent successful efforts to ban smoking in public places are an example of building network capitol. Megacommunities of associations, business, and government successfully lobbied state policy makers to enact smoke free legislation. This was directly related to years of relationship building, joint strategy formulation, and problem solving.

Public health policy advocacy involves many of the basic tenets of a megacommunity. The first tenet is that, in order to influence from a position of strength, it is necessary to convince partners that the proposed policy will be a win–win situation. Another tenet is that you must understand the needs of the constituents affected by the policy in order to provide the information needed to either support or remain neutral during the political process. Cultural sensitivity is a megacommunity tenet that stresses avoiding stereotyping to navigate successfully political, economic, and social changes that can sabotage your advocacy efforts (Gerencser et al., 2008).

Another megacommunity tenet is continuous environmental scanning. This is done to forecast and anticipate opportunities for and potential barriers to effective policy formulation. Success is inexorably tied to timing and adapting to current events (Gerencser et al., 2008).

In this information age, the megacommunity tenet of transparency is critical to policy success. This transparency is also important in developing trust, another Megacommunity tenet. As Steven Covey (2006) discusses, trust can create immeasurable success and prosperity in all dimensions of our lives. After trust is broken, partners frequently become adversaries, making policy acceptance extremely difficult (Gerencser et al., 2008).

The foundation of an effective megacommunity is based on four guiding principles. These principles are inherent in public health policy formulation and advocacy. These principles are as follows (Gerencser et al., 2008):

- Respect the autonomy and opinions of all partners
- Share a commitment to continuous communication, engagement, and resource sharing
- Be dedicated to taking action
- Embrace conflict and practice effective conflict resolution

The health problems this nation and the world are facing are complex. Public health is charged with planning, acting, and evaluating strategies to address these problems. The idea of megacommunities is an innovative 21st century model that can be used to solve these complex problems by facilitating effective policy formulation and advocacy.

References

Aldrich, S., & Newcomb, J. (2005). *Thinking ahead: Anticipating early impacts of an avian influenza pandemic.* Cambridge, MA: Bio Economic Research Associates.

American Heart Association. (2003). *Heart disease and stroke statistics: 2003 update*. Dallas, Texas: Author.

American Obesity Association. (2008). *AOA fact sheets*. Retrieved December 31, 2008, from http://obesity1.tempdomainname.com/subs/fastfacts/Health_Effects.shtml

Armour, B. S., Woollery, T., Malarcher, A., Pechacek, T. F., & Husten, C. (2005). Annual smoking-attributable mortality, years of potential life lost, and productivity losses—United States, 1997–2001. *Morbidity and Mortality Weekly Report, 54*(25), 625–628.

Association of State and Territorial Health Officials. (2006). *The built environment, physical activity, and health* (fact sheet). Retrieved February 12, 2010, from http://www.govinstitute.org/policyguide/pdfs/health.pdf

Association of State and Territorial Health Officials. (2008a). *States of preparedness: Health agency progress*. Arlington, VA: Author. Retrieved February 12, 2010, from http://www.astho.org/WorkArea/DownloadAsset.aspx?id=674

Association of State and Territorial Health Officials. (2008b). *2007 State public health: workforce survey results*. Arlington, VA: Author. Retrieved February 12, 2010, from http://www.astho.org/WorkArea/DownloadAsset.aspx?id=500

Awofeso, N. (2004). What's new about the "new public health"? *American Journal of Public Health, 94*(5), 705–709.

Benjamin, G. C. (2006). Putting the public in public health: New approaches. *Health Affairs, 25*(4), 1040–1043.

Bernhardt, J. (2006). *Director's blog: Health marketing musings*. Retrieved December 30, 2008, from http://www.cdc.gov/healthmarketing/blog_071306.htm

Bunton, R., & Crawshaw, P. (2006). Representing public health. *Critical Public Health, 16*(1), 1–4.

Centers for Disease Control and Prevention. (1993). Cigarette smoking-attributable mortality and years of potential life lost—United States, 1990. *Morbidity and Mortality Weekly Report, 42*(33), 645–649.

Centers for Disease Control and Prevention. (1994). *10 Essential public health services*. Retrieved December 31, 2008, from http://www.cdc.gov/od/ocphp/nphpsp/essentialphservices.htm

Centers for Disease Control and Prevention. (1999). Ten great public health achievements—United States, 1900–1999. *Morbidity and Mortality Weekly Report, 48*(12), 241–243.

Centers for Disease Control and Prevention. (2004). *The burden of chronic diseases and their risk factors: National and state perspectives 2004* (No. 2008). Atlanta, GA: U.S. Department of Health and Human Services.

Centers for Disease Control and Prevention. (2005). *Hepatitis C fact sheet*. Retrieved February 12, 2010, from http://www.doh.wa.gov/cfh/Hepatitis/Documents/cfact.pdf

Centers for Disease Control and Prevention. (2006a). *CDC injury fact book*. Atlanta, GA: Author.

Centers for Disease Control and Prevention. (2006b). State specific prevalence of obesity among adults: United States, 2005. *Morbidity and Mortality Weekly Report, 55*(36), 985–988.

Centers for Disease Control and Prevention. (2008a). *Key facts about seasonal influenza (flu)*. Retrieved February 12, 2010, from http://www.cdc.gov/Flu/keyfacts.htm

Centers for Disease Control and Prevention. (2008b). *Celebrate life: World AIDS day 2008*. Retrieved December 18, 2008, from http://www.cdc.gov/Features/WorldAidsDay

Centers for Disease Control and Prevention. (2008c). *National public health performance standards program: Overview*. Retrieved August 7, 2009, from http://www.cdc.gov/od/ocphp/nphpsp/overview.htm

Cohen, H. W., Gould, R. M., & Sidel, V. W. (2004). The pitfalls of bioterrorism preparedness: The anthrax and smallpox experiences. *Am J Public Health, 94*(10), 1667–1671.

Covey, S. (2006). *The speed of trust: The one thing that changes everything*. New York: Free Press.

Cowie, C. C., Rust, K. F., Ford, E. S., Eberhardt, M. S., Byrd-Holt, D. D., Li, C., et al. (2009). A full accounting of diabetes and prediabetes in the U.S. population, 1988–1994 and 2005–2006. *Diabetes Care., 32*(2), 287–294.

DeVol, R., Bedroussian, A., Charuworn, A., Chatterjee, A., Kim, I. K., Kim, S., et al. (2007). *An unhealthy America: The economic burden of chronic disease*. Santa Monica, CA: Milken Institute.

Dietz, W. H. (1998). Childhood weight affects adult morbidity and mortality. *The Journal of Nutrition, 128*(2 Suppl), 411S–414S.

Federal Emergency Management Agency. (2008). *Annual major disaster declarations totals*. Retrieved December 18, 2008, from http://www.fema.gov/news/disaster_totals_annual.fema

Fontaine, K. R., Redden, D. T., Wang, C., Westfall, A. O., & Allison, D. B. (2003). Years of life lost due to obesity. *Journal of the American Medical Association, 289*(2), 187–193.

Gerencser, M., Van Lee, R., Napolitano, F., & Kelly, C. (2008). *Megacommunities: How leaders of government, business and non-profits can tackle today's global challenges together*. New York: Palgrave Macmillan.

Heishman, H., & Dannenberg, A. L. (2008). Influencing the environment in your built community. *Journal of Environmental Health, 70*(4), 66–67.

Institute of Medicine, Committee for the study of the Future of Public Health. (1988). *The future of public health.* Washington, DC: National Academy Press.

Institute of Medicine. (2001). *Who will keep the public healthy? educating public health professionals for the 21st century.* Washington, DC: The National Academies Press.

Kaiser State Health Facts. (2007). *United states: Health coverage & uninsured.* Retrieved January 1, 2009, from http://www.statehealthfacts.org/profileind.jsp?sub= 40&rgn=1&cat=3

Keppel, K., Bilheimer, L., & Gurley, L. (2007). Improving population health and reducing health care disparities. *Health Affairs (Project Hope), 26*(5), 1281–1292.

Lambrew, J. M. (2007). *A wellness trust to prioritize disease prevention* (discussion paper). The Hamilton Project. Retrieved February 12, 2010, from www3.brookings. edu/views/papers/200704lambrew.pdf

Lee, K. (2003). *Globalization and health: An introduction.* New York: Palgrave Macmillan.

Mays, G. P. (2004). *Can accreditation work in public health? Lessons from other service industries.* Working Paper Prepared for the Robert Wood Johnson Foundation, November 30, 2004.

McInnes, C. (2005). Health, security and the risk society. *The Nuffield Trust.* Retrieved February 12, 2010, from http://www.nuffieldtrust.org.uk/ecomm/files/ HSecrisksoc.pdf

Morland, K., Diez Roux, A. V., & Wing, S. (2006). Supermarkets, other food stores, and obesity: The atherosclerosis risk in communities study. *American Journal of Preventive Medicine, 30*(4), 333–339.

National Center for Environmental Health: Office of Global Health—Programs—Air Pollution/CDC. Retrieved August 5, 2009, from http://www.cdc.gov/ nceh/globalhealth/projects/airpollution.htm

National Public Health Performance Standards Program. *National public health performance standards program frequently asked questions.* Retrieved December 17, 2008, from http://www.cdc.gov/od/ocphp/nphpsp/PDF/ FAQ.pdf

Nolte, E., & McKee, C. M. (2008). Measuring the health of nations: Updating an earlier analysis. *Health Affairs, 27*(1), 58–71.

Office of Minority Health & Health Disparities. (2004). *Highlight 4/04 national minority health month.* Retrieved January 1, 2009, Retrieved from, http://www.cdc.gov/ omhd/Highlights/2004/HApr04.htm

Office of Minority Health and Health Disparities. (2008). *Disease burden and risk factors.* Retrieved December 18, 2009, from http://www.cdc.gov/omhd/AMH/dbrf.htm

Office of the Surgeon General. (2001). *The Surgeon General's call to action to prevent and decrease overweight and obesity.* Rockville, MD: U.S. Department of Health and Human Services.

Olshansky, S., Jay, D. J., Passaro, R. C., Hershow, J. L., Carnes, B. A., Brody, J., et al. (2005). A potential decline in life expectancy in the United States in the 21st century. *New England Journal of Medicine, 352*(11), 1138–1145.

Pallansch, M. A., & Sandhu, H. S. (2006). The eradication of polio—progress and challenges. *The New England Journal of Medicine, 355*(24), 2508–2511.

Perlino, C. M. (September, 2006). The public health workforce shortage: Left unchecked, will we be protected? Washington, DC: American Public Health Association. Retrieved February 12, 2010, from http://www.apha. org/NR/rdonlyres/597828BF-9924-4B94-8821- 135F665E9D45/0/PublicHealthWorkforceIssueBrief.pdf

Pfizer Facts. *Racial differences in cancer: A comparison of black and white adults in the United States.* Retrieved August 9, 2009, from http://media.pfizer.com/files/products/ Racial_Differences_in_Cancer.pdf

Public health and environment. Retrieved January 1, 2009, from http://www.who.int/phe/en

Robert Wood Johnson Foundation. (2006–2007). *Exploring accreditation: Final recommendations for a voluntary national accreditation program for state and local public health departments.* Retrieved February 12, 2010, from http:// www.rwjf.org/files/research/explore_accreditation.pdf

Shattuck, L. (1850). *Report of the sanitary commission of Massachusetts 1850* (No. 37). Boston: Dutton & Wentworth. Retrieved July 28, 2008, from http://www. deltaomega.org/shattuck.pdf

Smith, B. J., Tang, K. C., & Nutbeam, D. (2006). *WHO health promotion glossary: New terms.* Retrieved July 31, 2009, from http://www.who.int/healthpromotion/ about/HP%20Glossay%20in%20HPI.pdf

The Millennium Project. (2009). *State of the future 2009.* Retrieved August 5, 2009, from http://www.millennium-project.org/millennium/SOF2009-English.pdf

Thorpe, K., & Howard, D. (2006). The rise in spending among Medicare beneficiaries: the role of chronic disease prevalence and changes in treatment intensity. *Health Affairs, 25*(5), 378–388.

Trust for America's Health. (2007). *Pandemic flu and the potential for U.S. economic recession.* Retrieved August 7, 2009, from http://healthyamericans.org/reports/ flurecession/FluRecession.pdf

Trust for America's Health. (2008a). *A healthier America: 10 top priorities for prevention.* Retrieved August 9, 2009, from http://healthyamericans.org/assets/files/ 10ThingsBook.pdf

Trust for America's Health. (2008b). *F as in fat 2008.* Retrieved December 18, 2008, from http:// healthyamericans.org/reports/obesity2008

Trust for America's Health. (2008c). *Blueprint for a healthier America.* Retrieved December 18, 2008, from http://healthyamericans.org/assets/files/Blueprint.pdf

Trust for America's Health. (2008d). *Ready or Not? Preparing for potential health emergencies and bioterrorism attacks.* Retrieved December 18, 2008, from http://healthyamericans.org/reports/bioterror08

Turnock, B. J., & Barnes, P. A. (2006). *Director's blog: Health marketing musings.* Retrieved December 30, 2008, from http://www.cdc.gov/healthmarketing/blog_071306.htm

World Health Organization. (2002). *The world health report 2002.* Geneva: Author.

World Health Organization. (2005). *The Bangkok charter for health promotion in a globalized world* (11 August 2005). Retrieved July 30, 2009 from, http://www.who.int/healthpromotion/conferences/6gchp/bangkok_charter/en/index.html

World Health Organization. (2006). *Preventing disease through healthy environments: Towards an estimate of the environmental burden of disease.* Retrieved December 15, 2008, from http://www.searo.who.int/en/Section316/Section503/Section2141_11776.htm

World Health Organization. (2007a). *International spread of disease threatens public health security.* Retrieved December 18, 2008, from http://www.who.int/mediacentre/news/releases/2007/pr44/en/index.html

World Health Organization. (2007b). *The World Health Report 2007: A safer future: Global public health security in the 21st century.* Retrieved July 30, 2009 from http://www.who.int/whr/2007/whr07_en.pdf

World Health Organization. (2008a). *Impact of the global financial and economic crisis on health.* Retrieved February 12, 2010, from http://www.who.int/mediacentre/news/statements/2008/s12/en

World Health Organization. (2008b). *WHO regional office for Europe: Public health services.* Retrieved February 12, 2010, from http://www.euro.who.int/publichealth

CASE STUDY

Policy Tools for Helping People at Risk for or Living with Cancer

Alison P. Smith, BA, BSN, RN

The bad news is that the lifetime probability of developing cancer is one in every two men and one in every three women (National Cancer Institute, 2005). Cancer remains the second most common cause of death by disease, claiming the lives of more than half a million people per year (American Cancer Society, 2007). As the population ages, cancer rates are expected to increase (U.S. Cancer Statistics Working Group, 2003). Disparities in health outcomes persist among minority populations (Agency for Healthcare Research and Quality. 2008).

The good news is that for the first time since 1999 the incidence and mortality rates for all cancers combined decreased for both men and women. Similarly, death rates decreased, on average, 1.8% per year from 2002 through 2005 (CDC, 2005a). The 5-year cancer survival rate has risen to 64% for adults (CDC, 2005b).

The hope is that nearly one third of cancer deaths are preventable. Health policy is a powerful and evidence-based tool for preventing, detecting early, and successfully treating cancer. Although not all of these policy levers are currently being put to their fullest use, the discussion here provides an overview of how and where policy at the federal, state, and local level can effect outcomes for people at risk for and living with cancer. These examples span the continuum of cancer research and care. These examples encompass policy vehicles such as the creation, expansion, and appropriation of funding for programs and services; taxation for users and tax credits for developers; and incentives for or restrictions on personal behavior.

Cancer Prevention

Smoking is the number one cause of preventable cancer deaths (CDC, 2005). Although smoking rates have dropped in recent years, the CDC reported that in 2004 approximately 20.9% of U.S. adults were current smokers. Although health education has proven somewhat effective in reducing tobacco use, other policy interventions have been more directly linked to healthy behaviors, namely, smoke-free air ordinances, tobacco taxation, and provision of evidence-based smoking-cessation services.

Today, males are twice as likely to die from lung cancer in Kentucky as they are in California (Figure 1), or as Tim Byers, MD, MPH, University of Colorado, put it, "Children face wildly different prospects in terms of mortality based solely upon the chance of their geo-political place of birth." Since 1986, California has pursued a coordinated,

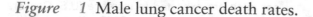

Figure 1 Male lung cancer death rates.

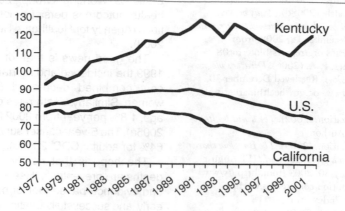

aggressive, multipronged approach to reduce tobacco use through education, user taxation, and clean-air legislation. By applying evidence-based policy and practice intervention from tobacco research, California has realized a steady decline in tobacco use and in deaths caused by lung cancer as well as healthcare cost savings.

In 2006, the Surgeon General Richard Carmona published a report on second-hand smoke that accelerated the adoption of smoke-free air ordinances across the country. As of April 2008, 24 states have passed smoke-free laws that cover restaurants and bars. Hundreds of cities and counties across the country have also taken action in some form. These ordinances not only protect nonsmokers from the deleterious effects of smoke, but they support smokers in their efforts to quit. Of note, smoke-free policies do not have an adverse economic impact on the hospitality industry—a counter argument commonly posed by opponents of smoke-free laws.

Tobacco taxation at the federal and state level has also proved effective in reducing smoking (Husten, 2008). Adults and particularly youth are sensitive to price increases (Chaloupka et al., 2002). For adults, a 10% price increase decreases consumption by 4% and increases cessation by 1.5% (Task Force on Community Preventive Services, 2005).

Finally, policies driving tobacco cessation services are an important component of cancer prevention (Husten, 2008). Seventy percent of smokers want to quit, and more than 40% try to quit each year; however, most tobacco users do not use treatments shown to be effective when trying to quit (Fiore et al., 2008). Access to cessation services can be provided through private and public policy decisions (e.g., employer insurance benefits, publicly funded health insurance plans like Medicare and Medicaid). In addition, publicly funded quit lines are available in the United States through a national network via 1-800-QUIT NOW (Husten, 2008). This network routes callers to their state's quit line service, which is funded by the state and/or the CDC. Coverage for nicotine replacement therapy also varies by state (North American Quitline Consortium, 2010).

Other cancer-preventing policies are currently being tested, evaluated, and debated. With the link between colon and other cancers with obesity, a variety of polices targeting obesity reduction are being debated, including "fat taxes" for unhealthy foods, mirroring tobacco taxes, mandatory calorie reductions in public school lunch programs or increased physical activity requirements, and food content bans such as the New York City Board of Health's action to ban artificial trans fats in restaurants. Similarly, the discovery and approval of vaccines to prevent human papilloma virus (HPV), a common cause of cervical cancer, has stimulated more discussion on policy opportunities to prevent cancer. Just as the hepatitis vaccination policies mandate immunization for school entrance, mandatory HPV vaccination is also being debated (Wells, 2008).

Cancer Screening and Early Detection

Scientific discovery is rapidly evolving to achieve better screening and earlier detection of cancer through advances of the fields of radiology imaging, pathology, genetics, and others. As screening and early detection methods become perfected and Food and Drug Administration approved, the U.S. Preventive Services Taskforce (USPSTF) evaluates and grades the evidence supporting the wide spread use of these methods. The USPSTF was first convened by the U.S. Public Health Service in 1984 and, since 1998, is sponsored by the Agency for Healthcare Research and Quality. This independent panel of experts in prevention and primary care rigorously reviews "impartial assessments of the scientific evidence for the effectiveness of a broad range of clinical preventive services, including screening, counseling, and preventive medications" (Agency for Healthcare Research and Quality, 2008). The USPSTF recommendations routinely trigger changes in Medicare and Medicaid, which routinely trigger changes in private insurance coverage benefits. In this example, access to cancer screening and early detection is significantly affected by the role of a federal agency influencing public and private health policy decisions.

In addition to effecting standards of coverage and care, federal and state public health policy has also been put in place to administer screening and early detection programs. In the case of cervical and breast cancer, the federal government funds public health programs such as the National Breast and Cervical Cancer Early Detection Program through the CDC. States also play a role in administering these programs through local and state health departments. Federal and state policy makers determine the scope of such programs the degree to which they are funded (Wells, 2008).

Other states have pursued cancer-specific program policies. Using Arizona tobacco tax revenues authorized through Proposition 303, the state funds the AZ Well Woman HealthCheck Program aimed to improve the early detection of breast cancer. Through Amendment 35, a portion of Colorado's to-

bacco excise taxes are directed through the Department of Public Health and Environment to fund programs that raise awareness and provide screening for breast, cervical, and colorectal cancer. Similarly, Wyoming passed in 2007 a Cancer Control Act that funded the creation of a the Wyoming Colorectal Cancer Early Detection Program in hopes of addressing the state's second leading cause of cancer death, colon cancer (C-Change, 2007).

Cancer Treatment

The Institute of Medicine (IOM) report "Care Without Coverage: Too Little, Too Late" states that uninsured patients get about one half the health care of insured patients and, consequently, die sooner than insured patients, largely because of delayed diagnoses (IOM, 2002). Another IOM report, "Ensuring Quality Cancer Care," cites concerns about lapses in care that can lower the chances of survival and can compromise the quality of life of cancer patients (IOM, 2004). The number of uninsured and underinsured Americans coupled with the high and rising costs of cancer treatment makes access to health services through private or public health insurance essential. In fact, half of personal bankruptcies are attributed to illness and medical bills (Himmelstein et al., 2005). Without insurance, some individuals choose not to be screened, delay screening, or refuse treatment do to financial constraints. Federal healthcare reforms have the potential to change cancer outcomes dramatically by providing better access to screening, early detection, and treatment services.

At a point when patients and their families are facing the challenge of cancer, they must navigate an extremely complex healthcare system. As the 2001 President's Cancer Panel (PCP, 2001) report "Voices of a Broken System: Real People, Real Problems" stated, many patients "must fight their way into and through a dysfunctional system even as they struggle to save their very lives." The often-devastating personal hardships of the cancer experience were noted in the 2004 PCP report "Living Beyond Cancer: Finding a New Balance: Medical, Psychosocial, Insurance, Employment and Educational Issues." Patient navigation in cancer care refers to individualized assistance offered to patients, families, and caregivers to help overcome healthcare system barriers and facilitate timely access to quality medical and psychosocial care, from prediagnosis through all phases of the cancer experience. Cancer patient navigation services can and should take on different forms in different communities. In 2005, the H.R. 1812 Patient Navigator Outreach and Chronic Disease Prevention Act was signed into law authorizing appropriations for the Department of Health and Human Services to award grants to programs designed to facilitate access to health services. Limited appropriations have restricted the impact of this act.

In 2004, Delaware was the first state to provide treatment for qualified individuals who do not have health insurance and who are not eligible for Medicaid. The Delaware Cancer Treatment Program helps to pay for cancer treatment for a period of 1 year for Delaware residents between the ages of 0 and 64 years who have been diagnosed with cancer on or after July 1, 2004, were a resident of Delaware at the time of diagnosis, have no comprehensive health insurance, and have a household income that meets qualification guidelines, which are 650% of the Federal Poverty Level (e.g., the income for a family of four must be less than $122,525) (C-Change, 2007).

Cancer Research

Continuing to research aspects of cancer prevention, early detection, treatment, and quality of life issues remains a top scientific and policy priority for the cancer community. Although research is carried out by academic institutions and pharmaceutical and biotech companies, the NCI drives a significant portion of cancer research within its walls and through its grant programs to NCI-designated cancer centers and others. The effects of advocacy and policy actions are illustrated in this recent chain of events. In 1998, cancer patients, survivors, caregivers, scientists, and advocates marched on the National Mall in Washington, DC to renew the Nation's commitment to fighting cancer. Congress responded by doubling the National Institute of Health budget for the following 5 years beginning in fiscal year 1999. The NCI budget was increased by 80% over this period. The direct result of this funding infusion was a 30% increase in R01 grant dollars to individual investigators. University researchers and administrators responded by becoming more involved in cancer research and investing more heavily in their scientific programs and facilities (Niederhuber, 2007).

Enabling the promise of cancer research through policy actions extends beyond funding the NCI. For example, chemoprevention, the development of agents to prevent or halt cancer, is an emerging field that faces several major systemic barriers currently delaying progress in research and development. Specifically, the limited life of patents, the uncertainty of reimbursement, and an uncharted clinical trial design and regulatory approval process deter scientific and financial investment in this area. In order to recoup investment in drug development, pharmaceutical companies require patent and intellectual property protection and data exclusivity. In the case of chemopreventive drugs, which take far longer to evaluate their efficacy and safety, extended protection/exclusivity or other tax incentives would likely stimulate investment in this field (Grabowski & Moe, 2008). Similarly, federal policy actions to value and cover preventive therapies would reduce the uncertainty of agents being paid for by Medicare, Medicaid, and other private payers once they are developed (C-Change, 2008). Additional legislative encouragement and agency level action by the Food and Drug Administration to define further the procedures for evaluating agents developed using biomarkers and other new scientific techniques would accelerate the research process.

Other Key Policy Issues

The ability to fight cancer depends on the health of the cancer workforce. A critical shortage of cancer specialists threatens the nation's ability to provide cancer care across the continuum from prevention to survivorship. Nearly all of the professional disciplines who play a role in the delivery of comprehensive cancer services are experiencing a shortage, including physicians, nurses, social workers, pharmacists, public health workers, researchers, scientists, technologists, and cancer registrars (American Public Health Association, 2007; American Society for Therapeutic and Radiation Oncology, 2004; American Society for Clinical Oncology, 2007; Buerhaus, 2006; Oncology Nursing Society, 2005; National Association of Social Workers, 2006; National Cancer Registrars Association, 2006). For example, the demand for oncologists is expected to exceed supply by 25% to 30% by 2020 (ASCO, 2008). Advocacy efforts to attract students; better fund scholarships, education, and training; and improve or adapt reimbursement mechanisms are underway to bolster the field. Without a healthy workforce, achievement of any national goals to improve cancer research, prevention, and care will be difficult.

Policy Landscape

The policy landscape for affecting the hope of people at risk for and living with cancer is vast. These examples demonstrate a variety of ways in which funding, restrictions or allowances, and programs at the federal, state, and local level can affect some aspect of the cancer problem. Because cancer is more than one disease, affects so many people, and relies on so many interconnected systems to be prevented and treated, the policy challenges are equally complex; however, the growing body of evidence-based policy and practice outcomes offers another source of hope for fighting cancer.

References

Agency for Healthcare Research and Quality. (2008). *2007 National Healthcare Disparities Report.* Rockville, MD: U.S. Department of Health and Human Services, Agency for Healthcare Research and Quality; February 2008. AHRQ Pub. No. 08-0041.

American Cancer Society. (2007). *Cancer facts & figures 2007.* Atlanta, GA: Author.

American Public Health Association. (2007). *Strengthening the public health workforce.* Retrieved February 10, 2007, from http://www.apha.org/NR/rdonlyres/0E0166BC-2D70-4352-9FC1-98DF8520861E/0/PublicHealthWorkforceFactSheet.pdf

American Society for Clincal Oncology and Association of American Medical Colleges. (2007, March). *Forecasting the supply of and demand for oncologists: A report to the American Society of Clinical Oncology from the AAMC Center for Workforce Studies.* Retrieved December 8, Downloads/Cancer%20Research/Oncology%20Workforce%20%Report%20FINAL.pdf

American Society for Therapeutic and Radiation Oncology. (2004). Grants, internet helping improve oncology workforce shortage. *Cancer/Oncology News.* Retrieved August 28, 2004, from http://www.medicalnewstoday.com/medicalnews.php?newsid=12598

Buerhaus, P., Donelan, K., Ulrich, B. T., Norman, L., & Dittus, R. (2006). State of the registered nurse workforce in the United States. *Nursing Economic$, 24*(1), 6–12.

Campaign for Tobacco-Free Kids. (2009). A decade of broken promises: The 1998 state tobacco settlement ten years later. Retrieved November 18, 2008, from http://www.tobaccofreekids.org/reports/settlements/2009/fullreport.pdf

C-Change. (2007). Increasing access to cancer care: A guide for comprehensive cancer control coalition action. Washington, DC: Author.

C-Change. (2008). Considering reimbursement for cancer preventive agents. Washington, DC: Author.

Centers for Disease Control and Prevention. (2005a). Annual smoking attributable mortality, years of potential life lost, and productivity losses—United States, 1997–2001. *MMWR, 54*(25), 625–628.

Centers for Disease Control and Prevention. (2005b). *Morbidity and Mortality Weekly Report, 53,* 528.

Chaloupka, F. J., et al. (2002). Tax, price and cigarette smoking: evidence from the tobacco documents and implications for tobacco company marketing strategies. *Tobacco Control, 11,* i62–i72.

Fiore, M. C., & Jaén, C. R. (2008). A clinical blueprint to accelerate the elimination of tobacco use. *Journal of the American Medical Association, 299*(17), 2083–2085.

Grabowski, H., & Moe, J. (2008). Impact of economic, regulatory, and patent policies on innovation in cancer chemoprevention. *AACR's Cancer Prevention Research, 1*(2), 84–90.

Himmelstein, D. U., Warren, E., Thorne, D., & Woolhandler, S. (2005). Illness and injury as contributors to bankruptcy. *Health Affairs.* Retrieved February 12, 2010, from http://content.healthaffairs.org/cgi/reprint/hlthaff.w5.63v1

Husten, C. G. (2008, October). Tobacco use: Ending the epidemic. *MedSurg Nursing, 17*(5), 345–354.

Institute of Medicine, Board on Health Care Services. (2002). *Care without coverage: Too little, too late.* Washington, DC: National Academy of Sciences.

Institute of Medicine. (2004, January). *Ensuring quality cancer care.* Washington, DC: National Academy of Sciences.

Jemal, A., Thun, M. J., Ries, L. A. G., Howe, H. L., Weir, H. K., Center, M. M., et al. (2008). Annual report to the nation on the status of cancer 1975–2005, featuring trends in lung cancer, tobacco use, and tobacco control. *Journal of the National Cancer Institute.* Retrieved February 12, 2010, from http://jnci.oxfordjournals.org/cgi/content/full/djn389v1

National Association of Social Workers, Center for Workforce Studies. (2006). *Assuring the sufficiency of a* frontline workforce: A national study of licensed social workers executive summary. Washington, DC: Author.

National Cancer Institute. (2005). DevCan: Probability of Developing or Dying of Cancer Software, Version 6.0 Statistical Research and Applications Branch. Retrieved December 8, 2008, from http://srab.cancer.gov/devcan

North American Quitline Consortium. Quitline facts. Retrieved January 19, 2010, from http://www.naquitline.org/?page=quitlinefacts

National Cancer Registrars Association. (2006, June). Frontline workers Workforce analysis study of the cancer registry field. San Francisco, CA: University of California at San Francisco Center for Health Professions.

Niederhuber, J. (2007). Perspectives in cancer research: A look inside the National Cancer Institute Budget process: Implications for 2007 and beyond. Cancer Research, 67, 856–862.

Oncology Nursing Society. (2005, March). The impact of the national nursing shortage on quality cancer care—ONS position. Pittsburgh, PA: Author.

President's Cancer Panel. (2001, September). Voices of a broken system: Real people, real problems, 2000–2001. Bethesda, MD: National Cancer Institute, National Institute of Health.

President's Cancer Panel. (2004, May). Living beyond cancer: Finding a new balance, 2003–2004. Bethesda, MD: National Cancer Institute, National Institute of Health.

Task Force on Community Preventive Services. (2005). Tobacco. In S. Zaza, P. A. Briss, K. W. Harris (Eds.), The Guide to Community Preventive Services: What Works to Promote Health? (pp. 3–79). Atlanta, GA: Oxford University Press.

U.S. Cancer Statistics Working Group. Department of Health and Human Services, Centers for Disease Control and Prevention and National Cancer Institute. (2003). United States cancer statistics: 2000 incidence. Atlanta, GA: Author.

Wells, S. (2008). Cervical cancer: An overview with suggested practice and policy goals. MedSurg Nursing, 17(1), 43–50.

Photo Credits

The History of Health Insurance in the United States

Leah Curtin
and
Franklin A. Shaffer

OVERVIEW

This chapter provides an overview of the growth of the insurance within the healthcare industry. The major trends and merits of public and private insurance are described. The major stakeholders are presented with their role in the evolution of healthcare insurance including the government at the state and federal level, insurance companies, employers and the consumer. The major features of various insurance plans are described. An overview of the major features and aims of healthcare reform is presented as well as a look towards the future relative to existing political influence.

OBJECTIVES

- To describe the evolution of the insurance industry in the healthcare sector
- To identify the role of the stakeholders such as federal and state government, employers, and private insurance companies in the evolution of healthcare insurance

- To analyze the various types of insurance accompanied with their major features
- To explain role and choice relative to the type of insurance selected by an individual
- To analyze the nurse's role as an advocate and its important impact on healthcare insurance and the voice for the consumer

KEY TERMS

- ❏ Benefits
- ❏ Blue Cross and Blue Shield

- ❏ Civilian Health & Medical Program for Uniformed Services (CHAMPUS)

(continues)

- ❏ Consolidated Omnibus Budget Reconciliation Act (COBRA)
- ❏ Disability insurance
- ❏ Employees Retirement Income and Security Act (ERISA)
- ❏ Employer coverage
- ❏ Government regulation
- ❏ Health Information Technology for Economic and Clinical Health Act (HITECH)
- ❏ Health insurance
- ❏ Health Insurance Portability and Accountability Act (HIPAA)
- ❏ Healthcare reform
- ❏ History of healthcare reimbursement
- ❏ Managed care
- ❏ Market economics
- ❏ Medicaid
- ❏ Medicare
- ❏ Private coverage

The rudimentary state of medical technology before 1920 had one thing going for it: Most people had very low medical expenditures because there was not much on which to spend any money. A 1918 Bureau of Labor Statistics survey of 211 families living in Columbus, Ohio, found that the chief cost associated with illness was not the cost of medical care, but rather the fact that sick people could not work and did not get paid (Starr, 1982). A 1919 State of Illinois study reported that lost wages because of sickness were four times larger than the medical expenditures associated with treating the illness (State of Illinois, 1919). As a result, most people felt they did not need health insurance. Instead, households purchased "sickness" insurance—similar to today's "disability" insurance—to provide income replacement in the event of illness.

Thus, health insurance in the United States is a relatively new phenomenon. The first *individual* insurance plans to cover accidents or illness began during the Civil War (1861–1865). These offered coverage against accidents related to travel by rail or steamboat. The plans did, however, pave the way for more comprehensive coverage of all illnesses and injuries. The first *group* policy giving comprehensive benefits was offered by Massachusetts Health Insurance of Boston in 1847. Insurance companies issued the first individual disability and illness policies in about 1890. The first employer-sponsored group disability policy was issued in 1911 (Scofea, 1994).

The precursor to modern group health insurance plan was formed in 1929. A group of teachers in Dallas, Texas contracted with Baylor Hospital for room, board, and medical services in exchange for a monthly fee (Starr, 1982). As the demand for hospital care increased in the 1920s, this new payment innovation revolutionized the market for health insurance. The Baylor Plan provided 21 days of hospitalization for a fixed $6.00 payment. Among other things, Baylor Hospital embraced the plan as it helped ensure that people paid their bills. Prepaid hospital service plans grew over the course of the Great Depression. Prepaid hospital care was mutually advantageous for subscribers and hospitals: The prepaid plans enabled (healthy) consumers to afford hospital care. They also benefited hospitals by providing them with a way to earn income during a time of falling hospital revenue.

The demand for health insurance increased with advances in medical technology and as government policies encouraged the popularity of health insurance as a form of employee compensation. In 1932, the nonprofit Blue Cross was the first to offer group health plans (Reed, 1947). The American Hospital Association designed the Blue Cross guidelines so as to reduce price competition among hospitals. Prepayment plans seeking the Blue Cross designation had to provide subscribers with free choice of physician and hospital given a requirement that eliminated single-hospital plans from consideration. Blue Cross plans benefited from special state-level enabling legislation allowing them to act as non-profit corporations and enjoy tax-exempt status. They were also free from the usual insurance regulations. Originally, this exemption was provided because Blue Cross made benefits available to low-income individuals. Without the enabling legislation, Blue Cross plans would have had to organize under the laws for insurance companies. As for-profit companies, the plans would have had to meet reserve requirements to ensure their solvency. Organizing as commercial insurance companies meant that they either had to meet reserve requirements or be subject to assessment liability. Given that most plans had limited financial resources available to them; they would not have been able to meet the requirements.

The commercial insurance companies were initially reluctant to offer health insurance. They feared that they would not be able to overcome problems relating to adverse selection so that offering health insurance would not be profitable. The success of Blue Cross and later Blue Shield showed how easily adverse selection problems could be overcome by focusing on providing health insurance only to groups of employed workers. This allowed commercial insurance companies to avoid those most likely to become ill because they insured only relatively young, healthy people. The success of private health insurance was always based on avoiding adverse selection. (Adverse selection is a disproportionately large number of sicker persons enrolled in a health plan.) Over the years, the techniques for doing so improved. Insurance companies avoided

insuring the older population, disabled persons, and those at high risk to illness until eventually they were covered by governmental plans.

Several large life insurance companies entered the health insurance market in the 1930s and 1940s as the popularity of health insurance increased. These plans were not beholden to the hospitals like Blue Cross and Blue Shield. They were organized as indemnity plans meaning that cash payments were made for covered healthcare services. Individuals received the fixed payment and were responsible for the bill. These employee benefit plans gained popularity during World War II and into the late 1940s and 1950s. Strong unions bargained for better benefit packages, including tax-free, employer-sponsored health insurance. Wartime (1939–1945) wage freezes imposed by the government actually accelerated the spread of group health plans. Unable by law to attract workers by paying more, employers instead improved their benefit packages, adding health care.

Government Coverage (Public Insurance Programs)

Government programs to cover healthcare costs began to expand during the 1950s (federal matching for welfare recipients and the Veteran's Administration) and 1960s (Medicare and Medicaid). Disability benefits were included in social security coverage for the first time in 1954. The political atmosphere become favorable toward nationalized health insurance proposals after John F. Kennedy was elected to office in 1960, especially when the Democrats won a majority in Congress in 1964. Following Kennedy's assassination, Lyndon Johnson led the movement to pass Medicare and Medicaid. In 1965, Medicare passed with bipartisan support (70 House Republicans joined 237 House Democrats and in the Senate 13 Republicans joined 57

Democrats). Wilburn Cohen, Secretary of Health, Education, and Welfare under Johnson, is widely considered to be the architect of Medicare (U.S. Department of Health and Human Services, n.d.). It is a federal program with uniform standards that consisted of two parts: Part A is the hospital insurance program that the aged are automatically enrolled in on reaching age 65; Part B provides supplemental medical insurance, or subsidized insurance for physicians' services. One broadly held misconception is that Medicare provides free coverage for all Americans over the age of 65 years. This is not entirely true. To be eligible for Medicare, one must have worked and paid the Medicare tax for at least 10 years, and then one must pay the monthly premium for Part B.

Ironically, although the American Medical Association vigorously opposed Medicare, calling it socialized medicine, physicians and hospitals stood to benefit tremendously. They would both receive payment for services that were previously considered bad debt or charity. Fearing that physicians would refuse to treat Medicare patients, the government agreed to reimburse physicians according to their usual, customary,

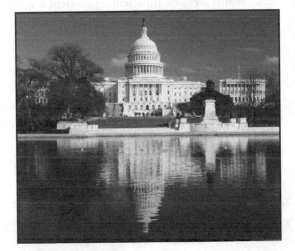

and reasonable rate. In addition, doctors could continue to bill patients directly so that the patients rather than the doctors had to deal with Medicare for reimbursement. Funding for Medicare comes from payroll taxes, income taxes, trust fund interest, and enrollee premiums for Part B. Medicare has grown from serving 19.1 million recipients in 1966 to 44.1 million in 2008, and projections are that it will cover over 70 million retirees by 2020 (Kaiser Family Foundation, 2009).

Part A of the Medicare benefit program covers hospital stays of at least 72 hours. It also will pay for limited stays in a nursing home, provided that the nursing home care is related to the hospital stay, the patient requires skilled nursing supervision in lieu of rehabilitation, and the Medicare benefit received in the nursing home is skilled rather than routine. Part A coverage is usually free, having been paid for by the beneficiary's periodic payroll tax deductions.

Part B of the Medicare benefit package is optional and offers medical insurance. It covers some of the medical providers and services not covered by Part A. Part B Medicare benefit can include a doctor's visit, a laboratory test, an X-ray, a flu vaccination, and certain outpatient procedures, to name a few. The Part B Medicare benefit is not free. Instead, the person must choose whether to pay for Part B when notice of Medicare benefit eligibility is received at the age of 65 years. In 2008, the Part B monthly premium was $96.40 (and more for seniors with higher incomes) (Kaiser Family Foundation, 2009).

In 1997, Part C of the Medicare Benefit system gave Medicare members the option to receive their care through private insurance plans. These private plans were in place of the Part A/Part B coverage of the original Medicare benefit plan. Regulations for these private plans were modified in 2003, and they became known as Medicare Advantage, or MA, plans (http://www.ms.hhs.gov).

The Part D Medicare benefit became effective on January 1, 2006. Anyone eligible for Parts A or B was automatically eligible to participate in the Part D prescription drug plan. Part D is confusing and complicated. In 2008, the standard benefit requires payment of a $275 deductible. The beneficiary then pays 25% of the cost of a covered Part D prescription drug up to an initial coverage limit of $2,510. Once the initial coverage limit is reached, the beneficiary is subject to another deductible, known officially as the Coverage Gap, but referred to more commonly as the "donut hole," in which they must pay the full cost of medicine. When total out-of-pocket expenses on formulary drugs for the year, including the deductible and initial coinsurance, reach $4,050 (now $4,350 in 2009), the beneficiary then reaches catastrophic coverage, in which he or she pays $2.25 for a generic or preferred drug and $5.65 for other drugs, or 5% coinsurance, whichever is greater. The $4,050 amount is calculated on a yearly basis, and a beneficiary who amasses $4,050 in out-of-pocket costs by December 31 of one year will start his or her deductible anew on January 1 (Kaiser Family Foundation, 2009). Most low-income subsidy patients are exempt from all or part of the donut hole and the deductible. This defined standard benefit is not the most common benefit offered by Part D plans for other beneficiaries. For further information on Medicare and all of its complexities, you are referred to visit Medicare's excellent and extremely informative Web site at www.medicare.gov.

The other major health insurance program that is offered as a partnership between the federal and state governments is Medicaid. Medicaid was passed at the same time as the Medicare legislation. It is an entitlement program that originally provided healthcare services to welfare recipients including the aged, blind and disabled. As currently designed, the federal government sets broad guidelines for the program in terms of eligibility and services, and states have discretion over implementation. The costs are primarily covered by the federal government. In 2008 Medicaid served 58 million persons and cost $319 billion dollars (Kaiser Family Foundation, 2010).

Medicaid eligibility covers two groups. Mandatory groups covered by the program include most persons who receive federally assisted income maintenance, low-income families and children who meet eligibility requirements for AFCD as of 1996, SSI recipients, low income pregnant women and children, recipients of adoption and foster care services and certain Medicare beneficiaries. Optional groups are populations that the states may include in the program. There is tremendous flexibility. For example, states have the option to cover distinct populations such as AIDS patients.

Medicaid is a comprehensive program because the population served by Medicaid is sickest and least able to pay. Every state must provide 10 basic health services: inpatient, outpatient hospital services, physician services, rural health clinics, other laboratory and X-ray, skilled nursing facility and home health for individuals 21 and over, EPSDT for individuals under 21, family planning, and nurse midwives. There are an additional 33 optional services that states may choose to provide including prescription drugs, dental, and optical. Nursing home and home health care fall under optional services under this category. As a result, Medicaid is best described as 50 different programs. The federal government matches state healthcare spending between 50% and 83% of costs based on the average per capita income in each state (Kaiser Family Foundation,

2010). States have tremendous discretion to specify income cut-off for eligibility and payment levels for services which impacts the cost of the program (Kaiser Family Foundation, 2010).

Medicaid serves three distinct populations. It is most clearly associated with the services provided to children. In fiscal year 2006, children accounted for 50% of Medicaid beneficiaries but only 19% of costs. The elderly for whom Medicaid pays long-term care services and Medicare Part B premiums for qualified individuals were 10% of beneficiaries and accounted for 24% of costs. Last, Medicaid is the primary source of healthcare coverage for the disabled. They comprise 15% of beneficiaries and 41% of costs (Kaiser Family Foundation, 2010). This is the fastest growing part of Medicaid in terms of numbers and costs.

In addition to Medicare and Medicaid, the federal government has extended health benefits to children through the SCHIP program that was created in 1997. This program allocated $40 billion over 10 years to expand child health insurance coverage. States could provide services using their Medicaid programs; they could develop separate plans that could limit benefit packages or require cost sharing; or they could develop plans with elements of both. States set eligibility guidelines for the program but could offer health insurance to children up to 19 who were not already insured (GovTrack, 2007).

The federal government's role extends over many areas of health care, including the Food and Drug Administration, Centers for Disease Control, and National Institutes of Health (the nation's research agency), for the public's benefit. The federal government not only provides insurance through the Medicare and Medicaid Programs, but it also serves as an employer and offers its own insurance through the Federal Employees Health Benefits Program. The government also covers the Department of Defense, ensuring that the active and retired service personnel receive their healthcare coverage. Also, the Department of Veterans Affairs covers civilian, current, and retired personnel's health care. The arm of the federal government extends beyond Medicare, even though Medicare is its largest public insurance. In 2008, national health spending was estimated to reach $2.4 trillion (Centers for Medicare and Medicaid Services, n.d.). The total public share of this amount, including state, federal, and local, was estimated at $1,108 trillion, or 46% of all national health spending. The federal share alone, through Medicare, Medicaid, and other programs and entities, was $810.6 billion, or 33.75% of the total national health spending. If tax subsidies that encourage provisions of health coverage and health care are added in, the total governmental share comes close to three fifths (60%) of all U.S. health spending (Centers for Medicare and Medicaid Services, n.d.).

Large Employer Coverage

Most private health coverage in the United States is employment based. Employer-sponsored health insurance originally was paid for by businesses on behalf of their employees as part of an employee benefit package. Today, the employer typically makes a substantial contribution toward the cost of coverage. In 2008, the average employee contribution was 16% of the cost of single coverage and 27% of the cost of family coverage. These percentages have been stable since 1999. Health benefits provided by employers are also tax favored. Employees can make contributions to health spending accounts on a pretax basis if the employer offers the benefits through a section 125 cafeteria plan. Although large companies are more likely to offer retiree health benefits than small firms, the percentage of large firms offering these benefits fell from 66% in 1988 to 34% in 2002 (Thomasson, 2002).

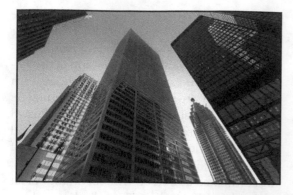

Employers are reticent to continue paying for retiree benefits because the costs for employer-paid health insurance are rising rapidly. Since 2001, premiums for family coverage have increased 78%, whereas wages have risen 19% and inflation has risen 17%, according to a 2007 study by the Kaiser Family Foundation. Employer costs generally have risen significantly per hour worked and vary significantly. In particular, average employer costs for health benefits vary by firm size and occupation. The percentage of total compensation devoted to health benefits has been rising since the 1960s. Average premiums, including both the employer and employee portions, were $4,704 for single coverage and $12,680 for family coverage in 2008.

Small Employer Group Coverage

According to a 2007 study, about 59% of employers at small firms (3 to 199 workers) in the United States provide employee health insurance; however, the percentage of small firms offering coverage has been dropping steadily since 1999 (Claxton et al., 2007). The study notes that cost remains the main reason cited by small firms who do not offer health benefits. Small firms that are new are less likely to offer coverage than ones that have been in existence for a number of years.

For example, using 2005 data for firms with fewer than 10 employees, 43% of those that had been in existence at least 20 years offered coverage, but only 24% of those that had been in existence less than 5 years did. The rates from year to year are volatile and appear to be higher for newer, small businesses.

The types of coverage available to small employers are similar to those offered by large firms, but small businesses do not have the same options for financing their benefit plans. In particular, self-insuring the benefits is not a practical option for most small employers. A RAND Corporation study published in April 2008 found that the cost of healthcare coverage places a greater burden on small firms, as a percentage of payrolls, than on larger firms. A study published by the American Enterprise Institute in August 2008 examined the effect of state benefit mandates on self-employed individuals and found that the larger the number of mandates in a state, the lower the probability that a self-employed person will be a significant employment generator (Eibner, 2008).

Beneficiary cost sharing is, on average, higher among small firms than large firms. For the last 30 years, health policy has been characterized by increasing cost sharing with beneficiaries

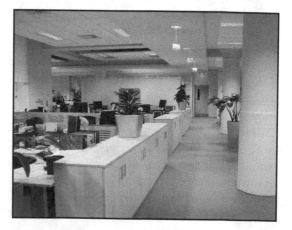

(deductibles, co-payments) and increasing determination to reduce usage of health benefits. This policy was supported by a surprisingly small number of studies on moral hazard, which have exerted a disproportionate influence on the thinking of policy makers (Nyman, 2003). The term *moral hazard* is defined as the additional healthcare coverage that consumers purchase when they are insured. With the advent of this theory, health insurance was transformed from a solution into a problem. Under this theory, insurance was socially valuable only if one could substantially curb the behavior of the insured. Otherwise, health insurance promoted overuse of health resources and contributed substantially to the growth in medical inflation. Managed care was born partially in response to this belief. Managed care is considered the systematic integration and coordination of the financing and delivery of health care performed by health plans that try to provide their members who are at least partly at risk for the cost of care.

When small group plans are medically underwritten, employees are asked to provide health information about themselves and their covered family members when they apply for coverage. When determining rates, insurance companies use the medical information on these applications. Sometimes they will request additional information from an applicant's physician or ask the applicant for clarification.

States regulate small group premium rates, typically by placing limits on the premium variation allowable between groups (rate bands). Insurers price to recover their costs over their entire book of small group businesses while abiding by state rating rules. Over time, the effect of initial underwriting "wears off" as the cost of a group regresses toward the mean. Recent claim experience—whether better or worse than average—is a strong predictor of future costs in the near term, but the average health status of a particular small employer group tends to regress over time toward that of an average group. Insurance brokers play a significant role in helping small employers find health insurance, particularly in more competitive markets. Average small group commissions range from 2% to 8% of premiums (Nyman, 2003). Brokers provide services beyond insurance sales, such as assisting with employee enrollment and helping to resolve benefits issues.

Health Insurance Regulation

Health insurance is regulated by both state and federal governments primarily to protect the public. The state is responsible for regulating the business or operations of insurance carriers. The federal government regulates the companies that cross individual state borders to ensure that they act in a similar and consistent manner. In 1945, the McCarran-Ferguson Act gave states the authority to govern the standards and oversee the business of insurance companies (Fernandez, 2005). The state requires that insurance carriers, with the exception of self-insured companies, be licensed by the state in order to conduct their business. The state also requires that companies provide certain benefits as stipulated by that state's regulations. Federal regulations focus more on ensuring that the right people get the right benefits (especially at-risk populations, including the poor and others). The three most notable federal laws regulating health insurance are the Employee Retirement Income and Security Act, the Consolidated Omnibus Budget Reconciliation Act, and HIPAA.

The Employee Retirement Income and Security Act (ERISA) was passed in 1974 in an effort to protect the retirement benefits of the public at large. ERISA has had a profound impact on health insurance as it supersedes state laws related to benefit plans (Kaiser Family Foundation, 2002). Therefore, companies that self insure as opposed to companies that purchase health insurance plans are exempt from state insurance regulation. Since the passage of ERISA, the number of employees covered by self insured plans increased to over 50%. This means there can be both federal and state regulation of health insurance in a given state. The question regarding exemption is whether or not weak state laws are being preempted by stronger federal law. Self insured plans tend to be less comprehensive than plans regulated by state insurance agencies. This impacts services such as prenatal care, well child care, and coverage of alternative medical providers such as chiropractors. In addition, self insured plans are not as expensive as companies do not pay premium taxes to state risk pools or reserves. Last, are problems sited in areas like the appeals process. The only remedy available to a covered person who has been denied benefits or dropped from coverage altogether is to seek an order from a federal judge (no jury trial is permitted) directing the plan (in actuality the insurance company that underwrites and administers it) to pay for "medically necessary" care. If a person dies before the case can be heard, however, the claim dies with him or her, as ERISA provides no remedy for injury or wrongful death caused by the withholding of care (Hall, 1994).

Even if benefits are improperly denied, the insurance company cannot be sued for any resulting injury or wrongful death. Many persons included among the 47 million people presently without healthcare coverage in the United States are former ERISA "subscribers" (insurance plan beneficiaries) who have been denied benefits— usually on grounds that the prescribed care is not medically necessary or is "experimental" or the beneficiary has been dropped from coverage, perhaps because he or she lost his or her job because of the very illness for which care was denied (Hall, 1994).

Another federal law is the Consolidated Omnibus Budget Reconciliation Act better known as COBRA which was passed in 1985 (Shaffer, 1986). COBRA applies to job-based plans with 20 or more employees. It allows workers the right to temporarily remain in their company's group health plan even if they lose their job or their dependent status. The protection offered by COBRA is important because group coverage cannot discriminate based on health status while individual coverage can. If an individual is sick and about to lose his or her job, COBRA assures the availability of coverage. The cost of coverage, however, discourages most persons from applying for coverage because there is no requirement that employers pay a portion of the premium.

The other federal statute governing the insurance industry is the Health Insurance Portability and Accountability Act (HIPAA). It was passed in 1996 and addressed employees' concerns over their inability to take their insurance from one employer to another (Fernandez, 2005, p. 7). HIPAA also limited the plan's ability to deny coverage for preexisting medical conditions to 5 years. HIPAA also protects the confidentiality of personal as well as business information. Recently, HIPAA's reach was expanded by the Health Information Technology for Economic and Clinical Health Act (HITECH) provisions of the American Recovery and Reinvestment Act which made important changes in privacy regulation in an effort to protect the confidentiality of the information housed in electronic records (Centers for Medicare and Medicaid Services, 2010). HITECH is a regulatory response to the data-mining efforts of many insurance companies as they seek to reduce their exposure to the effects of adverse selection. HIPAA and HITECH regulations require that practicing healthcare professionals protect the confidentiality of personal records of patients just like the insurance industry is obliged to protect the personal information of its enrollees and potential enrollees, regardless of the settings or the industry confidentiality of personal information.

Managed Care in the 1990s

Health insurance underwent major changes starting in the early 1990s, with the defeat of the Clinton Health Plan. The American public "chose" by default market-based reform as that strategy most likely to yield the highest quality service for the lowest cost. Universal coverage, indeed even provision of essential services to those in greatest need, was considered political "pie in the sky." The health insurance industry rapidly developed managed care products to replace its indemnity plans. Managed care never promised the American people universal coverage or even affordable health insurance coverage for all. Rather, it promised its investors a respectable return on investment and its beneficiaries the fulfillment of its contractual obligations: nothing more and nothing less. It did suggest that competition would control costs and increase quality. Managed care is an insurance or delivery mechanism that includes: limitation on the number of providers serving a covered population, either through direct ownership or employment, or through selective contracting or through some combination of these elements; adherence by providers to utilization management controls; incentives for patients to use only the providers designated by the managed care plan; some degree of financial risk for providers, ranging from HMOs that assume the full risk for the cost of care to contractual arrangements under which carriers and providers share risk (Center for Studying Health System Change, 1997).

Managed care demonstrates that health insurance is more than protection against risk. It is a highly profitable business. Market economics demands the adoption of strategies that optimize profit through gaining competitive advantage. Competitive edge is determined by meeting the demands of one's customers (i.e., the ones who buy your products/services). Today, that customer is almost always business or government, and their chief demand is for lower prices. These customers are fostering competition among health plans that, in turn, seek providers who underbid one another. Historically, the first managed care organizations (called health maintenance organizations) were nonprofit. They delivered services to clearly defined populations such as city employees (Health Insurance Plan in New York City), or cooperative members (Group Health in Puget Sound), or ship workers (Kaiser Permanente in California) (Center for Studying Health System Change, 1997). With federal incentives to expand this model, insurance companies developed managed care plans. These managed care organizations (MCOs), now dominate the market (Center for Studying Health System Change, 1997). The entry of for-profit insurance companies led to competition among health plans for members which was evidenced by mergers and hostile takeovers as MCOs sought greater market share and thus greater bargaining power with both their customers (business and government) and clients (healthcare providers) (Eckholm, 1994). The larger the MCO and the greater its market share in a given region, the tougher the strategies for controlling costs and the tighter is the squeeze on local providers. Managed care strategies, which exclude high-risk patients, limit access to high-cost care, and reward low-cost providers, encourage hospitals and health networks to

- Adopt economies of scale (form chains, expand established product lines, create group purchasing arrangements)

- Increase their market share (arrange mergers and acquisitions, bid aggressively for managed care contracts, purchase physician practices)
- Increase the efficiency of service delivery (develop outpatient services, streamline management, standardize care plans)
- Control costs (close unprofitable institutions and services, increase productivity through restructuring and re-engineering jobs, hire and incentivize physicians to encourage frugal decision-making)

Individual providers (physicians, in particular) responded to the pressures brought by both managed care entities and institutional providers by organizing large multispecialty group practices that gave them leverage in bargaining with local and even national health networks and managed care entities. Many have formed their own "managed care products" called individual practice associations; still others have bought stock in or received stock options as part of their agreements with existing publicly traded MCOs. Many physicians have become employees of hospitals and health networks and MCOs, often incentivized through profit sharing.

To put the matter succinctly, health insurance organizations (private and governmental) and the strategies they adopted and providers of all types (for-profit, nonprofit, personal, and institutional) and the strategies that they employ are more a function of market-based economics than of "managed care." The drive for profit, which is the sine qua non of the marketplace, is ipso facto a disincentive to ensuring high-risk populations (McCormick, 1998).

Employer coverage and age-dependent coverage virtually guarantee plan switching, which discourages long-term accountability because members do not stay in a plan over their lifetimes. Indeed, in the case of Medicare Advantage Plans (Part C), enrollees are almost encouraged to change plans when they are dissatisfied. As a result, (managed care) plan managers have no incentive to provide preventive care and may be tempted to ration access to care. Enrollees, on the other hand, have little incentive to take "lifetime benefit limits" seriously and make careful choices about the use of their benefit over the long haul.

Health Insurance in the Twenty-First Century

Since its initial uptake in the 1990s, there has been tremendous resistance to managed care. Patients resent their loss of choice. Physicians resisted the loss of autonomy that resulted from tightly structured managed care plans. Employers had difficulty controlling costs following the initial savings. The government found it difficult to develop managed care systems in either the Medicare or Medicaid systems. What has evolved are hybrid forms of organization that represent a loosening of the managed care model. MCOs now offer a range of products including indemnified products. For example, an enrollee can see a panel physician and only make a co-payment for services or an enrollee can go out-of-network and be reimbursed a fixed amount for the service. What has become more popular than MCOs are Point-of-Service Plans that have no gate keeping and Preferred Provider Organizations that offer discounted fee-for-service in a limited panel.

Consumer–driven plans are a relatively new insurance model, but many persons assume it will grow. They represent a fundamental shift in the provision of health insurance. The insurance industry understood the managed care mandate as constraining costs by modifying physician practice patterns. In contrast, the industry is redefining its mission as designing benefit packages to encourage cost conscious choices by consumers. By making consumers responsible for more of the purchasing decisions these plans transfer risk to individuals who will control demand for services. Existing health insurance products do not expose enrollees to financial risk. The lack of risk exposure leads enrollees to pay little attention to whether they genuinely need a health service before using it. This leads to extensive overuse and misuse of services and thus ever increasing costs. The solution is to put consumers at risk and provide them with extensive information and support to make wise decisions. The two components of consumer-driven plans are high deductibles and health savings accounts. High deductible for an individual are minimally $1,000 but may be much higher. Expenses subject to the deductible are covered by health savings accounts to which employers and employees have contributed. Recognizing that many persons will avoid preventive care if they have to pay out-of-pocket, these services are sometimes exempt from the deductible.

Problems and More Problems

The history of health insurance can also be understood as a history of expanding access to health care. This was the intent of the Baylor Plan, Blue Cross and Blue Shield, commercial health insurance, and Medicare and Medicaid. In 1993, President Bill Clinton presented to Congress a healthcare reform plan that guaranteed health insurance for all Americans. Fueled by well-funded opposition from the health insurance industry, the bill was soundly defeated, allegedly for its high cost and complexity. Despite various federal efforts such as the 1996 Mental Health Parity Act that required some employers to offer health plans with psychiatric benefits, or the Health Insurance Portability and Accountability Act whose purpose was to protect individuals from losing their health insurance when they changed jobs or became self-employed or the SCHIP program, the government has not ensured the overall quality or comprehensiveness of insurance offered by employers.

In 2007, more than 45 million people in the United States (15.3% of the population) were without health insurance for at least part of the year (Kaiser Family Foundation, 2010). The percentage of the non-older population who are uninsured has been steadily increasing since the year 2000. Among the uninsured population, some 37 million were employment-age adults (ages 18 to 64 years) and more than 27 million worked at least part time. About 38% of the uninsured live in households with incomes over $50,000. According to the U.S. Census Bureau (2007), nearly 36 million of the uninsured are legal U.S. citizens. Another 9.7 million are noncitizens, but the Census Bureau does not distinguish in its estimate between legal noncitizens and illegal immigrants (U.S. Census Bureau, 2007). It has been estimated that nearly one fifth of the uninsured population is able to afford insurance; almost one quarter is eligible for public coverage, and the remaining 56% need financial assistance (8.9% of all Americans). An estimated 5 million of those without health insurance are considered "uninsurable" because of pre-existing conditions (Kaiser Family Foundation, 2010).

A report published by the Kaiser Family Foundation in April 2008 found that the economic downturn of 2008 placed a significant strain on state Medicaid and SCHIP programs. The authors estimated that a 1% increase in the unemployment rates increased Medicaid and SCHIP enrollment by 1 million and increased the number uninsured by 1.1 million. State spending on Medicaid and SCHIP increased by $1.4 billion (total spending on these programs increased by $3.4 billion). This increased spending occurs at the same time state government revenues are declining. During the last downturn, the Jobs and Growth Tax Relief Reconciliation Act of 2003 included federal assistance to states, which helped states avoid tightening their Medicaid and SCHIP eligibility rules. The authors concluded that Congress should consider similar relief for the current economic downturn.

Many health professionals, tend to look at an aging society from the standpoint of its health; however, few of us consider the social, political, and clinical impact of a rapidly growing, heavily entitled cohort of aging people—the Baby Boomers—who already are characterized by political activism. Now this voting block, all 79 million, is more united than ever: rich or poor, educated or illiterate, of all races and of both parties and genders, over concerns surrounding entitlements, including Medicare.

2009 Insurance Reform Efforts

Once again, healthcare reform is on the table and Congress is considering how to expand access to health insurance. The value of health insurance is not difficult to establish. It helps restore both physical health for a person when he has an ac-

Content removed due to

copyright restrictions

cident, experiences a heart attack, or discovers a cancer. The benefits of health insurance in these circumstances underlie the public support for policies that subsidize health insurance or extend publicly provided health insurance to a large portion of Americans who are otherwise uninsured. Obama's health plan is currently stalled in Congress, but the complexity of making health care widely available was seen in the range of options considered by the House and Senate during 2009.

On June 19, 2009, the House Tri-Committee released a draft bill on health reform that included a public plan financed by premiums (American Nurses Association, 2010).

This bill initially reimbursed healthcare providers using Medicare's lower rates. The triggered responses were predictable, including those voiced from the American Medical Association, the health insurance industry, and House Republicans: (1) Doctors and hospitals say that a public plan that forces them to accept lower payments (Medicare rates) would shrink their incomes dramatically; (2) Insurance companies say that a public plan would have built-in advantages—that would allow it to "take over" the insurance market; (3) Republicans worry that a public plan would amount to a "government takeover" of health care that would cost untold trillions. In response, the House Republicans proposed individual tax breaks for buying health insurance and "pools" for states and small business to get lower cost healthcare plans. They also proposed increasing incentives for people to build health savings accounts, allowing dependent children to stay on parents' policies until the age of 25 years and encouraging employers to reward employees for improved health. This, of course, assumes that the uninsured/underinsured have the money to save, get tax refunds, and so forth.

On June 19, 2009, the Senate Finance Committee leaked a 10-page draft that contains the following four alternatives:

1. A Medicare-based plan in which providers would be paid the same rates as from Medicare. Premiums would be the lowest of any model, but government costs would be the highest.
2. A self-sustaining plan in which premiums would cover the cost of claims. Patients would pay more than under the Medicare model but less than for private insurance.
3. A triggered plan in which the "public plan" would kick in only if private insurers did not sufficiently expand coverage and lower costs to certain mandated levels at some as yet unspecified future date.
4. Regional co-ops that would be owned and operated by states/regions and that would collect premiums and provide coverage (keeping the federal government out of it).

In September of 2009, the Senate's "Bi-Partisan" Health Reform Plan was released (American Nurses Association, 2010). This effort, led by Senator Max Baucus, was supposed to construct a bipartisan plan. The Democratic chairman of the Senate Finance Committee (Baucus) eliminated the public option entirely and kept the insurance mandates, but to date, no Republicans are willing to vote for his bill. The public health insurance option as defined in both the Senate HELP bill and the House bill (H.R. 3200) was not a far-left liberal proposal. A far-left liberal proposal would actually have been a single-payer plan. The public option is a program that initially had broad based support.

If the Senate bill is enacted as is, citizens would have to buy a private insurance policy or

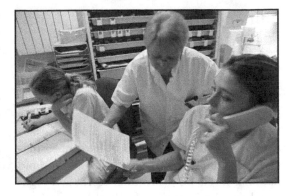

be penalized by the federal government. Thus, individuals would be forced to purchase insurance from the same companies that have refused to cover pre-existing conditions, canceled policies if someone does get sick, denied claims, or refused to pay for life-saving procedures. Penalties for failing to get insurance would start at $750 a year for individuals and $1,500 for families. Households making more than three times the federal poverty level—about $66,000 for a family of four—would face the maximum fine: $3,800 for families and $950 for individuals.

2009 began with a Democratic Administration that was determined to reform health care. To achieve health reform, lawmakers must stifle their reluctance to impose mandates and some form of taxation. But such action comes in the face of powerful lobbyists for the insurance and pharmaceutical companies who are fighting to protect their constituents' profits. Even the American Medical Association, although favoring reform, is not supportive of any plan that will cut physician reimbursement. So far, the hospital industry is the only one making any concessions. In August 2009, the hospital industry pledged to contribute $155 billion in Medicare and Medicaid savings in the next decade. But their support is not enough to move what is now a stalemated situation.

Nursing and Healthcare Reform: A Progressive Experience

Nursing, as articulated by its professional associations, has been deeply committed to addressing the inequities of the current healthcare system. Since the early 1980s, nursing organizations, particularly the American Nurses Association (ANA), have participated in representing, as well as informing, the profession at state and national levels on healthcare reform and organized nursing's agenda for healthcare reform (American Nurses Association, 2010). The ANA supported the Clinton Healthcare Plan and has been extremely involved at all levels with the Obama administration's current effort to reform "health insurance" in this country.

The American Nurses Association developed *Nursing's Agenda for Health Care Reform* when Clinton was president, and over 70 nursing organizations signed it (American Nurses Association, 1991). Its essential elements are providing access to care, ensuring universality of coverage, shifting resources more toward primary care, involving consumers in the decision process, and emphasizing quality. Clinton's major domestic agenda was to pass the Health Security Act. Clinton included nurses in task forces and coalitions with consumers and the business community as well as in the review process developing the Health Security Act. It is generally accepted that the Clinton plan was too complex to pass, but media and market forces were more influential in its defeat than any other single factor.

Since the Clinton era, nursing has become increasingly more visible as well as more vocal in positioning nurses within the policy formulation and implementation arena. This can be attributed to two major factors: first, the endorsement of a presidential candidate, and second, the success gained with obtaining reimbursement for advanced practice nurses. Certainly their endorsement of Barack Obama as a presidential candidate in 2008 brought nursing to the forefront of the public within the nation as well as around the world. Nursing indeed was highly visible during the Obama campaign and even more so after his election.

President Obama made it clear from the beginning that his domestic agenda would have healthcare reform as a major priority and that nursing was part of the solution. Senator Ted Kennedy was another strong proponent of nursing, and he too helped move nursing's agenda to the federal level. *Nursing's Agenda for Health Care Reform*, with some minor adjustments, continues to be the nursing platform. The agenda has also served to some degree to solidify nursing and nurses across specialties and area of practice settings.

Aspects of nursing's agenda were also addressed in several of the recent Institute of Medicine's research studies that addressed quality and safety as well as staffing and workforce preparation, Another factor that may have added to nursing's visibility is the American Nurses Credentialing Center's Magnet Recognition Program, which was recently included in The Joint Commission's accreditation processes (American

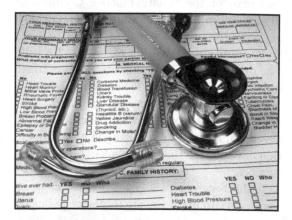

Nurses Credentialing Center, 2010). Thus, it is gratifying that H.R. 3200, to provide affordable, quality health care for all Americans and reduce the growth in healthcare spending, and for other purposes, goes further than any recent legislative initiative in recognizing nursing and its contribution to solving the "health insurance crisis" in this nation. The findings from the recent Gallup Survey, the first of its kind, *Nursing Leadership from Bedside to Boardroom: Opinion Leader's Perceptions,* conducted on behalf of Robert Wood Johnson Foundation, found that opinion leaders from diverse roles and industries believed that nurses have the expertise, knowledge and ability to influence health reform (Robert Wood Johnson Foundation, 2010a). "Nurses are highly trusted sources of healthcare information, but as we look to reform our health system, our nation is not taking advantage of all that nurses have to offer," said Risa Lavizzo-Mourey, MD, MBA, president and CEO of the Robert Wood Johnson Foundation. "This survey shows that opinion leaders recognize that we are squandering opportunities to learn from nurses and implement their ideas. We must build on the widespread trust of nurses' expertise as an essential component in leading and implementing reform" (Robert Wood Johnson Foundation, 2010b).

References

American Nurses Association. (1991). *Nursing's agenda for health care reform* [Brochure]. Washington, DC: Author.

American Nurses Credentialing Center. (2010). *ANCC Magnet recognition program.* Retrieved September 10, 2009, from http://www.nursecredentialing.org/Magnet.aspx

American Nurses Association. (2010). Health system reform. Retrieved February 12, 2010 from http://www.nursingworld.org/MainMenuCategories/HealthcareandPolicyIssues/HealthSystemReform.aspx

Annas, G. (1995). The market vs. medicine. *New England Journal of Medicine, 332,* 745–748.

Blecher, M. B. (1998). Burned on the street. *Hospitals and Health Networks, 72*(5), 22–26.

Center for Studying Health System Change. (1997). The trajectory of managed care. *Issues Brief, 9,* 1.

Centers for Medicaid and Medicare Services. (2010). *CMS information related to the Economic Recovery Act of 2009: Health information technology.* Retrieved February 16, 2010, from http://www.cms.hhs.gov/Recovery/11_HealthIT.asp

Centers for Medicaid and Medicare Services. (n.d.). *Research, statistics, and data systems.* Retrieved February 10, 2010, from http://cms.hhs.gov/home/rsds.asp

Claxton, G., Gabel, J., DiJulio, B., Pickreign, J., Whitmore, H., Finder, B., et al. (2007). Health benefits in 2007: Premium increases fall to an eight-year low, while offer rates and enrollment remain stable. *Health Affairs, 26*(5), 1407–1416.

Davis, M. M., & Rorem, C. R. (1932). *The crisis in hospital finance and other studies in hospital economics.* Chicago: University of Chicago Press.

Eckholm, E. (1994, December 18). The healing process . . . A special report: While Congress remains silent health care transforms itself. *The New York Times,* p. A11.

Eibner, C. (2008). *Economic burden of providing health insurance: How much worse are small firms.* Santa Monica, CA: Kauffman-RAND Institute for Entrepreneurship Public Policy, RAND Corporation. Retrieved February 16, 2010, from http://www.rand.org/pubs/technical_reports/2008/RAND_TR559.pdf

Emery, G., & Emery, J. C. H. (1999). *A young man's benefit: The independent order of odd fellows and sickness insurance in the United States and Canada.* Montreal, Québec: McGill-Queen's University Press.

Fernandez, B. (2005). *Health insurance: A primer.* Washington, DC: Congressional Research Service.

Flexner, A. (1910). *Medical education in the United States and Canada.* New York: Carnegie Foundation for the Advancement of Teaching.

Hall, M. A. (1994). Disclosing rationing decisions: A reply to Paul S. Applebaum. *Milbank Quarterly, 72,* 645.

Henderson, J. W. (2002). *Health economics and policy* (2nd ed.). Cincinnati, OH: South-Western.

Kaiser Family Foundation. (2007). *The Medicare Part D coverage gap: Costs and consequences in 2007.* Retrieved September 20, 2009, from http://www.kff.org/medicare/7811.cfm

Kaiser Family Foundation. (2009). *Kaiser fast facts.* Retrieved September 20, 2009 from http://facts.kff.org

Kaiser Family Foundation. (2010). *State health facts.* Retrieved February 8, 2010, from http://www.statehealthfacts.org/mfs.jsp?rgn=2&rgn=1&x=9&y=10

Kaiser Family Foundation and Health Research and Educational Trust. (2002). *Kaiser/HRET survey of employer-*

sponsored health benefits, 2002. Retrieved February 12, 2010, from http://www.kaisernetwork.org/health_cast/uploaded_files/ACF4D95.pdf

McCormick, R. (1998). The end of Catholic hospitals? *America, 179*(1), 5–12.

Madden, J. M. (2008). Cost-related medication nonadherence and spending on basic needs following implementation of Medicare Part D. *Journal of the American Medical Association, 299*(16), 1922–1928.

Marmor, T. R. (2000). *The politics of Medicare* (2nd ed.). New York: Aldine de Gruyter.

Newhouse, J. P., Manning, W. G., Duan, N., Morris, C. N., Keeler, E. B., Leibowitz, A., et al. (1987). The findings of the Rand Health Insurance Experiment—a response to Welch et al. *Medical Care, 25,* 157–179.

Numbers, R. L. (1978). Almost persuaded: American physicians and compulsory health insurance, 1912–1920. Baltimore, MD: Johns Hopkins University Press.

Nyman, J. A. (2003). *The theory of demand for health insurance.* Stanford, CA: Stanford University Press.

Reed, L. S. (1947). *Blue Cross and medical service plans.* Washington, DC: U.S. Public Health Service.

Robert Wood Johnson Foundation. (2010a). *Nursing leadership from bedside to boardroom: Opinion leaders' perceptions.* Retrieved February 10, 2010 from http://www.rwjf.org/pr/product.jsp?id=54350

Robert Wood Johnson Foundation. (2010b). *Opinion leaders say nurses should have more influence on health systems and services.* Retrieved February 16, 2010, from http://www.rwjf.org/healthreform/product.jsp?id=55091

Scofea, L. A. (1994, March). The development and growth of employer-provided health insurance. *Monthly Labor Review, 117,* 1–10.

Shaffer, F. A. (1986). *Patient and purse strings.* New York: National League for Nursing.

Starr, P. (1982). *The social transformation of American medicine: The rise of a sovereign profession and the making of a vast industry.* New York: Basic Books, Inc.

State of Illinois. (1919). *Report of the health insurance commission of the state of Illinois.* Springfield, IL: Illinois State Journal Co. Retrieved September 20, 2009, from http://openlibrary.org/works/OL10306882W/Report_of_the_health_Insurance_Commision_of_state_of_Illnois

Thomasson, M. A. (2002, July). From sickness to health: The twentieth-century development of U.S. health insurance. *Explorations in Economic History, 39,* 233–253.

U.S. Census Bureau. (2007). *Health insurance coverage: 2007.* Retrieved February 16, 2010, from http://www.census.gov/hhes/www/hlthins/hlthin07.html

U.S. Congress. Medicare, Medicaid, and SCHIP Extension Act of 2007, S.2499-110th (2007). Retrieved February 11, 2001, from http://www.govtrack.us/congress/bill.xpd?bill=s110-2499&tab=summary

U.S. Department of Health and Human Services. (n.d.). *Medicare.gov.* Retrieved February 16, 2010, from http://www.medicare.gov

CASE STUDY

Public Mores and the "Business of Health Care"
Leah Curtin and Franklin A. Shaffer

The "business of health service delivery" is at odds with long-held and highly cherished public perceptions of health care as a humanitarian service—a resource for individuals and communities in times of need. Case law as well as generally accepted codes of professional ethics support this assumption. Thus, one of the most pervasive and significant problems that providers face vis-à-vis managed care involves public expectations that access to the providers' services will be determined by an individual's need rather than a contractual arrangement between two business entities (or between a business entity and the government). Moreover, the public assumes that once access is gained, treatment is determined by professional assessments of services needed to correct (or at least ameliorate) the patient's medical condition when, in fact, treatment options often are influenced by an intricately worded list of limited benefits and exclusions.

So pervasive is the influence of the market ethos that business language and metaphors have replaced those of medicine among health administrators, physicians, and even nurses (Annas, 1995):

The market metaphor leads us to think about medicine in already familiar ways: emphasis is placed on efficiency, profit maximization, customer satisfaction, the ability to pay, planning, entrepreneurship, and competitive models. The ideology of medicine is replaced by the ideology of the marketplace. Trust is replaced by caveat emptor. There is no place for the poor and uninsured in the metaphor of the market. Business ethics supplant medical ethics as the practice of medicine becomes corporate. Nonprofit medical organizations tend to be corrupted by adopting the values of their for-profit competitors. A management degree becomes at least as important as a medical degree. Public institutions, which by definition cannot compete in the for-profit arena, risk demise, second-class status, or simply privatization.

This language gap—and the distance it connotes between the person who is a patient and the person who is the professional—becomes ever more apparent as the language of managed care evolves. It is the language of a coldly complex business, which confuses patient and professional alike almost as thoroughly as it changes the climate within which they receive and give care (California Medical Association, 1996). The power of language to alter attitudes is unchallenged: This in and of itself is a serious issue for all healthcare professionals (who now are called "providers"). At the very least, changes in language and metaphors presage a change in culture: the collective manifestations of a collective value system.

The social and political aspects of the current situation are defined in terms of the national debate over the economic nature of healthcare services: Are they social goods to be distributed equitably, or are they commodities to be bought and sold in an open market? Although most Americans tend to think of health care as a service necessary for personal well-being, they also tend to support a capitalist ideology that treats health services like any other commodity. Even if healthcare services are

commodities, the only valid reference point for evaluating them needs not be the market place. It is possible to conceptualize a compromise. That is, health service delivery's primary purpose need not be solely the generation of wealth (secondary to customer satisfaction, of course)—it could be similar to that of the nation's utility, education, and transportation systems. Their primary function is to support the nation's activities and only secondarily to generate wealth. Public access is protected by law and provided by tax monies, and their quality is both a benefit and a concern for all. In all of these sectors, one can find both not-for-profit and for-profit service providers—some publicly traded, and others not.

If access to healthcare services is in the public's best interests—and few would argue in the contrary—should their provision remain primarily in the private sector? Government has been contracting with the private sector for provision of health services for many years (Medicare and Medicaid) and in recent years has dismantled much of its own delivery system (public health hospitals, the Veteran's Administration, Civilian Health & Medical Program for Uniformed Services [CHAMPUS, a healthcare plan for military dependents and retirees operated by the DoD]). One might question if this is appropriate in view of the unprofitability of many of the most essential services: control of infectious diseases, immunizations, health screening, care of the chronically ill, indigent care, neonatal intensive care, trauma centers for the severely injured, chronic psychiatric care, and so forth. In terms of the competition inherent in a market-based system, is it appropriate for government to contract with low-cost providers who do not subsidize research, who do not educate health professionals, and who do not provide indigent care and/or other costly social burdens? Is it fair to make public hospitals and teaching hospitals and health networks compete for contracts with agencies that have no social duty to absorb the costs of teaching, researching, or caring for the poor?

The California Medical Association reported that California's seven top for-profit managed care organizations (HMOs) spent an average of 74% of premiums on patient care in 1995, whereas their nonprofit counterparts California Kaiser and Group

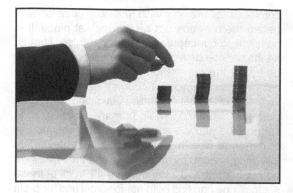

Health of Puget Sound spent 98% and 94%, respectively (Langley, 1998). Few publicly traded health organizations (whether they are managed care entities or for-profit hospital chains) subsidize either education or research, and very few provide indigent care—while they commonly eliminate their unprofitable "product lines." For example, CNN reported on July 7, 1998, that several for-profit HMOs have pulled out of their Medicaid contracts because of unacceptable medical-loss ratios, and this when the nation's 130 public hospitals are in crisis; they have been forced to cut or even eliminate some services entirely, and many will soon be forced to close, despite the disproportionate share funds they receive. *The New York Times* (April 7, 1996) predicted that "cash poor public hospitals and private hospitals serving large numbers of uninsured or those on Medicaid" will most likely be forced to close their doors in the next few years.

This is not to say that nonprofit institutions necessarily do provide unprofitable care: The Daughters of Charity closed all of their inner-city (unprofitable) hospitals while sitting on $2 billion in liquid cash reserves (Warren, 1999). As a people, we are somewhat hypocritical in our attitudes toward for-profit medicine. We complain about for-profit MCOs, but most of us have been quite comfortable with for-profit insurance companies. We resent the profits made by publicly traded managed care and hospital corporations, but we accept with equanimity the profits made by pharmaceutical firms and medical equipment companies. We are alarmed about the growing influence of for-profit hospitals and accept with equanimity, the prevalence, indeed the dominance of, for-profit nursing homes. Is the problem

defined in terms of tax status (for-profit *versus* not-for-profit), or is the problem *profiteering* under either tax status? Is the problem far more fundamental—one that pits our ideals against one another: the ideal of care for the sick as a work of charity and the ideal of entrepreneurial capitalism as a function of rugged individualism?

Professional Ethics as a "Provider" Issue

It is perhaps only human to think that the problems faced by one's own generation are unique to it. In some rare cases, this may be so, but in almost anything that has to do with money, there truly is nothing new under the sun. In fact, *The Encyclopedia of Bioethics* devotes considerable space to money, medicine, and conflicts of interest, and the British Medical Association in its 1974 document *Medical Ethics* succinctly summarized the wisdom of the ages on this subject: "A general ethical principle is that a doctor should not associate himself with commerce in such a way as to let it influence, or appear to influence, his attitude toward the treatment of his patients" (Hall, 1994).

Few would disagree, but what is unique about contemporary managed care in the United States is its institutionalization of conflict of interest. For example, Hall contends that managed care plans should be permitted to give physicians financial incentives for rationing resources, even though he stipulates that the incentives should be "reasonable" and that plan participants should be informed of them. Most likely, Hall's argument is based on his previous contention that people who make informed decisions to purchase less expensive health insurance waive their right to be informed of particular decisions not to treat them (Burton, 1998).

Although there is little doubt that the cumulative financial impact of fee-for-service medicine is staggering, few before have suggested that we give physicians and nurse practitioners financial incentives not to treat people. The cumulative impact of common MCO strategies (paying a reduced fee-for-service tied to year-end profit sharing) is just coming to light. A study by the nation's largest managed care company, United HealthCare Corporation, found that many of their doctors routinely fail to prescribe essential drugs and diagnostic tests (Burton, 1998).

Paying healthcare professionals for improving systems, piloting innovative approaches to care delivery, researching less invasive diagnostics and therapeutics, and even doing something really revolutionary such as engaging in prevention and health promotion might save money. "Incentivizing" professionals does not save money; it merely shifts it around (Blecher, 1998). Paying caregivers to ration care at the bedside more than implies that professionals will make clinical decisions based on personal gain rather than on patient need—it relies on it.

Advocacy Versus Stewardship?

If, in fact, many care decisions in the past were based *less* on improving the patient's health than on increasing the provider's wealth leading to massive overutilization, it seems reasonable to assume that creating financial incentives for professionals not to do things for patients will result in equally enormous underutilization—but not necessarily savings. Cost per case has been going up every year, and managed care premiums are going up (even operating revenues among the nation's top HMOs went up an average of 22% last year) (Aaron, 2004), whereas access among the insured and uninsured alike has been going down and public programs such as Medicaid are under financial duress. Critics claim that incentivizing professionals not to treat will lead to a situation in which the money that would have been spent on care will end up in the provider's pocket rather than the public's purse appears to be justified.

Now, in an interesting move, some bioethicians are suggesting that the advocacy model of professional ethics be modified to reflect contemporary circumstances. The primary ethical obligation of the professional would move from patient advocacy to responsible stewardship of society's resources, thus legitimizing the subordination of the patient's best interests to what, in a market-driven economy, amounts to the providers' profit!

Managed Care's Issues

To summarize, the many issues managed care poses for providers and health networks are crystallized in the moral problems occasioned by its shifting of the financial risks of care from insurer to provider. The issues occasioned by market-based reform include the following:

- The problems presented by clashes between public expectations and payer restrictions
- The corporatization of health service delivery and the cultural shift from humanitarian endeavor to business enterprise
- The depersonalization of treatment as time and money constraints stretch resources and the culture rewards efficient "business-like" behavior
- The underfunding of care for the poor and uninsured, even as these populations grow
- The restructuring of care and re-engineering of healthcare roles as the emphasis shifts from quality of care to conservation of resources
- Rapid mergers of both health plans and institutional providers with all the turmoil that represents as rules change, services are eliminated, and support services are minimized to save money
- The unhealthy competition inherent in market-based reform that posits profit-taking and market-share as the measures of successful performance
- The undermining of the professional ethic of advocacy
- The use of incentives that pander to greed and self-interest

The costs of sophisticated technologies and the ongoing care of increasingly fragile patients have pulled many other elements into what previously were considered "privileged" professional interactions. The fact that very few citizens indeed could pay out of their own pockets for the treatment and ongoing care they might need led to social involvement (few people remember that both widespread health insurance and public programs are relatively recent phenomena); however, whether in tax dollars or insurance premiums, other people's money is being spent on the patient's care. Clearly, those "other people" never intended to give either the patient or the professional open-ended access to their collective pocketbooks. Just what form their involvement ought to take is being tested as "managed care" attempts to control the costs. What limits are acceptable to providers: lower profit margins? Quality controls? Acceptable risk levels? What are acceptable limits for patients: restricted choice? Restricted mobility? Restricted access to high tech? What about the general public: decreased access to high tech? Higher taxes? Underserved populations? Abandonment of the sick/poor?

Which "techniques" are acceptable, and which are not: risk sharing with providers? Financial incentives for decision makers? Rationing access? Imposing behavioral parameters? The issues posed by market-based managed care cannot be adequately addressed merely in terms of social resources, nor will answers be found in subordinating human rights to practical materialism. Negotiating ethical guidelines for the "safe" handling of such problems to the good of individuals and of society requires a revitalization of the "old" values: the old commitment to master craftsmanship and altruism, the old emphasis on patient advocacy and human rights. These old values, however, must be applied with the "new" knowledge of lifestyle choices (and thus personal responsibility), likely outcomes (and thus reasonable options), and the limits of success (and thus fair redeployment of health resources) (see Appendix B: Glossary of Managed Care Terminology).

Case Study References

Aaron, H. J. (2004, January 15). The good, the bad and the ugly. *The Washington Spectator, 30.*

Annas, G. (1995). The market vs. medicine. *New England Journal of Medicine, 332,* 745–748.

Blecher, M. B. (1998). Burned on the street. *Hospitals and Health Networks, 72*(5), 22–26.

Burton, T. M. (1998, July 8). United HealthCare Corp finds drugs, tests are often underutilized. *The Wall Street Journal,* p. A1.

California Medical Association. (1996). *Knox-Keene health plan expenditures summary: Fiscal year 1994–1995.* San Francisco, CA: California Medical Association.

Center for Studying Health System Change. (1997). The trajectory of managed care. *Issues Brief, 9,* 1.

Hall, M. A. (1994). Disclosing rationing decisions: A reply to Paul S. Applebaum. *Milbank Quarterly, 72,* 645.

Langley, M. (1998, January 7). Nuns zeal for profits. . . *The Wall Street Journal,* p. A1.

Rosenthal, E. (1996, April 7). Groups predict New York hospital closings. *New York Times,* A11. Retrieved on February 9, 2010, from http://www.nytimes.com/1996/04/07/nyregion/groups-predict-new –york-hospitals-closings.html?pageswanted=1

Warren, T. (Ed.). (1999). The history of bioethics. *The Encyclopedia of Bioethics.* London: MacMillan.

CASE STUDY

The Advocacy Imperative
Elizabeth Summy

The role of advocacy by organizations has evolved dramatically from the early days when friends would share opinions and resources. Today, advocacy—the act of arguing on behalf of a particular issue, idea, person, or animal—is a highly sophisticated practice and a multimillion dollar enterprise. It exists in many forms: grassroots, the act of engaging those with similar interests around a specific action or agenda; grass tops, the act of teaching those with similar interest (i.e., nurses) about organizing themselves and their message to enhance effectiveness; and net roots, the act/practice of taking an advocacy agenda to and through the Internet in order to spread the message and engage participation through online dialogue and influence. The proliferation of social networking sites is revolutionizing the way people connect. Hospital CEOs are blogging to link the executive suite with the OR suite. Surgeons are "tweeting" from the operating room, and their patients are posting stories about their recovery on Facebook. These are truly unprecedented times.

Although the Internet has flattened the world, just because someone says (or writes) so, does not make it so. In advocacy, influence is predicated on credibility. To be credible one has to have the experience and perspective to explain the facts and tell the stories that provide context to the situation. In healthcare settings, clinicians have tremendous influence among peers, administration, and patients. How and when they choose to use their influence is both learned (through clinical training) and observed (influenced by the culture of an organization). Likewise, institutional providers have influence shaping the context in which clinicians provide care.

With health care emerging as one of the most important national issues, how to address our healthcare challenges will dominate the Congressional agenda and that of state legislatures, to a certain degree, in the upcoming years. It will also be the driver of advocacy agendas for the organizations that represent the providers and consumers of health care. In this case, examples of advocacy related to hospitals will be given from an organization that takes a system perspective and from engaged practitioners who take are concerned with the provision of care.

The American Hospital Association: Advocacy for System Change

For organizations, influence is "peddled" in many different ways. One of the most important is associations that represent a constituency with a shared mission. The role of advocacy by such associations has grown dramatically as the stakes for resources, prestige, and influence have grown. The members of these associations count on them to track issues that may impact their profession or the industry in which they work. Likewise the associations count on their members as being among their greatest assets. The credibility of a nurse talking with a legislator about how a particular bill will impact his or her work is very powerful. When that same nurse speaks on behalf of thousands of nurses and thousands of healthcare organizations, the voice is magnified. Understanding the environment and representing the interests of the people served are at the core of advocacy.

The American Hospital Association (AHA) is one of the oldest representative organizations in the health care sector. Organized in 1898, by a small group of hospital "superintendents" (the original terms for hospital directors) the AHA was initially a venue for the group to share among its members information and gather new ideas. While many groups are formally organized and recognized for their efforts on behalf of hospitals, the AHA is the largest. The AHA membership includes 5,717 hospitals, health systems, and postacute care organizations. It represents the majority of the nation's hospitals (public, private, not-for-profit, and special).

For nearly 115 years, the AHA has been a leader or contributor for a number of key activities that have shaped the healthcare field and hospital environment. Since the 1930s when the AHA played a key role in the organization of hospital insurance through Blue Cross, to the 1960s when the AHA's support was critical to the passage of Medicare to the present discussion of health care reform, the AHA has been at the fore of most key changes in the financing and delivery of care. Many think of the AHA as an influential lobby, which it is, but it is also a convener of conversations and content. It has played a variety of roles over the years in the identification of practices to improve hospital care and delivery through dialogue, advocacy, and dissemination of best practices. A "society of healthy communities where individuals reach their highest potential for health" is the vision behind the work of professional staff in Washington, DC and Chicago. Staff in Washington is focused on policy, communications, and partnerships to advance the interests of hospitals before Congress and the Executive Branch. The Chicago presence, lesser known but no less significant, focuses on serving members, both institutional and personal, through education, research, and publishing. The hospital advocacy agenda is really a cycle of activities that span a continuum from practice to legislation back to practice.

Advocacy is the strong voice that the AHA lends to the field. At the core of any advocacy activity is the desire to shape legislation and regulation the implementation of which affects the operations of an organization that provides feedback to inform policy and, ultimately, influences legislative and regulation. To illustrate, the AHA advocacy agenda focuses on legislation (i.e., reauthorization of the Children's Health Insurance Program) or regulation (i.e., Schedule H implementation). After passed or implemented, the AHA prepares the field for implementation through education, tools, and resources. It stays close to the field through conversations and gathers feedback to identify and inform other conversations about policy. These insights from the field are synthesized and embedded in the policy, which is used to influence the legislative or regulatory landscape, and the cycle starts all over again. The AHA represents a strong future through work on long-term system reform. It builds stronger, more efficient, and more effective acute care delivery through performance improvement activities.

Nurses Transforming Care at the Bedside: Advocacy for Quality Care

Another approach to improving the delivery of care can be seen in the project, Transforming Care at the Bedside (TCAB) is a joint effort by the Robert Wood Johnson Foundation and the Institute for Healthcare Improvement. Begun in 2001, it is a deliberate effort to engage nurses at the bedside in improving the quality of care that they deliver. The approach is intended to address the many serious problems in health care that were identified in the Institute of Medicine report "Crossing the Quality Chasm."

At its core, TCAB is about transformation, innovation, and engagement—of nurses, patients and families, and healthcare leadership. The principles for engagement are rooted in the science of high reliability, which calls on organizations to actively "seek to know what they don't know." Organizations must place a priority on learning, communication, and systems thinking. This means tracking small failures, resistance to oversimplification, sensitivity to operations, capacity for resilience, and deference to expertise, even as it shifts in the organization (Weick & Sutcliffe, 2007). Highly reliable organizations know that they are vulnerable to failures, but they work hard and smart to avoid failure while preparing for it so that they can minimize the impact.

Since inception, the TCAB has relied on the nurses and staff closest to the process to redesign the work to reduce waste. By reducing waste, nurses are able to spend more time at the bedside. Comprised of nurses, TCAB teams focus on three things: (1) generating innovative ideas to improve the safety and reliability of care, increase patient-centeredness of care, and shift staff effort from work of low value to patients to work of high value; (2) focusing on building effective care teams; and (3) developing systems that enhance the timeliness, reliability, and efficiency of delivering quality care (Robert Wood Johnson Foundation and the Institute for Healthcare Improvement, 2005).

TCAB is just one example that highlights the influence of nurses and their contributions to the success of a hospital. Numerous associations represent the professional interests of the nursing profession. These concepts of quality must also become integrated into the agenda of large membership organizations like the AHA. At their formation, all associations were created to share and gather ideas from others about their professional interests. Associations affirm the notion that the influence of many is more powerful than the interest of one. It is in that collection of ideas and perspectives that change can take root. It is important for nurses to embrace the notion that they can "lead where they are."

The Future of Advocacy for Acute Care Delivery/Hospitals

In a 2008, the Joint Commission issued a report containing guiding principles and actions for hospitals of the future in meeting care delivery challenges. The report recommended action in five core areas: economic viability (i.e., need to align performance and payment systems to meet quality and efficiency related goals), technology (i.e., make the business case and provide sustainable funding to support the widespread adoption of health information technology, patient-centered care (i.e., make adoption of patient-centered care values a priority for improving patient safety and patient and staff satisfaction), staffing (i.e., develop professional knowledge and skills necessary in a more complex healthcare environment), and hospital design (i.e., improve safety with evidence-based design principles and design flexibility in to the building to accommodate advances in medicine and technology) (The Joint Commission, 2008).

We are at the crossroads of decisions that we have never had to make before. The growth in healthcare costs cannot be sustained. In the history of health care, fundamental change has come about because of consumer demand (access), environmental factors (post-WWII recovery and the current recession), or financial incentives (both market and government driven). The shape of these decisions requires advocacy on the part of those who best understand what is required to provide to provide quality care to patients in a context that can be sustained.

References

The Joint Commission. (2008, November). *Healthcare at the crossroads: Guiding principles for the development of the hospital of the future.* Retrieved from http://www.aramarkhealthcare.com/RelatedFiles/JC_Hosptal_Future.pdf

Robert Wood Johnson Foundation and the Institute for Healthcare Improvement. (2005). *A new era in nursing: Transforming care at the bedside.* Retrieved from http://www.rwjf.org/pr/product.jsp?id=15704&topicid=1252

Weick, K., & Sutcliffe, K. (2007). *Managing the unexpected: Resilient performance in the age of uncertainty.* New York: John Wiley and Sons.

Photo Credits

Health Services Research

Donna M. Nickitas,
Keville Frederickson,
and
Jonathan Small

OVERVIEW

Predicting and responding to the healthcare demands of the 21st century will require resources from many fronts. Interdisciplinary partnerships will be needed to coordinate healthcare needs, to develop models for future needs, to determine appropriate resources, and to measure quality outcomes with respect to cost.

Because health services research is centrally focused on the ability to build knowledge and generate the evidence needed to craft the delivery of high-quality, cost-efficient health care, it will be the heuristic that leads to informed answers. This type of research provides the facts for improving how, when, and where health care is to be delivered; however, determining what criteria constitute "good" research is critical. If the research evidence is valid and reliable, then it has the potential to direct health policy that is innovative and fair, and that has a high level of cost benefit. For the peak and best use of resources, healthcare practices and delivery systems must be tracked and analyzed to determine improvement, progress over time, and most importantly factors that affect both quality and cost.

OBJECTIVES

- To understand the formal definition of health services research
- To determine factors that contribute to research that can serve as the foundation for health policy decisions
- To describe methods and strategies for health services research

- To explain how performance measurement and reporting systems are currently used
- To recognize how performance measurement data influence health policy decisions on process improvements that lead to improved quality and patient safety

(continues)

KEY TERMS

- Agency for Healthcare Research and Quality (AHRQ)
- Care coordination
- Centers for Medicare & Medicaid Services (CMS)
- Chronic illness
- Evidence-based practice
- Health Care Financing Administration

- Health disparity
- Health inequality
- Health policy meta-analysis
- Health services research
- Large data sets
- Process-of-care measures
- Quality indicators
- Quality measurement and improvement

Definition

Health services research is the multidisciplinary field of scientific investigation that studies how social factors, financing systems, organizational structures and processes, health technologies, politics, and personal behaviors affect access to health care and ultimately our health and well-being. The definition of health services research is constantly evolving and has been defined differently by a variety of experts and organizations; however, the most comprehensive definition is one by the Agency for Healthcare Research and Quality (AHRQ). It defines health services research as the analysis of how people get access to health care, how much care costs, and what happens to patients as a result of this care. The main goals of health services research are to identify the most effective ways to organize, manage, finance, and deliver high-quality care, reduce medical errors, and improve patient safety (AHRQ, 2007). Its re-search domains are individuals, families, organizations, institutions, communities, and populations. To effectively reshape the U.S. healthcare system to focus on objective evidence and outcomes rather than physician preference as the basis for treatment decisions, healthcare clinicians must recognize the importance of evidence-based practice (EBP) to guide healthcare delivery and the movement toward patient-centered care for many of the improvements in healthcare quality and efficiency. Rousseau (2006) describes evidence-based practice as a paradigm for making decisions that integrate the best available research evidence with decision-maker expertise and client/customer preferences to guide practice toward more desirable results. For evidence-based practice to make a difference in client outcome, it must include care coordination as well.

Care coordination ensures that client's needs and preferences are understood and that those needs and preferences are shared between clinicians, clients, and families as the client moves from one healthcare arena to another. As the number of healthcare clinicians and treatments involved in a patient's care has increased, the coordination of care has become more challenging. Less attention is being paid to the care that patients receive as they move from one setting to another (Naylor, 2006). In fact, a recent analysis of Medicare beneficiaries discharged from hospitals with a diagnosis of heart failure showed a 27% readmission rate within 30 days, a 39% readmission within 60 days, and almost 50% within 90 days (Jencks et al., 2009). Research has shown that care must be well coordinated to avoid waste, overuse, underuse, or misuse of prescribed medications and conflicting plans of care (Bodenheimer, 2008). Care coordination has a significant impact on health status and an effect on quality of life, especially for hospitalized older adults (Naylor & Keating, 2008). Older adults who experience several changes related to their care settings are at higher risks for adverse outcomes because of the numerous health issues that persist beyond hospital discharge (Naylor, 2004).

Care coordination becomes an even more important issue given the increasing number of persons with chronic health conditions. Bodenheimer (2008) suggests that clients with chronic health conditions may see up to 16 different physicians a year. When patients receive care from multiple providers, they are at greater risk for fragmented care because of communication breakdown, which often results in poor handoffs (Coleman & Berenson, 2004; Krizner, 2009; Naylor & Keating, 2008). As life expectancy increases so will chronic illnesses. In 2000, 125 million people in the United States were living with at least one chronic illness, a number that is expected to grow to 157 million by 2020. The number of individuals with multiple chronic conditions is expected to reach 81 million by 2020 (Bodenheimer, 2008). As individuals with chronic ill-

ness attempt to navigate the complex healthcare system and transition from one care setting to another, they will be unprepared or unable to manage their care. Again, incomplete or inaccurate transfer of information, poor communication, and a lack of appropriate follow-up care can lead to confusion and poor outcomes, including often preventable hospital readmissions and emergency department visits.

The Institute of Medicine has identified care coordination as a priority for national action because of its great importance to improve care (Adams & Corrigan, 2003). In May 2006, the National Quality Forum (NQF) endorsed a definition and framework for care coordination. NQF has defined care coordination as a "function that helps ensure that the patient's needs and preferences for health services and information sharing across people, functions, and sites are met over time" (National Quality Forum, 2009b). This framework includes five key dimensions: healthcare "home"; proactive plan of care and follow-up; communication; information systems; and transitions or hand-offs. These represent essential components and subcomponents for which performance measures are developed if care coordination is to be comprehensively measured and improved (see Table 1).

In 2008, the National Priority Partnership made care coordination one of six national priorities and has committed to working toward the following goals (National Quality Forum, 2009b):

- Improve care and achieve quality by facilitating and carefully considering feedback from all patients regarding coordination of their care
- Improve communication around medication information; work to reduce 30-day readmission rates
- Work to reduce preventable emergency department visits by 50%

Table 1 FRAMEWORK FOR CARE COORDINATION

1. Healthcare "home"—a source of usual care selected by the patient (such as a large or small medical group, a single practitioner, a community health center, or a hospital outpatient clinic). The medical home functions as the central point for coordinating care around the patient's needs and preferences.

2. Proactive plan of care and follow-up—an established and current care plan that anticipates routine needs and actively tracks up-to-date progress toward patient goals.

3. Communication—available to all team members, including patients and family—shared plan of care. All medical home team members work within the same plan of care and are measurably co-accountable for their contributions to the shared plan and achieving the patient's goals.

4. Information systems—the use of standardized, integrated electronic information systems with functionalities essential to care coordination is available to all providers and patients. Important characteristics include seamless interoperability; an evidence-based plan of care management; efficient and effective integration of patient information, laboratory, imaging, referrals, medications, social and community services, and self-management support; patient registries and population-based data, especially those promoted by local, state, and federal public health agencies; support for quality improvement and safety; case/disease management; decision support tools; and provider alerts and patient reminders.

5. Transitions or "hand-offs"—transitions between settings of care are a special case because currently they are fraught with numerous mishaps that can make care uncoordinated, disconnected, and unsafe. Some care processes during transition deserve particular attention:

   - Medication reconciliation
   - Follow-up tests and services
   - Changes in plan of care
   - Involvement of team during hospitalization, nursing home stay and so forth
   - Communications with persons who do not speak English well or at all

Using Research for Changes in Health Services

Health services research attempts to focus on practices that have strong evidence that they are effective in reducing the likelihood of harming a patient, are generalizable (i.e., they may be applied in multiple clinical care settings and/or for multiple types of patients), are likely to have a significant benefit to patient safety if fully implemented, and are usable by consumers, purchasers, providers, and researchers.

The evidence emerging from health services research is predominantly centered on quality measurement and improvement. These findings from quality and performance measures have historical roots within the American healthcare system dating back to the early 1900s. In 1910, Ernest Codman, MD, became one of the first healthcare professionals to propose a quality method system when he introduced what was known as the end-result system of hospital standardization. Codman learned to track every patient to measure the effectiveness of his or her treatment. Later, Codman created the minimum standard for hospitals to help diminish and eliminate substandard care. Only 13% of 692 hospitals initially met the minimum standard of care (Anderson & Schulke, 2008).

Efforts to improve or quality-control healthcare delivery were impacted by the quality movement. This movement which began in the industrial sector is identified with W. Edwards Deming and Joseph M. Juran. Deming is considered the pioneer in the quality management movement. As an advocate for quality, he identified that 80% to 85% of problems are system related with the rest of 15% to 20% associated with human error or worker produced. He advocated and adopted principles of management that encouraged organizations to increase quality while simultaneously reducing costs (by reducing waste, rework, staff attrition, and litigation while increasing customer loyalty). The key, as suggested by Deming, is to practice continual improvement and to think of manufacturing as a system, not as bits and pieces.

Juran's philosophy of quality is focused on three premises: quality planning, quality control, and quality improvement. This quality trilogy (planning, improvement, and control) seeks to define quality as fitness to serve, correct service the first time to meet customer's need and freedom from deficiencies (Anderson & Schulke, 2008). Before 1966, improvements in healthcare quality focused primarily on structure and included such activities as evaluating staffing levels, facility attributes, licensing, and accreditation. With the quality management work of Avedis Donabedian, the concept of quality management expanded to include the evaluation of processes and outcomes. This three-pronged approach (structure, process, and outcomes) launched the development of standards of care and clinical guidelines used by healthcare organizations today. In fact, it is the Donabedian model that drives the IOM in performance measurement with their six aims of quality, including: safe, effective, patient-centered, timely, efficient and equitable (IOM, 2006). Implementation of IOM guidelines by healthcare organizations support the creation of a mission and vision, development of a quality management plan, support for quality, use of evidence-based clinical practice, and utilization management. Studies and reports are available at the IOM Web site, http://www.iom.edu/CMS/8089.aspx.

Public reporting on measurement and outcomes by hospitals is relatively new. The Health Care Financing Administration (now renamed the Centers for Medicare & Medicaid Services [CMS]) was the first to attempt to measure and publicly report hospital outcomes that were reported from 1986 to 1993. The Health Care Financing Administration was forced to withdraw its mortality measures because of the widespread criticism it received from hospital administrators. In 2006, CMS reintroduced outcomes reporting with risk-adjusted mortality rates for heart failure and heart attack. The process-of-care measure shows how often hospitals give recommended treatments known to get the best results for patients with certain medical conditions or surgical procedures. This is one way to compare the quality of care that hospitals give.

The precursors of today's process-of-care quality measures began with the development of a modest set of Medicare quality indicators under the supervision of officials at the Health Standards and Quality Bureau. Indicators reflected a perceived need to acknowledge that the available data focused on care processes and could not capture or describe most of the factors influencing patient outcomes. In addition, quality indicators were developed for self-assessment and internal use by providers, avoiding much of the political pushback associated with public reporting. The indicators themselves were constructed by expert consensus among leading clinicians, based on the strong scientific foundation of large-scale clinical studies such as the Physicians' Health Study—a January 1988 study affirming that aspirin therapy prevents heart attack—and the

August 1988 Second International Study of Infarct Survival, which showed that aspirin therapy reduced heart attack mortality by 23% at a cost of $13 per life saved (Krumholz et al., 1995). Studies showed that about a quarter of patients who appeared to be candidates for aspirin treatment were not receiving it.

In 1999, the Joint Commission on Accreditation of Healthcare Organizations (now simply The Joint Commission) began to develop a set of core measures for hospitals, announcing its measure sets 2 years later. The measures for heart attack, heart failure, and pneumonia were nearly identical to those in nationwide use for 5 years by the Medicare program, but varied slightly in their specifications. The Joint Commission added measures addressing pregnancy and related conditions, extending the reach of quality measures to a large, new population beyond the older and disabled. With two similar public and private measurement systems for care of older persons operating side by side, providers asked for the compromise of a common set of measurement specifications, but it took 2 years of negotiations to produce a single nationally standardized set of 10 core measures in 2002. Agreement on these core measures lessened inefficiencies in hospital data gathering and reporting and coincided with the launch of the public–private Hospital Quality Alliance that called on hospitals to report publicly their performance using the new unified measure set. The core measures were formally adopted by act of Congress in 2003 as the basis for a reimbursement incentive for voluntary performance reporting. Subsequent legislation has repeatedly expanded both the measure set and the extent of the incentive for hospital reporting. All of the Hospital Quality Measures used by The Joint Commission and the CMS are endorsed by the NQF. These measures are also used for the "Hospital Quality Alliance: Improving Care through Information," a voluntary public reporting initiative led by the American Hospital Association, the Federation of American Hospitals, and the Association of American Medical Colleges. This initiative is supported by The Joint Commission, the CMS, the NQF, the AHRQ, the American Federation of Labor and Congress of Industrial Organizations, and the AARP (formerly American Association of Retired Persons). Hospital quality measures and other core measure data are part of the priority focus process that is used by The Joint Commission to help focus onsite survey activities. These data are also publicly reported on The Joint Commission's Quality Check Web site (www.qualitycheck.org). The public availability of performance measurement data facilitates user comparisons of hospital performance and permits comparisons against overall national rates.

Evidence Based Practice

One source of health services research is EBP. This approach to patient care stresses decision making, which is based not only on the available evidence but also on patient characteristics, situations, and preferences. It recognizes that care is individualized and ever changing and involves uncertainties and probabilities. EBP develops individualized guidelines of best practices to inform the improvement of whatever professional task is at hand. EBP is a philosophical approach that is in opposition to tradition. EBP began in 1971 when Professor Archie Cochrane scolded medical practitioners for their approach to care by saying that only health care based on research evidence should be reimbursed (Cochrane, 1971). At the same time, he contended that the only research that should be conducted and used would be the randomized controlled trial (RCT). The RCT is the highest level of research that includes randomization (all participants have an equal chance for assignment to the control and the experimental groups) at all levels of the research design, control, and intervention groups and represents an experimental design for a quantitative study. The key elements for using EBP are to determine the clinical problem or situation requirements, the level of EBP to be used, and how the outcome or evaluation of the intervention will be measured. Levels of EBP range from the RCT to perceptions of factors that influence treatment success by experts.

One of the most powerful approaches in determining factors that affect health and the effect of policy on health is a meta-analysis. A meta-analysis is a type of research in which the results of multiple studies are combined and analyzed to synthesize and summarize the results. In this way, one statistical outcome is produced to indicate the effectiveness of such things as a treatment outcome or factors that place populations at risk for an illness or disease. In order to conduct a meta-analysis, the terminology and definitions need to be systematic and have common meanings. For example, in attempting to present research data on health disparities, there were at least five different definitions of the criteria that constitute a health disparity. As a result, when synthesizing data on health disparities, it is difficult to know which studies to include as well as the frame of reference used to establish the definition.

Systems to stratify evidence by quality have been developed, such as this one by the U.S. Preventive Services Task Force for ranking evidence about the effectiveness of treatments or screening (Melnyk et al., 2005):

- Level I: evidence obtained from at least one properly designed RCT.
- Level II-1: evidence obtained from well-designed controlled trials without randomization.
- Level II-2: evidence obtained from well-designed cohort or case-control analytic studies, preferably from more than one center or research group.
- Level II-3: evidence obtained from multiple time series with or without the intervention. Dramatic results in uncontrolled trials might also be regarded as this type of evidence.
- Level III: opinions of respected authorities, based on clinical experience, descriptive studies, or reports of expert committees.

EXEMPLAR OF EBP FROM A PRIVATE ORGANIZATION: THE COCHRANE LIBRARY

The Cochrane Library consists of reviews of research that are evaluated independently using rigorous criteria for evaluating research that is necessary for making informed decisions about practice by healthcare providers. This is an outstanding repository of seven databases with information that is categorized in many ways, including relevance for specific professions such as nursing, physical therapy, and medicine as well as according to illnesses, body systems, and health promotion/disease prevention. The databases also include research evidence related to patient safety issues, financial and economic reports, and assessment of technology and methodology for conducting EBP. Overall, there are almost 750,000 records related to EBP. By searching for "health policy," 60 entries were returned with titles such as "Policy interventions implemented through sporting organizations for promoting healthy behavior change," "Pharmaceutical policies: effects of cap and co-payment on rational drug use," and "Methods of consumer involvement in developing healthcare policy and research, clinical practice guidelines and patient information material." In summary, the Cochrane Library is an excellent source for research related to health and health services policy. The research is evaluated using high standards and reported in a way that can be applied to interventions by healthcare providers as well as used to guide and direct policy.

FEDERAL EXEMPLAR: AGENCY OF HEALTH CARE RESEARCH AND QUALITY

AHRQ is the lead Federal agency charged with supporting research designed to improve the quality of health care, reduce its cost, address patient safety and medical errors, and broaden access to essential services. AHRQ sponsors and conducts research that provides evidence-based information on healthcare outcomes; quality; and cost, use, and access. The information helps healthcare decision makers—patients and clinicians, health system leaders, and policy makers—to make more informed decisions and improve the quality of healthcare services.

One category of research supported by AHRQ is the Evidence-Based Practice Program. Twelve five-year contracts have been awarded to institutions in the United States and Canada to serve as EBP centers. The EBP centers develop evidence reports and technology assessments based on rigorous, comprehensive syntheses and analyses of relevant scientific literature, emphasizing explicit and detailed documentation of methods, rationale, and assumptions (http://www.ahrq.gov;/2009). Their publications are organized in three categories:

- Evidence reports/technology assessments
- Evidence reports/technology assessment summaries
- Technical reviews and summaries

Beginning in 1999, the first EBP report was published. This first report presented the evidence on systematic review of the literature regarding the diagnosis of sleep apnea (which is identified now as "out of date") and the most recent, number 177, published February 2009 on the topic of complementary and alternative medicine in back pain utilization. The standards for these publications are very specific.

EBP AND SOCIAL POLICY

There are increasing demands for social policy and other decisions related to programs run by government and non-government organizations (NGOs) to be based on sound evidence as to their effectiveness. This has seen an increased emphasis on the use of a wide range of evaluation approaches directed at obtaining evidence about social programs of all types. A research collaboration called the Campbell Collaboration has been set up in the social policy area to provide evidence for evidence-based social policy decision making. This collaboration follows the approach pioneered by the Cochrane Collaboration in the health sciences (Cochrane, 1971). Using an evidence-based approach to social policy has a number of advantages because it has the potential to decrease the tendency to run programs that are socially acceptable (e.g., drug education in schools) but that often prove to be ineffective when evaluated (Frederickson, 2007).

Quality of Care and Equality of Care

A primary area for health services research has been the quality of care provided by healthcare agencies. Healthcare providers are held accountable for the care that is rendered to the public through many mechanisms. Quality of care is evaluated by accrediting agencies, the federal government health-related programs, and the insurance companies. The Institute of Medicine defines quality as "the degree to which health services for individuals and populations increase the likelihood of desired health outcomes and are consistent with current professional knowledge." Attributes of patient care include improved safety, improved outcomes, and improved satisfaction.

In addition, standards for quality care are a priority for determining equality in health care. For example, in a large data set analysis of three states—California, Florida and New York—it was found that blacks were not afforded the same level of treatment for a myocardial infarction as non-Hispanic whites (Bennett, 2004).

One landmark study conducted by the RAND corporation (McGlynn et al., 2003) in collaboration with the Community Quality Index (a collateral study of the Community Tracking Study) determined the extent to which 439 indicators of quality of care were implemented for 30 acute and chronic illnesses and also included evidence of preventive care. In addition, participants were sampled in 12 large metropolitan areas throughout the United States to determine the extent to which recommended standards of medical care were actually implemented. Through a health history interview and an examination of health records, patient health assessments and interventions were analyzed.

The indicators of quality of care used parts of the RAND Quality Assessment Tools system. The leading causes of illness, death, and seeking health care for different age groups formed the basis for selecting the conditions to be studied, as well as preventive strategies for each of the study conditions. For example, the condition of hypertension had 27 medical care indicators and included interventions such as lifestyle modification for patients with mild hypertension and pharmacotherapy for uncontrolled mild hypertension.

The RAND study serves as an exemplar of health services research because the study exceeded most criteria for quality and reliable research. Beginning with sampling, the study included representative cities throughout the United States, accounting for geographic diversity. Reliability of the data was implemented through the use of two approaches for data collection. Participant interviews were conducted as well as the examination of their health records to corroborate interview data.

Health Disparity

Although there is no universal agreement on a definition of health disparities, the term is generally used to refer to gaps in health care along racial, ethnic, and socioeconomic lines. Health disparities do not encompass all variations in health or health care but, rather, specifically the experience in which less fortunate populations systematically experience worse health or increased health risks than more privileged communities (Braveman, 2006). As defined by The Health Resources and Services Administration, health disparities are "population-specific differences in the presence of disease, health outcomes or access to health care" (Goldberg et al., 2004).

In measuring health inequality, the most common method has been to take more and less advantaged social groups and compare the two. To determine where a social group is situated, socioeconomic advantages are often determined by educational achievement, employment characteristics, income/expenditures, net worth, health insurance, or geographical location. In the United States, because health inequality is most often associated with racial and ethnic differences, health disparities have long been measured by comparing minority groups with whites or non-Hispanic/Latino whites (Braveman, 2006).

The problem with measuring health inequality is the variations in defining terms such as health inequality, health disparities, and racial and ethnic disparities in health care. For research to be useful, a clear identification must be made of what makes a group of people quantifiably measurable against another social group. In order to do so, a proposed definition to guide measurement must be presented that encompasses the significance of social standing as well as comparisons made between groups with different social status. A more concise definition for health disparity than the one presented here might be this: Health disparities are possibly preventable discrepancies in health among groups of people who are more and less privileged socially—differences that systematically place communally less fortunate populations at additional inconvenience on health. This definition succeeds in identifying target populations for comparison and includes both similar and dissimilar social ranks (Braveman, 2006).

When measuring or defining health disparity/inequality, the certain conditions that produce illnesses in one population might not have the same effect in other populations. In addition, the course of an illness or disease differs between a person or a group with full health insurance as compared with those without a similar social safety net. The patient who does not have access to or has limited access to necessary treatment could be forced to pay for their treatments out of pocket, thus forcing them and their family into a state of poverty, bringing on even more lethal health consequences (Fiscella et al., 2000).

Although the term health disparity is used often in the field of public health, there remain many different attitudes on what the term actually means. Based on different dictionary definitions and long-held personal beliefs, these differences have continued to cause problems when surveying research over a wide spectrum. There is, however, no disagreement about what health disparity/inequality ultimately reflects—a problem that needs immediate attention and fixing.

Recognizing the Influence of Culture

Outcomes that either measure health disparities or factors that contribute to health disparities use criteria that are often culture bound. The work of Gilligan (1982) first identified the gender bias of instruments used to measure ethical development. Her work focused on the male orientation that was inherent in both the development and norming of Kohlberg and Lickona's instrument on Moral Development (1976). Gilligan's work represented an early acknowledgment that an important factor in measurement is the conceptual perspective of the instrument as well as the population of origin for instrument development and testing. The focus with health disparities and health policy is directed toward the outcomes and effects of measurement across cultures. For example, to measure health beliefs among Mexican immigrants, or blacks, the psychometric properties will differ according to the specific ethnic group or race, particularly when the instrument was developed and validated on white Americans. For example, Fillenbaum et al. (1990) examined seven cognitive screening or neuropsychological tests in relation to clinical diagnosis. The authors reported that most measures, when adjusted for race and education, had lower specificities for blacks than for whites. They suggested that most measures were culturally or educationally biased. Similarly, Teresi (2001) reviewed studies of Differential Item Functioning and item bias in the direct cognitive assessment measures with respect to race/ethnicity and education. Specifically, item performance varied across groups that differ in terms of education, ethnicity, and race (Jones & Gallo, 2002).

Another factor that influences the value of outcome measures is the validity and reliability of translations. Instruments that have been rated as highly reliable and valid may not be so, once translated. One example is the Mini-Mental State Exam (Teresi et al., 1995), which includes a question about certainty of a fact, stating "no ifs, ands, or buts." This item was more easily understood by Hispanics than by non-Hispanics because the translation into Spanish and the cultural context were more easily understood (Teresi, 2001). As a result, a Hispanic client may be identified as cognitively more coherent than he is, meaning that the Hispanic client would be less likely to receive treatment for confusion or dementia than the one who is non-Hispanic. Research that is based on instruments that have been translated is prone to findings that reflect differences based on subgroups such as race, ethnicity, education, or socioeconomic status.

Another bias that may occur emanates from cultural, ethnic, or differences in backgrounds when research methods include interviewers or raters. In this instance, the evaluators may identify cues that are not culturally congruent, or the evaluator may transmit cues that have very different meanings cross-culturally. van Ryn and Burke (2000) examined the impact of physicians' perceptions and beliefs on patient diagnosis and treatment. They reported that physicians (mainly white) were more likely to rate white patients as more educated and more rational than black patients even after controlling for patient's actual educational level. Although this finding can be simply explained by adherence to stereotypical beliefs that are inherently discriminatory, communication barriers such as differences in the patient's use of language when referring to symptoms or symptom expression and/or interpretation of health-related behavior could possibly influence physicians' ratings across racial groups.

In summary, research that is used to formulate health policies related to health disparities must take into account variables that may have affected outcome such as cultural/racial/ethnic biases in the development and norming of the instrument, translational inconsistencies, and interviewer bias. These inherent differences may account for differences and inconsistencies in diagnoses, treatment, and outcomes.

Chronic Illness

Encompassing a wide range of diseases, chronic refers to all disorders that are long lasting or recurrent. The term is used to specifically describe the track of a disease or its rate of inception and advance. Defined by the U.S. National Center for Health Statistics, a chronic disease is one lasting 3 months or more. Along with being identified by how long they last, chronic illnesses are also most often characterized by an inability to be cured with medication or prevented by vaccine. Each year, millions of Americans suffer through the negative effects of living with chronic illnesses; 133 million people, or almost half of all Americans, live with a chronic condition. That number is projected to increase by more than one percent per year by 2030, resulting in an estimated chronically ill population of 171 million.

Almost half of all people with chronic illness have multiple conditions. As a result, many managed care and integrated delivery systems have taken a great interest in correcting the many deficiencies in current management of diseases such as diabetes, heart disease, depression, asthma, and others (Wagner et al., 1996).

Those deficiencies include the following:

- Rushed practitioners not following established practice guidelines
- A lack of care coordination
- A lack of active follow-up to ensure the best outcomes
- Patients inadequately trained to manage their illnesses

Overcoming these deficiencies will require nothing less than a transformation of health care, from a system that is essentially reactive—responding mainly when a person is sick to one that is proactive and focused on keeping a person as healthy as possible (Wagner et al., 1996).

One approach to chronic illness based on research is the Chronic Care Model (CCM). This model focuses on information and strategies for the management of chronic illnesses and originated from a synthesis of scientific literature undertaken by The MacColl Institute for Healthcare Innovation in the early 1990s. The Robert Wood Johnson Foundation funded further work on the model, which included an extensive review by an advisory panel of experts and was then compared with the features of leading chronic illness management programs across the United States. In 1998, the model was again revised, and the Robert Wood Johnson Foundation incorporated the model as the basis for their program Improving Chronic Illness Care. This center offers research, practice, and dissemination guidelines as well as protocols for quality improvement. The value of the CCM is the utilization of EBP to evaluate current research and incorporate cutting-edge outcomes into the model. These have been identified as the Breakthrough Series Collaborative, which serves as the approach for quality improvement (http://www.improvingchroniccare.org/index.php?p=The_Chronic_Care_Model&s=2). According to the Improving Chronic Illness Care, a chronic condition is any condition that requires ongoing adjustments by the affected person and interactions with the healthcare system.

To speed the transition, Improving Chronic Illness Care created the Chronic Care Model, which summarizes the basic elements for improving care in health systems at the community, organization, practice, and patient levels.

Considering the serious nature of these illnesses, it is alarming to find that numerous reports on medical care have consistently found major holes in the course and result of chronic illness treatment. Whether the patients surveyed were receiving managed care or not, major deficiencies were found. According to evidence, patients suffering from chronic illnesses are often given limited help from their insurance providers as they struggle to keep up basic function and quality of life while managing their diseases. This limited care is sometimes caused, for example, by a doctor's failure to recognize their patient's level of understanding about their condition, ability to function, or their perception of self-management. A deficiency of such things can ultimately lead to a lack of useful care and the want for restorative, supportive, and instructive services. Although managed care continues to grow, at the core it remains a system that persists in delivering subpar treatment for the chronically unwell, threatening the integrity of the entire system.

Although many factors play a role in determining the lack of care a patient is going to receive, most often it is the acute care orientation of medical practice. This approach to medical care severely limits the ability of medical caregivers to adequately fulfill the quantifiable and self-coping requirements of chronically ill patients. Most medical practices are designed and trained to respond to acute medical disorders, which creates a method of diagnosing and treating based on patient initiated visits and goals. These quick meetings, usually lasting in the range of 15 minutes, target the relieving of symptoms rather than evaluation and recovery of purpose. Often physicians are untrained and too overloaded to take up the task of organizing care, advising, and following up treatment.

Conclusion

This chapter provides an introduction into health services research as a multidisciplinary field of scientific investigation that examines how social factors, financing systems, organizational structures and processes, health technologies, and per-

Figure 1 Model for improvement of chronic illness care.

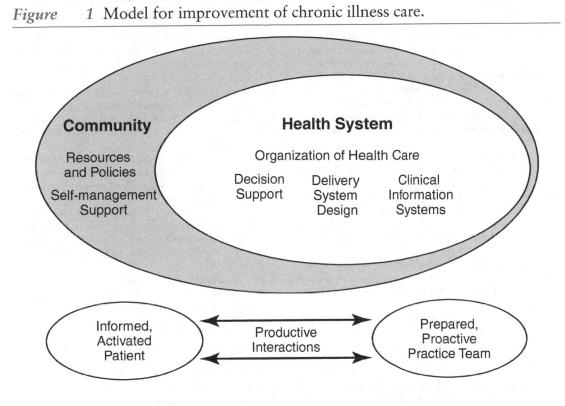

Functional and Clinical Outcomes

Source: Wagner, E. H. (1998). Chronic disease management: What will it take to improve care for chronic illness? *Eff Clin Pract, 1,* 2–4. Used with permission of the American College of Physicians.

sonal behaviors affect access to health care, the quality and cost of health care, and quantity and quality of life. The focus of research studies in health services are often centered on research issues that examine outcomes of the individual, family, organizational, institutional, community, and population level. For example health service research will seek to examine how people get access to health care, how much care costs, and what happens to patients as a result of this care.

While the primary goal of health services research is to identify the most effective ways to organize, manage, finance, and deliver high quality care; reduce medical errors; and improve patient safety. Health services research is grounded in theory and exists to perform research that can be applied by physicians, nurses, health managers and administrators, and other health professionals and stakeholders who make decisions or deliver care in the healthcare system. Finally, the findings and products that result from health services research can be used to improve the design of healthcare benefits, develop new policies to optimize the way health care is financed and paid for, facilitate access to healthcare services, and improve patient outcomes.

References

Adams, K., & Corrigan, J. (2003). *Priority areas for national action: transforming health care. Committee on identifying priority areas for quality improvement.* Board on Health Services, and Institute of Medicine. Washington, DC: The National Academies Press.

AHRQ, Agency for Healthcare Research and Quality. (2007). National Healthcare Quality & Disparities Report. Retrieved February 13, 2010, from http://www.ahrq.gov/qual/qrdr07.htm

Anderson, K. M., & Schulke, K. (2008). Linking public accountability to quality improvement. *Health & Hospital Network, 82*(11), 60–61.

Ashton, C. M., Haidet, P., Paterniti, D. A., Collins, T. C., Gordon, H. S., & O'Malley, K. (2003). Racial and ethnic disparities in the use of health services: bias, preferences, or poor communication? *Journal of General Internal Medicine, 18,* 146–152.

Bennett, K. (2004). *Individual hospital effects upon the measurement of racial disparities in the treatment of myocardial infarction.* Doctoral Dissertation, University of South Carolina.

Bodenheimer, T. (2008). Coordinating care: A perilous journey through the health care system. *New England Journal of Medicine, 358,* 1064–1071.

Braveman, P. (2006). Health disparities and health equity. *Annual Review of Public Health, 27,* 167–194.

Calkins, E., Boult, C., Wagner, E. H., & Pacala, J. (1999). *New ways to care for older people: Building systems based on evidence.* New York: Springer.

Cochrane, A. L. (1989). *Effectiveness and efficiency random reflections on health services* (Memoir Club Publications). New York: B M J Books.

Cochrane, A. L. (1971). *Effectiveness and Efficiency: Random Reflections of Health Services* (2nd ed.), London: Nuffield Provincial Hospitals Trust.

Coleman, E. A., & Berenson, R. A. (2004). Improving patient care. Lost in transition: Challenges and opportunities for improving the quality of transitional care. *Annals of Internal Medicine, 141*(7), 533–536.

Department of Health Services. (2009). *What is health services research?* Retrieved April 20, 2009, from http://depts.washington.edu/hserv/hs-research-definitions

Fillenbaum, G., Heyman, A., Williams, K., Prosnitz, B., & Burchett, B. J. (1990). Sensitivity and specificity of standardized screens of cognitive impairment and dementia among elderly black and white community residents. *Clinical Epidemiology, 43*(7), 651–660.

Fiscella, K., Franks, P., Gold, M. R., & Clancy, C. M. (2000). Inequality in quality. *Journal of the American Medical Association, 283,* 2579–2584.

Frederickson, K. (2007). Evidence-based practice: A reliable source to access interventions for youth risk behavior. *Research and Theory for Nursing Practice: An International Journal, 21*(3), 149–152.

Gilligan, C. (1982). *In a different voice.* Cambridge, Massachusetts: Harvard University Press.

Goldberg, J., Hayes, W., & Huntley, J. (2004, November). *Understanding health disparities.* Health Policy Institute of Ohio.

Jencks, S. F., Williams, M. V., & Coleman, E. A. (2009). Rehospitalizations among patients in the Medicare fee-for-service program. *New England Journal of Medicine, 360*(14), 1418–1428.

Jones, R. N., & Gallo, J. J. (2002). Education and sex differences in the Mini Mental State Examination: Effects of differential item functioning. *Journal of Gerontology Series B—Psychological Sciences and Social Sciences, 37,* P548–P558.

Kenny, S. J., Smith, P. J., Goldschmid, M. G., Newman, J. M., Herman, W. H. (1993). Survey of physician practice behaviors related to diabetes mellitus in the U.S. Physician adherence to consensus recommendations. *Diabetes Care, 16,* 1507–1510.

Kohlberg, L., & Lickona, R. (Ed.). (1976). *Moral stages and moralization: The cognitive-developmental approach. Moral development and behavior: Theory, research and social issues.* Holt, NY: Rinehart and Winston.

Krizner, K. (2009). Transitional care lacking in elderly. Managed healthcare executive e-news. Retrieved May 4, 2009, from http://managedhealthcareexecutive.modernmedicine.com/mhe/News+Analysis/Transitional-care-lacking-in-elderly/ArticleStandard/Article/detail/574706

Krumholz, H. M., Seeman, T. E., Merrill, S. S., Mendes de Leon, C. F., Vaccarino, V., Silverman, D. I., et al. (1995). Lack of association between cholesterol and coronary heart disease mortality and morbidity and all-cause mortality in persons older than 70 years. *Journal of the American Medical Association, 272*(17), 1335–1340.

McGlynn, E. A., Asch, S. M., Adams, J., Keesey, J., Hicks, J., DeCristofaro, A., & Kerr, E. A. (2003). The quality of health care delivered to adults in the United States. *New England Journal of Medicine, 348*(26), 2635–2645.

Melnyk, B. M. (2005). *Evidence-based practice in nursing & healthcare a guide to best practice.* Philadelphia: Lippincott Williams & Wilkins.

Naylor, M. D. (2004). Transitional care for older adults: a cost effective model. *LDI Issue Brief, 9*(6). Retrieved May 4, 2009, from http://www.commonwealthfund.org/usr_doc/LDI_issuebrief_Naylor.pdf

Naylor, M. D. (2006). Transitional care: A critical dimension of the home healthcare quality agenda. *Journal for Healthcare Quality: Promoting Excellence in Healthcare, 28*(1), 48–54.

Naylor, M. D., & Keating, S. A. (2008). Transitional care: moving patients from one setting to another. *American Journal of Nursing, 108*(9), 58–63.

National Quality Forum. (2009a). *NQF-endorsed definition and framework for measuring care coordination.* Retrieved April 2009, from http://www.qualityforum.org/pdf/ambulatory/txCareCoordination%20defandframe08-02-06.pdf

National Quality Forum. (2009b). *Endorsing preferred practices and performance measures for measuring and reporting care coordination.* Retrieved February 13, 2010, from http://www.qualityforum.org/projects/ongoing/care-coordination

Partnership for Solutions, Johns Hopkins University, for the Robert Wood Johnson Foundation. (2004). Chronic conditions: Making the case for ongoing care. Baltimore, MD: University of Maryland.

Perrin, J. M., Homer, C. J., Berwick, D. M., Woolf, A. D., Freeman, J. L., & Wennberg, J. E. (1989). Variations in rates of hospitalization of children in three urban communities. *New England Journal of Medicine, 320,* 1183–1187.

Raines, J. C. (2008). *Evidence-based practice in school mental health.* New York: Oxford University Press.

Ramirez, M., Ford, M., Steward, A., & Teresi, J. (2005). Measurement issues in health disparities research. *Health Services Research, 40*(5 Pt 2), 1640–1657.

Rousseau, D. M. (2006). Is there such a thing as 'evidence-based management'? *Academy of Management Review, 31,* 256–269.

Stockwell, D. H., Madhavan, S., Cohen, H., Gibson, G., & Alderman, M. H. (1994). The determinants of hypertension awareness, treatment, and control in an insured population. *American Journal of Public Health, 84,* 1768–1774.

Teresi, J. A. (2001). Statistical methods for examination of differential item functioning (DIF) with applications to cross cultural measurement of functional, physical and mental health. *Journal of Mental Health and Aging, 7,* 31–40.

Teresi, J. A., Golden, R. R., Cross, P., Gurland, B., Kleinman, M., & Wilder, D. (1995). Item bias in cognitive screening measures: Comparisons of elderly white,

Afro-American, Hispanic and high and low education subgroups. *Journal of Clinical Epidemiology, 48,* 173–183.

van Ryn, M., & Burke, J. (2000). The effect of patient race and socio-economic status on physicians' perceptions of patients. *Social Science & Medicine, 50*(6), 813–828.

Wagner, E. H., Austin, B. T., & Von Korff, M. (2001). Improving outcomes in chronic illness. *Managed Care Quarterly, 4*(2), 12–25.

Wagner, E. H., Austin, B. T., & Von Korff, M. (1996). Organizing care for patients with chronic illness. *Milbank Quarterly, 74,* 511–544.

Wagner, E. H. (1998). Chronic disease management: What will it take to improve care for chronic illness? *Eff Clin Pract, 1,* 2–4.

Wagner, E. H., Austin, B. T., Davis, C., Hindmarsh, M., Schaefer, J., & Bonomi, A. (2001). Improving chronic illness care: Translating evidence into action. *Health Aff (Millwood), 20,* 64–78.

CASE STUDY

Influence of Politics on Health Care Policy and Research

Carol F. Roye

In recent years, many barriers have been put in the way of women who simply want to obtain reproductive health care. These barriers are politically and ideologically driven. They have nothing to do with optimum health care. In fact, they often stand in the way of good health care. As I write, at the end of 2008, we have been living with increasing politicization of science and healthcare policy, to the detriment of patient well-being. This is not the first historical era when health care has been adversely impacted by politics, but it is certainly the worst that I have experienced.

A main concern for me was the Global Gag Rule. In 1984, President Reagan had implemented a policy at a world population meeting in Mexico City. Formally called the Mexico City Policy, the rule is often referred to as the Gag Rule because, in essence, the policy gags family planning providers. The Gag Rule is a ban on U.S. family planning aid—including shipments of free condoms and contraceptives—to foreign nongovernmental organizations and clinics that even mention the term abortion or advocate legalizing abortion in their country. In 1992, when Bill Clinton was elected, I felt tremendous relief because I knew patients and women around the world would benefit. We were not disappointed. President Clinton rescinded the Gag Rule, but President George W. Bush reinstated it on his first full day in office.

As a result, many clinics in underresourced countries have foregone U.S. aid. They gave up shipments of contraceptives, including condoms, which could have been used to curb the spread of HIV/AIDS and to prevent unwanted pregnancies. Many poor women around the world had come to depend on those shipments for family planning. The result of the Gag Rule has been, no doubt, more unwanted pregnancies, which leads to higher maternal and infant mortality and likely more cases of HIV/AIDS.

I was very acutely aware of the danger of the Gag Rule, as I had worked under what was essentially a domestic Gag Rule in the late 1980s. Between 1988 and 1993, Title X legislation prohibited doctors and nurses from providing information about abortion, even if the patient requested it. Although this domestic gag rule was not enforced nationwide, it was in effect in certain Title X funded clinics, including the inner-city clinic in New York City where I was a nurse practitioner.

Many of my patients were teen mothers. Sometimes they came to see me with a second unwanted pregnancy. When I asked representatives of the federal government who came to our clinic what I could tell a tearful, frightened 16-year-old who asked about abortion, I was told to say that it is "outside the purview of what I can discuss." Essentially, I was being told by representatives of the federal government that I would have to withhold information from my patients. I was not even supposed to refer pregnant patients to a prenatal clinic where a doctor or nurse might mention abortion as an option.

It was a good day for women's health when President Clinton rescinded the Gag Rule. Unfortunately, it was reinstated in January 2001 and has been in place ever since. Many professionals expect that President Obama will rescind the Gag Rule (Roye, 2009).

President Obama will have more health policy issues than the Gag Rule to contend with. President Bush left a parting jab at women's health. On December 18, 2008, just 1 month before the end of the Bush Administration, the Department of Health and Human Services introduced a regulation that was purportedly aimed at protecting workers with moral objections to abortion. The rule says that healthcare workers cannot be discriminated against for refusing to participate in procedures to which they object; however, the rule is so broad that the list of procedures can essentially be limitless, including provision of family planning or even vaccinations for that matter. Similarly, the definition of healthcare worker is so broad that it can include all workers and volunteers in a medical setting, including people who do not provide health care, such as janitors. The regulation went into effect 30 days after December 18, just a few days short of the Obama inauguration. Thus, if a woman goes to a federally funded clinic and requests contraception and the janitor objects to contraception and does not want to clean a facility where contraception is dispensed, his or her objections must be upheld, and the patient is denied care (Berger, 2009). Furthermore, there are already regulations that protect health workers' rights not to violate their religious beliefs.

The impact of this imposition of ideology on health policy is felt in the aggregate, as described previously here. Of course, it also has very personal ramifications for patients.

For example, recently I was sitting at the desk in my exam room in a large pediatric practice in a low-income neighborhood in New York City. The next patient to come in, Jasmine S., was an 18-year-old college freshman. She and her boyfriend had begun having intercourse. She told me that he is her first sexual partner. They use a condom most of the time, but she knows that she is at risk for pregnancy. After I examined her, we chatted about the birth control methods that are currently available. She decided that the vaginal ring would work best for her. I prescribed the ring and urged her to continue using condoms. I told her how to use both methods, and the important role of each in assuring her reproductive health.

Two weeks later, Jasmine came in for a scheduled appointment, to review the results of the laboratory tests we had done. When I asked her how she liked the ring, she told me she could not get it.

The pharmacist had written something on the back of the prescription. She handed it to me, and I saw that he had written "P/A." Not knowing what that meant, I called the pharmacist. He told me that she needed a prior authorization from her insurance company, and I thought I had heard incorrectly. Yes, we needed a prior authorization when my 6-month-old granddaughter needed neurosurgery and my 8-year-old daughter needed eye surgery. But is prior authorization to get the ring necessary? I called her insurance company, Fidelis, a Medicaid HMO in New York. The agent asked me whether the patient needed the ring for contraception or some other reason. I told her that I did not want to discuss the patient's private information with her. Indeed, that would have been violating the patient's confidentiality. She responded that without such information the patient could not get the medication.

Even with that information, the patient could not get the medication. I could have said that the patient has very irregular periods and I want to regulate them with the ring; however, I chose to be honest and, with Jasmine's permission, told the woman on the phone that it was for contraception. Fidelis is a Catholic company and therefore does not pay for contraception. The patient never asked to be put in a Catholic HMO. She was just assigned to that insurance plan. The Fidelis agent told me that another company pays for contraception for Fidelis patients. I spent a half hour on the phone with the other company. It was a long and difficult road to take to get a simple prescription. It was trying even for me, and I know how to navigate the healthcare system. Jasmine would probably never have gotten her contraception if I had not intervened. The barriers would have been insurmountable. Jasmine was not the only one of my patients to have difficulty filling her birth control prescription because of Fidelis.

Now, think about the plight of another patient, Marianna. She is typical of many of the patients I see. Marianna is 12 years old. She had her first period 6 months ago. This month her period has lasted for over 4 weeks and is still not going away. She comes into the clinic, and we check her for anemia. Her hemoglobin is 10.2. Marianna is anemic—no surprise given the fact that she has been bleeding for 4 weeks. How can we treat her? Of course, I will prescribe iron tablets for her, but that is a band aid.

We need to stop the bleeding. There is really only one way to stop the bleeding. She needs to take birth control pills. I give Marianna and her mother the prescriptions and sent them out. They are smiling, relieved to know that the bleeding can be stopped.

When they get to the pharmacy, however, the pharmacist wrote P/A on the back of the prescription because Marianna has Fidelis insurance. Perhaps he just refused to give her the birth control pills because he does not believe in contraception and is horrified at the thought that this 12-year-old needs birth control—and her mother is letting her use it. He will not give her the contraception, although he does give her the iron. Marianna's mother has to get to work and cannot afford to take any more time. She will not have a day off for 2 more weeks. Thus, Marianna continues to take her iron, and she continues to bleed; hopefully she will be okay until she can come back to the clinic.

The standards of good health care do not change every 4 to 8 years; however, health policy can change dramatically according to the theology or ideology of the presidential administration. As a result, Americans' health can be jeopardized or enhanced at the whim of the prevailing political winds.

The same holds true on a state-by-state basis, depending on the politics of the state. In New York State, for example, a teenager can obtain an abortion without parental knowledge or consent. The regulation is written that way so that teens are not afraid to seek health care when confronted by an unwanted pregnancy. In other states, however, things are quite different. In 34 states, teens must obtain parental consent. In some states, such as Mississippi, for example, consent of both parents is required. In Mississippi, there is only one clinic where women can obtain an abortion. Thus, women—adolescent or adult—who do not have the wherewithal to travel cannot get an abortion. Are they turning to back alley abortionists? Are they trying to do their own abortions—perhaps with information gleaned on the internet? Possibly. We do not know for sure.

Political winds and whims affect community health and individual health, to be sure; however, it does not stop there. Politics also affects health research. Research sets the stage for healthcare advances in the future; however, over the last 8 years, research into certain politically controversial topics such as HIV prevention in adolescents has been thwarted. For example, during the Clinton administration, I was awarded a grant by the National Institutes of Health to study the effectiveness of a program to promote condom use by sexually active teenage girls who were using hormonal contraception such as birth control pills.

While conducting that study, the Clinton administration ended and that of George W. Bush began. I read in the newspapers about something that was being called "the hit list," which listed several hundred federally funded studies that were considered morally questionable by a group on the far right of the political spectrum. The Traditional Values Coalition took credit for it. Sure that my study was not on the list, I still checked the list on the Internet. I was deeply offended to see my name and my study on the list. The list described my study and then said, in what was clearly meant to be an indictment, that the study promotes condom use. I was, of course, promoting condom use, not sexual activity. My program was aimed at reducing risk for sexually active girls who were at high risk for contracting HIV and other sexually transmitted infections. I knew that Nancy Reagan's "just say no" campaign was not going to prevent infections or pregnancy in this population. As it turns out, the "hit list" was the beginning of the end for my program of research (Roye, 2008). It seems likely that under the Obama Administration scientific inquiry into issues dealing with such "touchy" subjects as sexuality will again return to the United States.

My experience was not at all unique. Scientists whose research came under scrutiny as part of the "hit list" were surveyed and interviewed about the effect that experience had on their research. Most agreed that the controversy had a "chilling effect" on their research. The scientists also reported that they removed certain words from the title of their abstracts, such as anal sex, needle exchange, and harm reduction. Some researchers altered their research programs to be more politically correct, for example, deciding not to study adolescent sexual health. Others decided not to study certain stigmatized groups. The authors of the study concluded that politics can shape what scientists decide to study (Kempner, 2008).

As one of the "hit list" scientists, I expect that politics will have a minimal, if any, influence on scientific research in the near future. I presume that grant proposals will once more be judged solely on merit. In fact, I am planning a proposal investigating understudied areas of adolescent sexual health.

It is important for healthcare providers to understand the influence that politics can have on health care—in the aggregate, for individual patients and for health research. We must be vigilant about advocating for untarnished science and evidence.

References

Berger, M. E. (2009). *New health regulation permits "conscience" exceptions.* Retrieved January 6, 2009, from http://www.sltrib.com/faith/ci_11296447

Kempner, J. (2008). The chilling effect: How do researchers react to controversy? *PLoS Medicine, 5*(11), e222.

Roye, C. (2009). *Global Gag Rule must not be domesticated.* Retrieved January 6, 2009, from http://www.womensenews.org/article.cfm/dyn/aid/3648

Roye, C. (2008). Politics and nursing science: Not always a healthy combination. *Nursing Science Quarterly, 21,* 13–17.

Conclusion: A Policy Toolkit for Healthcare Providers and Activists

Roby Robertson and Donna Middaugh

OVERVIEW

What is the role of the healthcare professional in the political process? Given the range of issues addressed in this book, where does the political process begin and end? This healthcare policy book is centered on the notion that all healthcare providers require a fundamental understanding of the healthcare system that is not limited to the knowledge required to practice their discipline. No longer can healthcare professionals be prepared solely for clinical practice, but they must ready themselves to deal with the economic, political, and policy dimensions of health care because the services they provide are the outcome of these dynamics.

OBJECTIVES

- To define the role of the healthcare professional in policy advocacy and politics
- To describe processes for becoming a policy advocate within one's own organization and beyond
- To recognize the difference between expertise and internal and external advocacy in relation to stakeholders

- To apply the concepts of health policy to case study vignettes
- To develop one's own toolkit for becoming a health policy advocate

KEY TERMS

- ❏ Advocacy
- ❏ Constituent

- ❏ Expertise
- ❏ External stakeholder

(continues)

□ Internal stakeholder
□ Politics

□ Power
□ Stakeholder

This book offers an interdisciplinary approach to understanding healthcare practice and policy. Professional nurses and other allied health practitioners must have a seat at the policy table, but they must also understand the perspectives of their colleagues; therefore, we have used contributors from outside of nursing, including allied health professionals, activists, politicians, economists, and policy analysts who understand the forces of health care in America, to frame this textbook. The rationale behind an interdisciplinary approach is that no one person has the right solution to the challenges confronting health care in America. These challenges include high costs, limited access, medical errors, variable quality, administrative inefficiencies, and a lack of coordination.

It is not surprising that the healthcare system is under serious stress and that a host of actors both within and beyond the system have myriad solutions to the problem. This chapter suggests that politics is both necessary and critical to making changes, whether we are discussing system level reforms (e.g., national health insurance reform) or a local hospital improving health data access (e.g., electronic medical records). This textbook offers current and future healthcare practitioners who are committed to reducing health disparities and achieving healthcare equality insight into how clinical practice is derived from regulations and laws that are based on public policy and politics.

This book provides an overview of the essential elements that drive health policy in the United States. Within these pages, the reader has been given the following:

- A compelling rationale for engaging in health policy issues
- A thorough review of the healthcare delivery labor force

- An appreciation of the role of markets and government in the system of healthcare finance
- A description of how power, markets, and government affect healthcare organizations and the delivery of care
- Insight into key drivers of the organization of healthcare services, namely technology, quality, and research

This final chapter provides healthcare practitioners a toolkit or a working model of how to "do" policy advocacy within and beyond our organizational lines. This chapter answers these questions: "What is the health professional's role in policy advocacy and politics?" "What are the major distinctions in affecting policy through the two primary areas addressed in this book?" This chapter examines two broad components of policy change—the influence and power of stakeholders/constituencies and the power of expertise. These arenas overlap; of course, here we examine them separately to portray their specific roles more accurately.

What then is the healthcare practitioner's role in the political process? Where does that process take place? Many traditional views define the political process as external only, primarily defined at the policy-making levels of government or boards and commissions; therefore, the argument follows that professionals below senior-level decision makers are primarily reactive; that is, they respond to proposals from up the line and/or must calculate how to implement the changes that others have imposed on them.

In public administration, this has traditionally been defined as a politics/administration dichotomy; that is, political decisions are made by higher ups, and the administrator finds a way to carry out those decisions. In public administration and related policy fields, however, that dichotomy is no more because in actual decision-making and in the practicalities of day-to-day management, interactions at all levels of the organization are necessary to the practice of management/policy formulation and implementation. The administrators are trying to influence policy outcomes like those in the policy arena. And practitioners should do the same.

There is also another reason why practitioners must develop a political/policy toolkit. Politics and policy making are not a function only of the external environment of the organization. In fact, the most sophisticated and nuanced elements of such a policy/political role can be found also in the *internal environment* of the organization. Again, practitioners can play a role influencing these outcomes.

Imagine the following scenario. Your senior executive pulls you aside one day and says, "Do you know that proposal you've wanted to push forward about how we reallocate the staff here in the organization? Well, why don't you put together the budget, a time line, and what we need to do to move this forward in the next budget cycle?" You have been anxious to do so for some time, and you stay in the office every evening putting together the proposal (with fancy pie charts, a time line, personnel requirements, etc.), and you turn it in to your executive.

A week goes by and then two and then three. You are getting anxious; to do some of the time line issues you would need to get rolling soon, but you've heard nothing. You mention it to the executive and she nods, looks solemn, and asks you back into the office. She sits on the edge of the desk (not behind the desk, not a good sign) and pulls out your proposal. You can see it has been marked up with lots of red marks throughout. The executive shakes her head and says, "Well it really is a great idea; it really is the way

to go in the future, but I ran it up the line, and well, you know, 'politics got in the way.' It's just not going to fly!" She hands back your proposal. You return to your office and open the file cabinet of other projects that didn't get off the ground, and you think, politics!

Well? Why didn't it fly? What could have happened? Senior managers did not like the proposal? It competed with other proposed changes that could "fly." What kept yours from flying? Perhaps it was because you had not accounted for the politics of your own organization. Politics exist at the organizational level, not just at the policy-making level, and you sat back and allowed others to make the decision. Thus, our approach in this chapter is to suggest that the politics of the environment are both external and internal.

We suggest that the key to gaining more effective use of the policy environment, both inside and outside the organization, is to understand more effectively the *power* that one has to effect change. Unlike many analyses of power that are often based on the individual, our approach is to examine the organizational power that exists for the practitioner/advocate. We examine that power through two broad arenas—the power of stakeholder relationships and the power of expertise.

Figure 1 is a simple heuristic about power. This simple pyramid has been widely used in political science and policy fields for years. Power can be seen in the levels of the pyramid, with the narrowest (and thus the weakest type of power) at the top of the pyramid and becoming broader with more effective types of power moving down the pyramid. *Force* we all understand. The power to make others do things by forcing them to do so is obvious, from the actual use of force (including weapons) through the more common use of force in an organization which is the power of the organization to enforce rules, standards, and practices. *Influence* is more nuanced, but its role is also obvious—does the organization have the capacity to convince others that they should support or acquiesce to the organization's decision? There are many reasons why an organization may be able to influence a decision. Possibly the organization has shown in the past the capacity to be successful; maybe it is because the organization has demonstrated knowledge or connections to accomplish the tasks required. Nevertheless, the organization must convince others that its decisions are good. Finally, the broadest and most critical part of the power pyramid is *authority*. At the core of a lot of political theory about the state is authority—the acceptance of the organization to decide and the acceptance by others of its decisions without serious question. Expertise is one form of authority. We tend to accept the recommendations of those who are expert in a field.

One example of how all three elements of the power triangle work is driving your car late at night and stopping at a red light with nobody around. There you sit because a light bulb with a red cover over it is "on"! Now, that is power! Do you recognize why you stopped? Did you have to be convinced (well, maybe you think for a second that lights regulate traffic, but it is the middle of the night and there are no cars

Figure 1 Power pyramid.

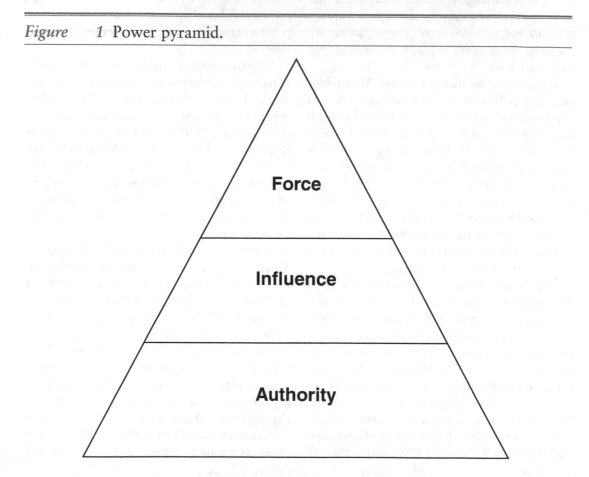

around!)? Do you run the light? Not right away because you first look around to see whether there is a police car around! Now, all three elements are in play, and you stopped at the light in the first place because? It turned red, and you stop at red lights!

Thus, how do we understand our power in organizations? Obviously, there are multiple elements in this—from the regulatory environment, the level of federalism, the growth of the state, and so forth. Here we summarize around two broad elements that undergird the organization's power: stakeholders and expertise. We are going to distinguish between internal and external power (power within the organization and beyond) (see Figure 2).

Stakeholder Power

For many in the healthcare arena, stakeholder power seems the most obvious political tool: A simple "who do you know, who is on our side" model of developing policy change is obvious. Too often, however, our approach is to simply add up the influentials on "our side" and on the "other side." The stakeholder list becomes a list of names, rather than a list of the nature of power relationships. Well, if it is just numbers, then

Figure 2 Focus and locus of organizational power.

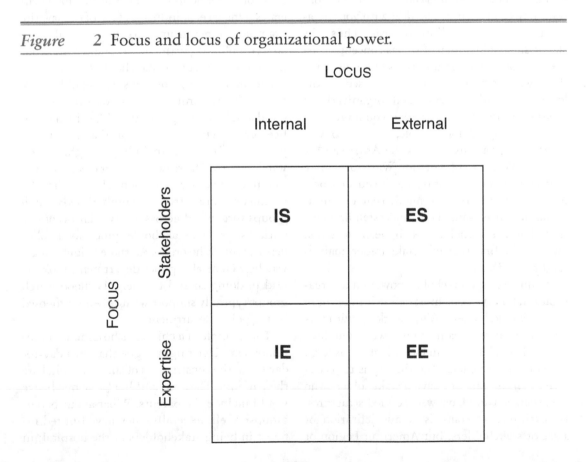

any policy supported by a greater number of individuals or organizations should prevail. Under those conditions, we would suggest that a national health system that is effective for the poor would be the easiest to pass, but somehow one knows that organizations representing low-income groups have less influence than those representing higher income groups. Right? So, it cannot be just numbers!

Thus, stakeholder analysis is tied to the network of stakeholders and which sets of stakeholders are closer to your organization and which are more distant. This close/distant issue is often defined in terms of natural and face-to-face relationships: ideally, what groups deal with your agency and/or policy arena on a routine and constant basis and what groups deal with your organization on a more limited basis. Thus, the classic stakeholder map often has concentric circles of groups and organizations closer and further away from the organization based on the level of interdependence and organizational closeness (Fottler et al., 1989). If you represent a Veterans' hospital, for example, members of veterans' organizations, such as the American Legion or Veterans of Foreign Wars, are more central to your organization, but if you are working from a children's hospital, that organizational tie is irrelevant. Thus, understanding how central other stakeholders are to the organization may be the first part of a stakeholder analysis (Figure 3).

To understand stakeholder power for an organization, however, one must define it in terms of *organized* stakeholders. When working with various healthcare organizations, we often hear stakeholders described in individual terms (e.g., patients or customers), but the key is to recognize the importance of having stakeholders who are organized and have well-defined structures. For example, "veterans" is a vague definition for a set of stakeholders, but American Legion or Veterans of Foreign Wars are two critical organized groups who represent veterans.

What if there is no organized set of stakeholders? The first question might be this: Why is that true? It might be that the stakeholders in the external environment that your organization deals with are too amorphous to be defined. In James Q. Wilson's (1989) terminology, you may represent a majoritarian organization that has no discernible set of constituents or stakeholders other than the public. If that is the case, stakeholder power will be more limited for your organization.

However, we have found that many organizations have developed stakeholder groups over time (often for nonpolitical reasons), which generates some level of influence. One of our favorite examples comes from outside the healthcare arena—police departments. If one thinks about natural constituents or stakeholders, then police departments' most obvious stakeholders are those who commit crimes—not sure how to build a stakeholder group there! Over time, police departments have developed a host of support organizations, including neighborhood watch groups. The reason for their creation is not to influence political decisions about police departments, but strong neighborhood watch groups (organized across a city) can become a critical secondary stakeholder group for a police department. Who organized those neighborhood watches? Generally, police departments took the lead in doing so and the neighborhood watch groups typically support what is being proposed by the police department.

The example of a children's hospital is appropriate here. One might argue that on a day-to-day basis, the constituents of such a hospital are the patients. They are children, but maybe we would include the parents. What about parent groups? Well, generally, they have limited interest in being stakeholders of the hospital; in

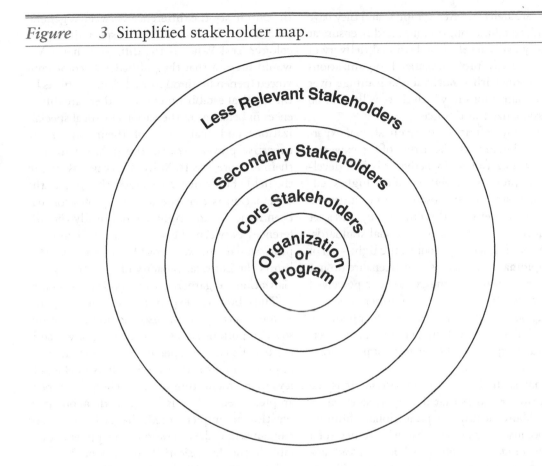

fact, they want to get their children well and leave the hospital. What about children suffering from a chronic illness or a long-term disease such as cancer? Most such hospitals have developed parent and children groups to get together from time to time to support each other (and to provide additional information to the hospital and to other patients and their families about coping with the illness). If the hospital's outreach department has helped organize the group so that it sets officers and meeting dates, then the group is now organized! Is it the same as a veterans' organization? Clearly not, but it would be wise to include such a group in any efforts to advocate for policy changes (inside and beyond the hospital).

Expertise

What is expert power in an organization? Some would define it in terms of knowledge acquisition and professionalism. Thus, an expert organization would have a high proportion of highly educated professionals, defined by advanced education, licensure, professional norms and ethical standards, and a lifetime of continuing education. The healthcare arena has a clear advantage here. The various professions within any existing healthcare arena are often complex, and they have specialized education, training, and licensure at virtually every level of professional delivery of services. Such professionalized organizations often begin with a noticeable advantage over other organizations in which there is little or no professionalized work force.

Thus, any definition of organizational expertise must begin with the nature of the expertise of the organization and whether it is well developed and professionalized and of the highest educational standards; however, one must be careful about defining this power simply as a set of acquired educational/professional standards. In the end, it is a bit like our traffic light—all of the diplomas, certificates, and licensure do not necessarily mean that the expertise is perceived as powerful. Similar to the number of stakeholders not being as important as the proximity of stakeholders to the decision makers, not all experts carry equal weight when it comes to organizational decisions.

What is the key to this expertise? It is the perception of others that the expertise is legitimate. Many healthcare professionals blunder here because they believe that achievement of a variety of graduate/professional degrees leads automatically to support of their expertise. To put it in simple terms, many occupations (especially in the healthcare arena) are licensed, certified, and with advanced education but thus do not have equal expertise power. Why? Maybe because the public or the broader political/policy environment does not differentiate the various specializations, or the expertise of the profession is recognized strongly only by the profession itself. The best example today is the widespread public agreement about the need for more nurses. How does that translate generally? Does the public differentiate well between LPN, RN, diploma, AD, BSN, MSN, NP, CRNA, CNS, or advanced practice nurses? No! Why not? Does

the public see the difference between a general practitioner in medicine and a specialist in oncology? Yes! What is the difference here? We would suggest that the public has become convinced (generally through well-defined efforts by the medical establishment) that there are differences in behavior in the various medical specializations and that some of them have more expertise power because the public perceives them as more expert. Why is that not as true in the field of nursing? We suggest that part of the explanation is that the nursing profession has been reluctant to emphasize publically the differences between the various areas of nursing professionalism. We would suggest that this limits the political capacity of the various specializations to garner separate political support.

Thus, building expertise power in an organizational setting must also include addressing some important issues, not the least of which is the belief that the expertise of the particular set of professionals is desired by others in the policy environment. Internally, in a hospital, for example, when policy is being made about how practices are implemented, changed, evolved, or reorganized, is the profession you represent at the table in the discussion? If not, why not?

Thus, as we develop the toolkit for expert power, we must ask a critical question: "Who believes this expertise is valued and should be represented in the decision making process (both within and beyond the organization)?"

Toolkit Case Studies

The case studies included in this toolkit chapter are designed to aid the reader in understanding the politics of organizational power. They are divided based on four categories: external stakeholder, internal stakeholder, external expertise, and internal expertise. Each of these real-life case studies illustrates how health professionals have applied the tools as highlighted within this chapter. The case study authors have included references for the reader's use, when applicable. To guide your comprehension and application of the toolkit, the authors have included several thought provoking questions at the end of each case study. Readers are encouraged to critically analyze the political methods and power used in each case study, exploring the stakeholders and type of expertise involved. The questions following each case study are helpful for group discussion, as well as individual analysis. This chapter concludes with one additional case study that has not had any sort of political result to date, and readers are asked to analyze that case in terms of how one might build the necessary political stakeholder and expert power.

External Expert Power

The first two cases presented here are doubtless well known to readers, but what may not be well known is the history of the development of policy in these areas. As you examine these two case studies, remember that their purpose is to show the role of expertise in affecting policy.

CASE STUDY

Margaret Sanger as Nurse and Public Health Advocate

Ellen Chesler

"No Gods, No Masters," the rallying cry of the Industrial Workers of the World, was her personal and political manifesto. Emma Goldman and Bill Haywood, Mabel Dodge, and John Reed were among her earliest mentors and comrades. Allied with labor organizers and bohemians, Margaret Sanger first emerged on the American scene in those halcyon days at the turn of the 20th century when the country seemed wide open with possibility, before world war, revolution, and repression provided a more sober reality.

She organized pickets and protests and pageants in the hope of achieving wholesale economic and social justice. What began as a callow faith in revolution quickly gave way to a more concrete agenda for reform. Working as a visiting nurse on New York's Lower East Side, she watched a young patient die tragically from the complications of a then-all-too-common illegal abortion and vowed to abandon palliative work and devote herself instead to single-minded pursuit of reproductive autonomy for women.

Sanger proudly claimed personal freedom for women. She also insisted that the price women pay for equality should not be the sacrifice of personal fulfillment. Following in the footsteps of a generation of suffragists and social welfare activists who had forgone marriage in order to gain professional stature and public influence, she became the standard bearer of a less ascetic breed, intent on balancing work and family obligations.

The hardest challenge in writing this history for modern audiences, for whom these claims have become routine, is to explain how absolutely destabilizing they seemed in Sanger's time. Even with so much lingering animus toward women's rights today, it is hard to remember that reproduction was once considered a woman's principal purpose, and motherhood, her primary role—that women were assumed to have no need for identities or rights independent of those they enjoyed by virtue of their relationships to men—and that this principle was central to the long-enduring opposition they have faced in seeking rights to work, to inheritance and property, to suffrage, and most especially to control of their own bodies.

Sanger needed broader arguments. By practicing birth control, women would not just serve themselves, she countered. They would also lower birthrates, alter the balance of supply and demand for labor, alleviate poverty, and thereby achieve the aspirations of workers without the social upheaval of class warfare. Not the dictates of Karl Marx, but the refusal of women to bear children indiscriminately would alter the course of history, a proposition ever resonant today as state socialism becomes an artifact of history, while family planning, although still contested, endures with palpable consequences worldwide.

In 1917, Sanger went to jail for distributing contraceptive pessaries to immigrant women from a makeshift clinic in a tenement storefront in the Brownsville section of Brooklyn. Classic elements of modernization, including urbanization, industrialization, and secularization, were already driving down the nation's birthrate as a result of private contraceptive arrangements and a healthy underground trade in condoms, douches, and various contraptions. Sanger's contribution was to demand services for the poor that were available to the middle class. Her heresy, if you will, was in bringing the issue of sexual and reproductive freedom out in the open and claiming it as a woman's right. She staged her arrest deliberately to challenge New York's already anachronistic obscenity laws—the legacy of the notorious Anthony Comstock, whose evangelical fervor had captured Victorian politics, in a manner eerily reminiscent of our time—and led to the adoption by the federal government and the states of broad criminal sanctions on sexual speech and commerce, including all materials related to contraception and abortion. Zealous protector of traditional values and "savior" of vulnerable single women, Comstock had himself authorized as a special agent of the U.S. Post Office, with the power to undertake searches and make arrests. He died of pneumonia in 1915, after repeated confrontations with Sanger and her supporters that generated widespread publicity and sympathy for her cause, transforming it from a radical gesture to a cause célèbre.

Direct action tactics served Sanger well, but legal appeal of her clinic conviction also established a medical exception to New York's Comstock Law. Doctors—although not nurses, as she originally intended—were granted the right to prescribe contraception for health purposes, and under that constraint, she built the modern family planning movement with independent, free-standing facilities as the model for distribution of services, a development that occurred largely in spite of leaders of the medical profession, who remained shy of the subject for many years and did not formally endorse birth control until 1937, well after its scientific and social efficacy was demonstrated.

By then, Sanger and Hannah Stone, the medical director of her New York clinic, had also achieved another legal breakthrough. They prevailed in a 1936 federal appellate court decision in New York that licensed physicians to import contraceptive materials and use the federal mails for their transport. The ruling effectively realized years of failed efforts to achieve legislative reform in Congress, although it did formally override prohibitions that remained in several states until the historic ruling in Griswold with its claim of a constitutional doctrine of privacy, later extended so controversially to abortion in Roe v. Wade.

Sanger had long since jettisoned political ideology for a more reasoned confidence in the ability of education and science to shape human conduct and in the possibility of reform through bold public health initiatives. Her most prominent mentor through this passage was H.G. Wells, the renowned British man of letters and influence, who foresaw the development of states that would mix free markets with centralized planning for social welfare. Both became tribunes for the rational, scientific control of the world's population and its resources, with Wells giving Sanger international credibility and enhancing her stature.

With hard work and determination, she was able to mobilize men of influence in business, labor, academia, and the emerging professions. No less critical to her success was her decision to invest in the collective potential of women, many of whom had been oriented to activism by the suffrage movement and were eager for a new cause after finally winning the vote in 1920. She also lobbied the churches, convincing the clerical establishments of the progressive Protestant and Jewish denominations of the virtue of lifting sexuality and reproduction from the shroud of myth and mystery to which traditional faiths had long consigned them. She even won a concession from the hierarchy of the American Catholic Church, which overruled the Vatican and endorsed natural family planning, or the so-called rhythm method, as a way of countering the secular birth control movement and reasserting religious authority over values and behavior.

With an uncanny feel for the power of well-communicated ideas in a democracy, Sanger moved beyond women's rights to put forth powerful public health and social welfare claims for birth control. She proved herself a savvy public relations strategist and an adept grass-roots organizer. Through the 1920s and 1930s, she wrote best-selling books, published a widely read journal, crisscrossed the country, and circled the globe, giving lectures and holding conferences that attracted great interest and drove even more publicity. She built a thriving voluntary movement to conduct national and state-level legislative lobbying and advocacy work and to work in communities on the ground, sustaining affiliate organizations that organized and operated pioneering women's health clinics. Offering a range of medical and mental health services in reasonably sympathetic environments, many of these facilities became laboratories for her idealism.

Yet the birth control movement stalled during the long years of the Great Depression and World War II, stymied by the increasing cost and complexity of reaching those most in need and overwhelmed by the barrage of opposition it engendered. The issue remained mired in moral and religious controversy, even as its leadership determinedly embraced a centrist politics and a sanitized message. When hard times encouraged attention to collective needs over individual rights and when the New Deal legitimized public responsibility for economic and social welfare, Sanger cannily replaced the "birth control" moniker with the more socially resonant content of "family planning." Both were terms she invented and popularized after consulting allies and friends. These strategies of accommodation, however, did nothing to stop officials of the National Catholic Welfare Conference and other opponents from making the most scandalous accusations that birth control was killing babies, waging war on poor families, even causing the depression itself by slowing population growth and lowering consumer demand, a proposition that some economists of the day also endorsed.

Having enjoyed Eleanor Roosevelt's enthusiastic support and personal friendship in New York, Sanger went to Washington in the 1930s hoping that Congress would overturn the Comstock law and legalize contraceptive practice as a first step to her long-term goal of transferring responsibility and accountability for services from small, privately funded clinics to public health programs with appropriate resources and scale; however, she failed to anticipate that the success of the Roosevelt's would depend on a delicate balancing of the votes of conservative urban Catholics in the north and rural, fundamentalist Protestants in the south. There would be no invitations to tea at the White House and no government support, at least until Franklin was safely ensconced in a third term.

What is more, the ever-fragile alliance Sanger built with the country's elites itself became a liability. Sanger resigned from the American Birth Control League she had founded, severing official ties with others in the movement who boldly advanced contraception as a means of slowing birthrates among the poor. Her own politics had long tended to the left, and she became an enthusiastic New Dealer. She offered family planning not as a panacea but as a piece of a broader package of health and social welfare policies that would also provide economic and social safety nets. She framed poverty as a matter of differential access to resources, including contraception, not as the immutable consequence of low inherent ability or bad character, a view held by many conservatives. She spoke out against immigration restrictions, held advanced views on race, and enjoyed enthusiastic support for her work from W.E.B. Dubois, from many others in the progressive black community, and eventually from Mrs. Roosevelt, whose commitments to civil rights were well known.

Like other well-intended social reformers of her day, Sanger also endorsed eugenics, the then ubiquitous and popular movement that addressed the manner in which biological factors affect human, health, intelligence, and opportunity. She took away from Darwinism the essentially optimistic lesson that man's common descent in the animal kingdom makes us all capable of improvement, if only we apply the right tools. Believing that ability and talent should replace birthright and social status as the standard of mobility in a democratic society, she endorsed intelligence testing, an enduring legacy of this era, and she did not repudiate the infamous Supreme Court decision of 1929 in *Buck v. Bell* that mandated compulsory sterilization on grounds of feeble-mindedness. She also supported the payment of bonuses to women who volunteered for sterilization because they wanted no more children.

These compromised views placed her squarely in the intellectual mainstream of her time and in the good company of many progressives who shared these beliefs. Still, her failure to consider the validity of standard assessments of aptitude or the fundamental rights questions inherent in these procedures has left her vulnerable in hindsight to attacks of insensitivity and bigotry. The family planning movement at home and abroad has long been burdened by the charges that it fostered prejudice, even as it delivered welcome services and relief from unwanted childbirth to women in need.

Embittered by these controversies and disenchanted with the country's increasing pronatalism after World War II, Sanger turned her attentions abroad. In 1952, she founded the International Planned Parenthood Federation, with headquarters in London, as an umbrella for the national family planning associations that remain today in almost every country in the world.

By the time of her death in 1966, the cause for which she defiantly broke the law had achieved international stature. Although still a magnet for controversy, she was widely eulogized as one of the great emancipators of her time. She lived to see the United States Supreme Court provide constitutional protection to the use of contraceptives in *Griswold v. Connecticut*. She watched Lyndon Johnson incorporate family planning into America's social welfare and foreign policy programs, fulfilling her singular vision of how to advance opportunity and prosperity, not to speak of human happiness, at home and abroad. A team of doctors and scientists she had long encouraged marketed the oral anovulant birth control pill, and a resurgent feminist movement gave new resonance to her original claim that women have a fundamental right to control their own bodies.

In the years since, however, further controversy has surrounded the practices of what developed as often alarmist global population control efforts that adopted rigid demographic targets and imposed harsh, unwelcome, and culturally insensitive technologies on women. Population policy makers and service providers have been fairly criticized for abusing rights by ignoring or downplaying the risks of providing costly technologies where health services are inadequate to cope with potential complications and where failure rates have been high, even though these products are medically benign when properly administered.

In 1994, the United Nations International Conference on Population and Development in Cairo created a framework for state responsibility to ensure programs allowing women to make free and informed decisions about family planning, but also obligating access to comprehensive, reproductive health services of high quality, including birth control. The benefit of effective family planning to the well-being of individuals, families, and communities was officially acknowledged, despite continued resistance from the Vatican and some conservative Islamic states. Population and development professionals, however, also committed to a doctrine that weds policies and practices to improvements in women's status—to education, economic opportunity, and basic civil rights for women subject to culturally sanctioned discrimination and violence—just as Margaret Sanger first envisioned.

Hundreds of millions of women and men around the world today freely practice some method of contraception, with increasing reliance again on condoms, in light of the epidemic spread of HIV-AIDS and other sexually transmitted infections. This represents a sixfold increase since rates of population growth peaked in the 1960s.

Still, half the world's population today—nearly 3 billion people—are under the age of 25 years. Problems associated with widespread poverty, food insecurity, and environmental degradation are widespread. There remains considerable unmet need for family planning and tragically insufficient funding for research on new methods and for new programming to meet ever-increasing demand. Funding for both population and development programs has slowed dramatically, as other needs compete for funds and as concern now spreads instead about an aging and shrinking population in many countries in the global north and south where birthrates have declined sharply. The cycles of history repeat themselves.

Case Study Questions

At what points did the science of birth control precede any change in policy/practice in this area? Why do you think that was the case? Why was the expertise of effective birth control not widely shared, and why did it take the medical establishment so long to endorse policy change in this area? Clearly, the women's movement was part of the opening of change in this area, but how did it contribute to the creation of knowledge? What happened to the policy of birth control after the American Medical Association supported it in the 1930s? Why did it take another 30 years for birth control to be widely available to women in America? Have there been changes in recent years in the broader environment that are analogous to the early adoption of birth control programs (e.g., RU 487 or the "morning after" pill)? Have these changes increased or limited access to birth control? Think through the acceptance of the expertise in this area and the ways in which it has contributed (or limited) the change in policy in this environment and the ways in which it has not been taken into account. Can you illustrate how expertise is still about perception, both within professional fields as well as in the broader public?

CASE STUDY

The Centers for Disease Control's 2006 Recommendations on Screening for HIV Infection

Kathleen M. Nokes

HIV is the virus that causes AIDS. Because this diagnosis is consistent with severe immune depression, a person can be infected with HIV for many years before AIDS develops (Centers for Disease Control [CDC], 2007). Except for newborns, all persons who test positive for the antibody to the HIV are diagnosed with HIV infection. Antibody testing is cheaper than direct viral testing for genetic evidence of HIV. HIV antibody testing first became available in 1985 and was primarily used to increase the safety of the blood supply; by 1987, the United States Public Health Service issued guidelines making counseling and testing a priority as a prevention strategy. Extensive guidelines structured the counseling session before persons agreed to consent to HIV testing, and it was emphasized that infected persons needed to avoid transmitting the virus and at-risk persons needed to adopt behaviors to decrease their risk. In 1993, the CDC recommended voluntary testing for hospitalized patients as well as outpatients in acute-care hospitals and emergency departments. Hospitals with high incidence rates were encouraged to adopt a policy of offering voluntary HIV counseling and testing routinely to all patients aged 15 to 54 years (CDC, 2006). The CDC focused on screening pregnant women and did not turn their attention back to hospitalized patients again until 10 years later, in 2003. Over that period, HIV infection transitioned from a terminal to chronic illness because of the development of effective strategies to control the infection and immune damage caused by HIV.

HIV infection is a stigmatizing condition. In order to encourage persons to learn their HIV status, extensive confidentiality laws were enacted that required that persons *choose* when and if they will be screened for HIV infection. Written informed consent was mandated in some states, including New York State, so that persons would be aware that their blood was being tested for HIV infection. When persons learned that they were HIV positive, not only were they concerned about their physical health, but there were consequences impacting relationships, personal safety, and economics as well as mental health. Because HIV infection can persist for years before significant symptoms are manifested, many persons chose to avoid the stress of learning their HIV status and continued in their day-to-day activities. Because HIV is transmitted from one person to another, there is also a sense of betrayal and anger that an intimate interaction resulted in danger, reflecting a lack of caring.

By 2003, the CDC acknowledged that hospitalized patients were not being routinely offered voluntary screening and cited lack of reimbursement for HIV screening, inadequate time for healthcare providers to conduct risk assessments and adequate counseling, and lack of explicit information about HIV prevalence as reasons for the low screening rates. After extensive consultation with key stakeholders, the CDC issued the *Revised Recommendations for HIV Testing of Adults, Adolescents, and Pregnant Women in Health-care Settings* in 2006. This case study examines components of these recommendations from a policy perspective. This policy analysis focuses on the two sections of the recommendations related to screening for HIV infection and consent and pretest information for nonpregnant women. To quote from page 7 of the *Morbidity and Mortality Weekly Report* of September 22, 2006:

In all health-care settings, screening for HIV infection should be performed routinely for all patients aged 13-64 years. Healthcare providers should initiate screening unless prevalence of undiagnosed HIV infection in their patients has been documented to be less than 0.1%.

In 1993, the CDC recommended screening persons aged 15 to 54 years, compared with the 2006 recommendation of ages 13 to 64 years. The lower age limit of 13 reflects the pediatric classification of AIDS, in which it is believed that infection occurred perinatally from the HIV infected mother to the fetus and/or infant. The decision to establish any upper age limit for routine screening in healthcare facilities, however, seems arbitrary. Of course, although it can be clearly established by looking at the 2006 prevalence data that while the highest percentage (22%) of persons living with AIDS were aged 40 to 44 (CDC, 2008), the number of persons older than age 64 diagnosed with HIV/AIDS increased only from 570 to 618 between the years 2003 and 2006 (CDC, 2008, Table 1) or less than 1% of the cases diagnosed in those years.

Nevertheless, the underlying rationale of the CDC for the 2006 recommendation is that approximately one quarter of the persons infected with HIV are unaware of their infection and therefore are not accessing treatment or engaging in preventing the spread of HIV infection. With any arbitrary upper age limit for routine HIV screening in healthcare facilities, we will never know the number of older persons who are living with HIV/AIDS. An argument for creating an upper age limit might be to avoid the cost associated with widespread HIV screening in very low-incidence populations, but the second part of the screening recommendations addresses this by instituting routine screening only in prevalence areas of more than 1%. New York has the highest prevalence case rate for adults with HIV infection (not AIDS) in the United States (261.7 per 100,000) (CDC, 2008, p. 8), and most of those New York cases live in New York City.

New York City reports the age category of 60 years or older and 8% of all the persons living with HIV or AIDS in NYC as of December 31, 2006, were in that age category compared with 24.5% of persons aged 50 to 59 years. From the time of HIV infection to the development of AIDS, as many as 10 to 12 years can elapse. There is thus every possibility that the numbers of cases of older persons are underreported, especially in an area with an established epidemic and high prevalence; nevertheless, the policy makers in New York are mirroring CDC recommendations to provide routine screening for persons only up to age 64 years. If the purpose of routine screening is to uncover persons who do not know they are HIV infected, then one wonders why an upper age limit for routine screening was recommended and implemented in high-incidence areas such as New York City.

The Federal Older Americans Act, amended in 2006, states that

The Congress hereby finds and declares that, in keeping with the traditional American concept of the inherent dignity of the individual in our democratic society, the older people of our Nation are entitled to . . . (2) The best possible physical and mental health which science can make available and without regard to economic status.

Is the CDC policy of establishing an upper age limit on the public health recommendation for routine HIV screening an example of ageism and a deviation from the promises of the Older Americans Act?

The second component of the 2006 revised recommendations relates to consent and pretest counseling. Specifically, the recommendation states this:

Screening after notifying the patient that an HIV test will be performed unless the patient declines (opt-out screening) is recommended in all health-care settings. Specific signed consent for HIV testing should not be required. General informed consent for medical care should be considered sufficient to encompass informed consent for HIV testing.

The assumption underlying this policy is that a competent person is seeking the services of a healthcare provider, and those services include screening for HIV infection. An opt-out option has been defined by CDC as

Performing HIV screening after notifying the patient that 1) the test will be performed and 2) the patient may elect to decline or defer testing. Assent is inferred unless the patient declines testing.

The American Cancer Society (2008) provides an explanation of the difference between implicit and written consent. They explain that all medical care requires the patient's consent, but in cases with low risk, such as having a blood test, a simple consent is adequate. They go on to say that in cases in which there are larger possible risks, written consent is necessary. The amount of blood needed for the HIV screening is easily included in the tubes of blood routinely drawn during a visit to a healthcare facility and the amount of time that the person drawing the blood takes to fill one more tube is negligible since access has already been attained.

The CDC recommendation supports that drawing blood for HIV is a low-risk procedure and simple consent is sufficient; however, the identification of an opt-out option recognizes that this screening requires special consideration. Persons are not given an opt-out option for other screening tests such as syphilis or hereditary issues such as sickle cell or other anemia. After admission into healthcare facilities, persons sign general consent forms and then explicit consent forms for specific procedures such as surgery. In the past, HIV screening has been handled as requiring an explicit consent form. With this new recommendation, HIV screening will be transferred to the general consent for medical treatment standard. Thus, why is an opt-out option being made available? If HIV is not a special case, why are persons being alerted that they can choose not to have this specific test? If HIV is a special case, what is the rationale? Could it be that, as cited by the CDC in 2003, healthcare providers do not want to spend the time doing the necessary counseling before the testing.

If healthcare providers do not want to take the time to counsel persons about HIV infection, will they be competent to handle newly diagnosed persons with HIV infection? Some persons will be surprised and perhaps devastated at learning that they are infected. By identifying the 25% of the cases that the CDC believes are infected and unaware, will

networks of knowledgeable and sensitive health-care providers also be identified? Will more resources be made available to stage and treat these newly diagnosed persons with HIV/AIDS? Does this public health policy focus on the needs of the group and harm the individual?

Because one of the reasons for the removal of a written consent is that healthcare providers do not have the time to counsel persons before testing for HIV, alternate methods of counseling could be developed. Persons could complete a simple true/false quiz while waiting to see the healthcare provider that addresses the key components of HIV counseling such as safer sex recommendations, the fact that HIV is a treatable condition, and that blood will be routinely tested for HIV but that clients can decline this testing. All clients would be required to complete five to six true/false questions in a format similar to that used in providing information about their health insurance. Clients would be able to review their answers with the healthcare provider and be more aware of their opt-out option, and healthcare providers would not need to spend excessive time in counseling. In situations in which computer access is available, these quizzes could be taken online and the responses made part of the client's electronic health record.

Policies related to HIV infection are often influenced more by politics and economics than public health considerations. Healthcare providers should not assume that new policies are based on sound practices but, rather, explore the motivation behind these policies, especially in situations in which marginalized populations are particularly impacted by the health issue. Healthcare providers should be vocal in their feedback about the proposed policy and provide clinical insights that might be helpful for legislators as they create laws.

Case Study Questions

In this second case, there are some very specific changes in hospital policy dealing with HIV. What are they? In what ways is the adoption and/or acceptance of those policies tied to expertise power? In the change in policy about HIV screening, what was the role of expertise, both within and beyond the medical community? How was expert knowledge balanced against our broader understanding of HIV throughout society? The expertise on these issues preceded the change in policy: what does that tell us about expertise and power?

Case Study References

American Cancer Society. (2008). *Making treatment decisions*. Retrieved May 11, 2008, from http://www.cancer.org/docroot/ETO/content/ETO_1_2X_Informed_Consent.asp

Centers for Disease Control and Prevention. (2006). Revised recommendations for HIV testing of adults, adolescents, and pregnant women in health-care settings. *Morbidity and Mortality Weekly Report, 55*(RR-14), 1–17.

Centers for Disease Control and Prevention. (2007). *Living with HIV/AIDS*. Retrieved May 11, 2008, from http://www.cdc.gov/hiv/resources/brochures/livingwithhiv.htm#q2

Centers for Disease Control and Prevention. (2008). *HIV/AIDS surveillance report, 2006*. Retrieved February 16, 2010, from http://www.cdc.gov/hiv/topics/surveillance/resources/reports

Older Americans Act Amendments of 2006. Title I—Declaration of Objectives; Definitions. Declaration of Objectives for Older Americans. Section 101. Retrieved May 11, 2008, from http://www.aoa.gov/AoARoot/AoA_Programs/OAA/oaa_full.asp

CASE STUDY

External Stakeholder Power: Successful Efforts to Pass Advanced Practice Nurse Legislation

Claudia J. Beverly

The Arkansas State Legislature meets every other year to conduct the business of the state. In the year preceding the legislative session, the Policy Committee of the Arkansas Nurses Association (ArNA) examines the healthcare needs of the state and designs a strategic health policy plan for nursing that will be introduced in the upcoming session. The work is always initiated with a clear understanding of the needs of the citizens of the State of Arkansas. In this rural state, 69 of the 75 counties are medically underserved. The poverty level is one of the worst in the country. The health statistics of Arkansans are in the bottom four states. and several counties do not have a single primary care provider. Given the many healthcare challenges facing the

state, nursing is in a key position to address these needs and is expected to do so by society.

In the early 1990s, the ArNA, which represents all nurses in Arkansas, concluded that advanced practice nurses were best prepared to address the primary healthcare needs of Arkansans. At that time, however, there was no standardization or clear regulation for this level of nurse other than national certification and the registered nurse (RN) license that is basic for all levels of registered nurses.

The ArNA's first attempt to address the primary healthcare needs of the citizens was in 1993. Their attempt to pass legislation that would allow prescriptive authority by advanced practice nurses failed. After this failure, the ArNA, with the assistance of its lobbyist, began to develop legislation to be introduced in the 1995 legislative session to provide a mechanism for advanced practice nurses to practice to the extent to which they were academically prepared. Additionally, a mechanism whereby society could be assured of safe practice by all providers needed to be in place.

The process began when a legislator from a rural area where the need was greatest introduced a "study bill." This study bill provided the opportunity for the ArNA to educate legislators about advanced practice nursing and how this type of nurse could address the healthcare needs of Arkansans. The study bill was assigned to the Interim Public Health, Welfare and Labor Committee of both the House of Representatives and the Senate. Several public hearings were held by the committee, and various groups and individuals both in support and in opposition were given the opportunity to voice their opinions.

During the hearings, there were opportunities to provide correct information supported by the literature. Clarification of the proposed legislation was also always on the agenda. At one point, concern was raised about the use of the term "collaboration with medicine," as some persons preferred to use "supervision" or a definition that would limit the practice to one being supervised. The task force initiated a process to define the term collaboration. A review of the literature showed that collaboration had already been defined in the seventies by both medicine and nursing. Armed with that information and definitions given by other sources, the task force reported their findings at the next hearing and the definition jointly developed by medicine, and nursing was incorporated in the proposed legislation.

Process for Success

The leadership of the ArNA understood the monumental task and the many challenges and barriers to addressing the healthcare needs of Arkansans. The association decided that appointing a special task force to lead its efforts was the best strategy. This strategy provided a mechanism for focusing on this issue while ensuring that the health policy committee would continue to focus on broader policy issues.

The association selected a chair, included the chair in selection of the members by ArNA leadership, and established the first meeting. As the process evolved, two co-chairs, a secretary, and a treasurer were named. The task force was representative of nursing broadly and included members of the Arkansas State Board of Nursing, master's prepared advanced practice nurses (midwives, certified registered nurse anesthetists, nurse practitioners, and clinical nurse specialists), registered nurses, faculty from schools of nursing preparing advanced practice nurses, and representatives from other nursing organizations. The task force met every other week during the first 6 months of the 2-year preparatory period and then weekly for the remaining year and a half.

The first order of business was to develop a strategic plan that included establishing a vision, mission, goals and objectives, strategies, and a time line. The vision was critical as a means of keeping task force members focused on the vast needs of Arkansans, particularly those in rural areas. The vision statement also served to keep the broader ArNA membership focused. A literature search on advanced practice nursing and health policy issues was conducted, and articles were distributed to all task force members. The assumption was that all of the members needed information to expand their current knowledge. Subcommittees were developed based on goals and objectives and the operational needs of the task force. Chairs were assigned for each subcommittee, and thus began the 2-year journey.

The American Nurses Association played a vital role in the process. The legal department was available to assemble and provide information, offer guidance, and identify potential barriers and challenges. The support provided by the ANA was pivotal to our success.

The work of the task force focused on external and internal strategies. External strategies focused on stakeholders, which included the Arkansas Medical Society and the Arkansas Medical Board and the Pharmacy Association. Understanding the views of our colleagues in other disciplines and identifying the opposition to our plans were critical to our success. Many meetings focused on educating those disciplines about the legislation we were seeking. Often this was a balancing act, providing the right information, but not too much of our strategy while attempting to keep our "enemy" close to us. We valued the process of negotiation and participated in many opportunities to negotiate with colleagues.

Throughout this process, the ArNA did have a "line in the sand," defined as the point at which there was no negotiation. Our line in the sand included regulations of advanced practice nurses by the Arkansas State Board of Nursing and reimbursement paid directly to the nurses. These two points were never resolved until a vote on the legislation occurred.

The good news is that the APN legislation passed successfully in 1995. The legislation was successful in that the criteria for an APN to be licensed in the State of Arkansas were written by nursing, APNs were to be regulated by nursing, and the legislation acknowledged national certification and educational requirements. Prescriptive authority was granted, and selected scheduled drugs could be ordered by an APN. Reimbursement to APNs was lost at the last minute. For APNs practicing in the field of geriatrics, Medicare passed reimbursement regulations in 1997. Medicaid reimburses geriatric nurse practitioners according to national guidelines. Reimbursement is critical to meeting Arkansans' needs and is a topic that is continuing to be discussed.

Many individuals participated in this successful campaign. A clear vision, legislation based on evidence and current literature, a comprehensive strategic plan, education of all parties, including those in opposition and those in support, and well-informed legislators were critical to success. Probably the most critical message in health policy legislation is to focus on the needs of the citizenry and what nursing needs to contribute.

Case Study Questions

We suspect that most nursing professionals can expand on this case; however, the key question is what is the nature of the building of a stakeholder network here? Who were the critical "first" players in this movement and why? As the network expanded, which other professional groups were involved? Why those? Do you see why some professions were the logical next parts of the coalition for adopting change? Who was most likely to oppose advanced practice nursing? Obviously, you do not include likely opponents in the initial development of the network of stakeholders, but why is that? How did the coalition eventually succeed through this inclusive network? What would you have done differently in a different practice arena? What does this case study tell you about building stakeholders for advancing practice? What would you need to do to apply this policy to advancing roles in your healthcare setting?

CASE STUDY

Internal Expertise Power: The Politics of Moving to an Electrical Medical Record

Pamela Trevino

Making significant change in an institution is a long and tedious process. It is essential to get support and buy in from all levels of the organization and often requires fancy footwork. For example, moving to an electronic medical record is a substantial process change for all who use it, and even small portions of the change can be daunting.

After learning the benefits and safety of bedside medication verification (BMV) using barcode technology, an executive safety committee at a 310-bed hospital decided to implement the technology and an electronic medication administration record. In the earliest stages of development, an executive-level committee included representatives from the following divisions: medicine (physicians), pharmacy, and nursing. They discussed the theoretical

and technological needs for the system to work within an existing technological framework and began evaluating systems.

As the executives began to evaluate the use of the system, it was decided that a front-line bedside staff member needed to be part of the decision making body, as the changes would directly affect those at the bedside. A nurse from an elite team trained to work in every hospital area was chosen to join the committee for her referent power, credibility, and knowledge of multiple hospital areas. Although the nurse was unsure about the necessity of the change, she joined the committee to represent the interests of the bedside staff. In the first weeks on the committee, the nurse was presented with the literature and evidence related to the increased safety of the barcode technology and asked to compare the new technology to the current standard of practice. As the bedside nurse became immersed in the literature, evaluated the current process, and was included in site visits, she became a strong advocate for the safety of the new technology.

As the process continued, a product was purchased, and the implementation process began. Interdisciplinary subcommittees, including all of the disciplines either affected or with a stake in the process, were formed to discuss the ways the system would change current practice. Medicine, nursing, pharmacy, respiratory therapy, information technology, quality management, billing, discharge planning, and fiscal administration were involved in building the system to meet all of the institution's needs, discuss the change in practice, and make policy and procedural changes.

To combat resistance to the product and related changes in process, the system was designed to look as much like the current paper forms as possible. A "BMV Fair" was held in which all front-line respiratory and nursing staff could see and use the technology prior to the official education and implementation. Staff members were encouraged to give feedback on the product, ways to improve the process, and their personal opinions of the technology. The system was then evaluated and changed to accommodate staff preferences where possible, to help remove barriers to acceptance, although the system was still not popular among front-line staff.

The "BMV Fair" also brought to the forefront the lack of basic computer skills in some members of the team. A basic computer competency was developed for all front-line staff members, and classes were offered for those team members who did possess basic computer skills. Staff members were advised early that they would be expected to be able to use the system, and they would not be allowed to work if they could not use the computer-based medication system.

With the move to computer-based charting, computers needed to be available at every bedside. Because of the diversity of the hospital, all units were asked to determine whether they would like mounted computers in every room or computers on wheels (COWs) that could be moved throughout a unit. Because patient rooms are fairly busy, all of the units decided on COWs because of their mobility and flexibility. Each unit was able to borrow several different models and "test drive" them in their area. Nurses were encouraged to give their feedback and suggestions to the purchasing team, and then to decide on a COW. Interestingly, all of the units chose the same COW, which then could be maintained in a central location by information technology personnel.

As the go-live dates approached, training was developed and taught by a member of the information technology staff with a nursing background and by the original bedside nurse on the committee. The bedside nurse shared her initial hesitancy to adopt the system as well as her change to advocacy. Because the institution had a culture geared toward patient safety, front-line staff were told that the process would feel clumsy and take longer initially than current practice but in the end would be safer for the patient. The education highlighted those things that had been added into the system for the convenience of the front-line staff, such as customized computers on wheels, the system "extras" that would save time and effort, and area-specific ways to incorporate the system into everyday practice. Because the hospital chose a staggered roll out, education for each area was held in the 2 weeks before the go-live date. Area-specific questions and concerns were anticipated and addressed with each class.

Within 30 minutes of going live, the system caught the first medication error. Initially, the staff member believed that the system was not working correctly but then learned that the system was correct and that he was attempting to give the wrong medication. This initial user became a strong advocate for the system, and without giving specifics, the information was shared with each subsequent group during their education to show the validity of the system. As more units began using the system, more events occurred, and the information was shared with all the staff members in the hospital. A centralized e-mail account was set up to allow staff to share successes, suggest improvements, and ask questions and feel they were part of the ongoing process.

The implementation was surprisingly smooth, and the system has become part of the culture of the hospital. There are still several committees related to different aspects of the system that meet on a regular basis to address issues that were not foreseeable during the original implementation; however, through careful planning, politics, and change agents, the implementation and enculturation have been a definite success.

Case Study Questions

Based on what you just read, what is the expertise being developed here? What is the challenge to others accepting this expertise? What is it in this case that indicates acceptance of the expertise? What were challenges? What role does process play in making changes such as these? Is there a danger that electronic records will define the questions rather than those involved in direct care?

CASE STUDY

Expanding Newborn Screening in Arkansas
Ralph Vogel

Advances in technology have created great advances in how we can provide services to families and their children. A prime example of this is the expansion of newborn screening, which has dramatically increased the number and type of genetic conditions that can be detected immediately after birth. Historically, most states have screened for hemoglobinopathies (like sickle cell anemia), thyroid, phenylketonuria, and galactosemia. These conditions, along with newborn hearing screening, were relatively easy to assess at a cost effective rate. With advanced laboratory and computer technology, we can now add multiple genetic conditions that are identified during a single run. In 2004, the March of Dimes proposed expanding the genetic conditions for which newborns are screened to their "List of 29," including several enzyme deficiency conditions and cystic fibrosis. The cost of the limited newborn screening was approximately $15 per newborn, and this would rise to about $90 with the expanded list. Insurance companies would cover the cost of adding the additional conditions. The value of newborn screening is in identifying genetic conditions early and implementing treatment plans from birth. Over the life span, this greatly reduces the morbidity and mortality associated with later diagnosis. With some conditions, the care can be as simple as a dietary change that is implemented from birth. Early diagnosis also allows for genetic counseling with families about the risk that additional children will have the condition.

Many states adopted this recommendation quickly, although the process has been slower in others. In Arkansas, a committee, titled the Arkansas Genetics Health Advisory Committee (formerly Service), has existed for several years. Their mission is to monitor health care related to genetics in the state. This diverse committee includes several members of the Arkansas Department of Health (ADH) involved in the newborn screening program administration and laboratory testing, the physicians from Arkansas Children's Hospital genetic clinic, and interested parties that either work in the area of genetics or are parents of children with genetic conditions.

The main purpose of the committee has been to coordinate care and to try to educate the public about genetic conditions and screening for newborns. The ADH receives samples from about 95% of the newborns in the state and does screening at their central location in Little Rock. When an infant is identified with a newborn genetic condition, the ADH then notifies the community hospital and the assigned pediatrician, who does the counseling with the family and develops a plan for care and follow-up.

Expanding the screening program to the existing March of Dimes List of 29 created several problems.

The committee, however, felt strongly that it should take an advocacy role to address these concerns. The first problem was the cost of increased screening. Although most of the individual cost for each child could be absorbed by insurance or Medicaid reimbursement, as in other states, the initial financial support would need to be provided by the state. The ADH had no provision for increasing funding but estimated that the increased cost would be as follows:

- Two million dollars for equipment and supplies
- The addition of at least two more laboratory technicians to do the increased testing
- The addition of at least one more public health nurse to coordinate the increased number of identified genetic cases
- Training for new and current personnel on the new equipment
- Personnel time to develop and coordinate the expansion of the program
- Development of an education program to make parents and professionals aware of the changes

Overall, the estimated cost for startup was approximately $3 million, some of which could be recouped after billing for the tests was established.

The committee and ADH decided that we would outline a plan for expansion with estimated costs and submit it to the director of the ADH, Dr. Faye Bozeman. With his approval, we would then approach legislators and ask for the needed funding to be included in the upcoming budget. Because the state legislature for Arkansas only convened every 2 years, it would be critical to move forward over the next 6 months. We prepared a letter to Dr. Bozeman that the committee approved on a Friday with the intention of mailing it on the following Monday. On the next day, Saturday, Dr. Bozeman was killed in an accident on his farm; therefore, we were in a quandary about who should receive the letter and whose approval would be needed in the ADH. Over the next 6 months, there was an interim head who was thrust into the position and did not want to approve anything at this level of expense. Basically, we were on hold until a permanent director was named. After about 3 months, we decided to take another tack and develop a plan to seek legislative approval for funding and then approach the new ADH director after the person was named. We developed a list of legislators to contact and identified members of the committee who had worked with the legislators in the past and could approach them.

By this time, we were 2 months from the legislature convening and knew that once it convened nothing new would be introduced; therefore, we had to get support before their convening. We approached some legislators and received tacit support, but none was willing to introduce a new bill or request funding at this time without a permanent head of ADH. We had lost the opportunity for funding until the next legislative session in 2 years.

The committee decided to continue to seek support from the legislators and ADH with the idea of gaining funding in 2 years. Meanwhile, we began to look at other states and what newborn screenings they were currently doing to make sure that politicians were aware of national standards. We had identified that Arkansas was one of the last five states to not expand newborn screening, and all of the surrounding states in the region had incorporated all or a large part of the March of Dimes List of 29. Making legislators aware of this became one of our goals, and once they realized that the states surrounding Arkansas were already doing expanded screening of newborns, they were more receptive to our plan.

After we started to discuss funding with legislators during the legislative session, they seemed willing to support newborn screening; however, then we had a surprise: They stated that it did not require any special legislation or special funding. They stated that the ADH could expand newborn screening without their approval because this was already within their realm of responsibility. Funding could be obtained by submitting a budget request to cover the cost of expansion.

The interim head of ADH was willing to support this since the head of the newborn screening section, was on our committee. By fall, we had the budget expansion approved and support for newborn screening expansion. The decision was then made to target July 1, 2008, as the date for starting the expanded program.

After we knew that the finances and political support were confirmed, we developed a timeline that involved acquisition of the equipment, training for ADH staff, an education program for the public, and a plan for making community hospitals and professional healthcare providers aware of the expansion. At this point, the ADH contacted members of the media that it had worked with in the past and developed a plan for public information advertisements to be run on television and radio. These began running in early May, 2 months before the July 1 start date. Because the media members had worked with ADH in the past, it was much easier to develop the advertisements. Print media advertisements were also started, and the local chapter of the March of Dimes provided funding and brochures that were distributed to OB/GYN physicians in the state to make expectant mothers aware of the testing to be done on their newborns. One of the members of the committee also wrote an article that appeared in the March issue of the *Arkansas State Board of Nursing Update* magazine, which is distributed to 40,000 healthcare providers in the state.

In July, the expanded screening was begun, and it has been continued with a relatively smooth transition, largely because of the preparation of the ADH staff in the laboratory and the outreach nurses. Because of the public awareness campaign, there has been little voiced concern from parents, and there seems to be an awareness of the value of the expanded screening.

Lessons learned from the process are these:

- Preparation is the key to a smooth transition.
- Know exactly what is required to proceed and who needs to approve new or expanded plans of action. If we had approached the legislature first to find out what they wanted, we could have saved time.
- Plan for the unexpected. We could not have anticipated Dr. Bozeman's death, but it did cause about a 6-month delay.
- Educate everyone who is going to be involved. This includes administrators, healthcare providers, laboratory staff, parents, and professionals in the communities impacted.
- Discuss with the media exactly what they need and use their expertise in terms of length of announcements and the best ways to distribute information.

Although the entire process took over 2 years, in the end, the transition has been very smooth, and few problems have been identified at any level. Having a diverse group on the committee was a strength because different members had different perspectives. This gave us much greater ability to anticipate problems and coordinate care, and in the end, the program in place will benefit newborns in Arkansas for years to come.

Case Study Questions

This case is a good example of how the stakeholders adapted as the intended policy change moved from internal adoption of policy to legislation back to internal adoption of policy within an existing organization. Can you see how the nature of the stakeholders defined for a legislative change is different from stakeholders for an adaptation of existing policy? The initial group involved in this process was established primarily as an informational group but changed to one advocating change. How did the group evolve to influence policy differently? If the initial group had been more broadly defined at the start, would it have made the same mistake about requiring legislative change to adopt the policy? Why or why not?

Final Case Study

This final case study is presented to stimulate the reader's political thinking. We encourage you to read the case carefully and then consider how you would go about creating an environment for policy change.

CASE STUDY

Workplace Violence

Steven L. Baumann and Eileen Levy

In the wake of the terrorist attack of September 11, 2001, and a series of tragic school shootings, workplace violence has gained national attention in the United States. Although nurses and other healthcare workers are generally well educated and regularly reminded to practice good hand washing and infection control, there is little attention given to the potential for violence in hospitals and other healthcare settings, even though it is common and can have devastating long-term consequences (Department of Health and Human Services, 2002; U.S. Department of Labor, 2004). According to Love and Morrison (2003), nurses who sustain injuries from patient assaults, in addition to suffering psychological trauma, are often out of work for periods of time, have financial problems, show decreased work productivity, make more errors at work, and report a decreased desire to remain a nurse. In addition to these problems, nurses who have been assaulted report feeling less able to provide appropriate care to their patients (Farrell et al., 2006) and are reluctant to make formal complaints (Love & Morrison, 2003). As was the case with needle stick injuries in the past, many organizations do not openly discuss organizational problems that increase the risk for violence, nor do they adequately prepare for episodes of violence, leaving nurses more likely to blame themselves for its occurrence.

The National Institute for Occupational Safety and Health (NIOSH), the same organization that requires hospitals to be attentive to infection control strategies and proper handling of hazardous materials, also provides clear definitions and guidelines to reduce the potential for violence in the workplace. According NIOSH, workplace violence includes acts of physical violence or threats of violence directed toward people on duty or at work (Department of Health and Human Services, 2002). NIOSH has recognized employer responsibilities in mitigating workplace violence and assisting employees who are victims (Love & Morrison, 2003). The U.S. government has required employers to provide safe workplaces since 1970 (U.S. Department of Labor, 2004). These federal guidelines call for hospitals and other organizations to incorporate written programs to assure job safety and security into the overall safety and health program for their facilities. Violence prevention, they suggest, needs to have administrative commitment and employee involvement.

This case study is of a moderate-sized, nonprofit community hospital in the New York Metropolitan area. As in many parts of the United States, this hospital and the communities it serves are becoming increasingly crowded and diverse. In this environment of change and tension, the hospital is a meeting place of people, many not by choice but in crisis, bringing together dramatically different histories, backgrounds, educational attainment, and cultures. The hospital and its clinics have become increasingly stressful, unpredictable, and at times hostile places. For example, the use of hospitals as holding tanks for acutely disturbed and violent individuals, the release of mentally ill persons from public hospitals without adequate outpatient programs and follow-up services, and the accessibility of handguns and drugs in communities all contribute to hospital and community violence. A failure of leadership at various levels, as well as inadequate reimbursement from payers, has contributed to violence that can occur on its premises.

The case study hospital, like most in the United States, has dramatically reduced the number of public psychiatric beds. Many of these former psychiatric patients have to rely on outpatient mental health services supported by community hospitals with a limited number of beds on one or two psychiatric units. In addition, the case study hospital reduced inpatient and outpatient addiction services. New research suggests that actively psychotic patients with schizophrenia and patients with schizophrenia who had a premorbid conduct problem or exposure to violence are more likely to be violent than less acutely ill patients and those without substance abuse or antisocial personality co-morbidity (Swanson et al., 2008). Nevertheless, it is a mistake to consider persons with mental illness or substance abuse as the only individuals who can become agitated or violent in healthcare settings. It is also shortsighted to solely blame any single policy, such as the deinstitutionalization of the chronically mentally ill, for workplace violence in the United States.

At the same time that the case study hospital has cut beds and programs for persons in distress, the case study hospital has a clear mission/vision/value statement that puts professional nurses in leadership positions and has taken steps to address workplace violence. It has made efforts to reduce violence in high-risk areas, such as the emergency department and psychiatric unit by restricting access to these areas, using surveillance equipment, panic buttons, and a strict requirement for all staff to wear identification, as other hospitals have. Community hospitals, like the one in this case study, however, often do not provide the kind of ongoing self-defense and violence prevention education and training that many psychiatric hospitals provide. In addition, all hospitals should have a task force and regularly meeting committee consisting of management, human resources/employee relations, employee assistance program staff, security and the office of chief counsel with the sole purpose of developing policies and procedures to prevent and address workplace violence.

Following The Joint Commission's (2008) lead, the case study hospital and nursing administration have hospital wide discussions and training on "behaviors that undermine a culture of safety." In addition, the hospital requires workplace violence risk assessment, hazard prevention and control, and safety and health training, as well as careful record keeping and program evaluation (U.S. Department of Labor, 2004). Hospitals need to keep in mind the malpractice crisis in this country. The move to put patients first does not turn over control of the hospital to patients or their families. Indeed, to understand Friedman (2007) correctly, in order to put patients' health and satisfaction first, the hospital needs effective leadership at the top and from its professional nurses. To prevent violence in the workplace, nurses need to strive to be as authentic in their patient contact as possible and to avoid detached impersonal interactions (Carlsson et al., 2006). The case study hospital provides considerable avenues of reward for individual nurses and other staff members to advance themselves and stand out as innovative, which helps mitigate the tendency for workers to "herd," to use Friedman's (2007) term—that is to say, to avoid developing themselves and improving the institution for the sake of togetherness with selected coworkers.

The case study hospital does provide a psychiatric nurse practitioner on staff and onsite one day a week as an employee assistance provider. Having this person onsite provides an opportunity for hospital staff to have counseling to become less reactive to emotionally intense environments, as recommended by Friedman (2007). Healthcare organizations also need to provide referral information such as employee assistance program or clinicians experienced in trauma care for employees who may exhibit more serious and persistent reactions to perceived violence and aggression (Bernstein & Saladino, 2007). Nurses and nursing organizations should become more familiar with national guidelines and recommendations and persuade their hospitals to adopt and implement them. The process for nurses is to focus more on taking responsibility for their own condition, practice self-regulation, and have a wide repertory of responses to stressful situations. Although this does not guarantee that violence will be avoided, it does make it less likely to happen and makes nurses better able to keep it in perspective. Friedman (2007) described this as being able to turn down the dial or volume. Nurses need to be just as effective in managing "toxic" emotional environments, as in handling toxic chemicals and infections. Nurses' interpersonal effectiveness is increased when they look for and support strengths in others. Postincident debriefing helps transform the experience into a team building and learning opportunity. Leaders should involve all staff and review events, including what precedes and follows an incident.

Case Study Conclusion

A community hospital in the New York metropolitan area is presented as a case study of an organization struggling to carry out its mission in a way that facilitates the growth and well-being of its employees. The hospital is experiencing different pulls. On the one hand it has had to cut back on essential programs. On the other hand, the nurses and the central leadership in the hospital need to work together to avoid quick-fix solutions and suffer the failure of nerve that Friedman (2007) talked about. The busy hospital environment in a changing society is stressful and at times a hostile and violent one. Nurses need to be effective leaders to help protect the integrity of the hospital as an organization—that is to say maintain its self-definition. They can best do this by becoming as self-defined as they can and

by consistently implementing federal guidelines to prevent and manage workplace violence.

Case Study Questions

In this last case you have a need for policy change—which we suspect is a need in many healthcare organizations—the need for workplace violence policies. Here is our challenge to the reader. Can you take our two components, both an internal and external role, and define what needs to be done to accomplish this policy change? We suggest that you define the work in terms of your most likely environment, whether a psychiatric facility or a hospital or clinic. How would you go about creating an environment for policy change here?

Some core questions should guide you. First, what key stakeholders are in the initial stakeholder group (i.e., those most likely to feel the strongest need for the policy)? Are they organized around various professional lines within your organization? How do you begin to create a networked shared view among these stakeholders? As you begin to broaden the network, which groups should be brought into the discussion? Let us give you an example: The human resource specialists in your organization will need to be involved at some point in creating a policy about the elimination/reduction of workplace violence. Should they, however, be in your initial set of stakeholders? Why or why not?

Now . . . the more difficult question: What is the expertise needed to make such a policy change? What are the kind of facts (someone has to gather the data in a systematic way), that need to be gathered? Are we discussing violence between patients and those providing medical services, or are we also talking about violence between fellow professionals within the organization? What kind of violence/danger are we discussing here—physical or verbal violence or both? What about safety issues (including other types of danger to employees and patients)? Would you agree that an emergency room might see these questions a bit differently from those handling financial claims (although both have real needs here)? How do you build expert power here? Who shares it, and who might be expert in defining these issues over time?

Case Study References

Bernstein, K. S., & Saladino, J. P. (2007). Clinical assessment and management of psychiatric patients' violent and aggressive behaviors in general hospital. *Medsurg Nursing, 16,* 301–309.

Carlsson, G., Dahlberg, K., Ekcbergh, M., & Dahlberg, H. (2006). Patients longing for authentic personal care: A phenomenological study of violent encounters in psychiatric settings. *Issues in Mental Health Nursing, 27,* 287–305.

Department of Health and Human Services. (2002). *Violence: Occupational hazards in hospitals.* Centers for Disease Control and Prevention/National Institute for Occupational Safety and Health. Document # 2002-101. Cincinnati, OH: National Institute for Occupational Safety and Health.

Farrell, G. A., Bobrowski, C., & Bobrowski, P. (2006). Scoping workplace aggression in nursing: findings from an Australian study. *Journal of Advanced Nursing, 55,* 778–787.

Friedman, E. H. (2007). *A failure of nerve: Leadership in the age of the quick fix.* New York: Seabury (originally published in 1999).

Love, C. C., & Morrison, E. (2003). American Academy of Nursing expert panel on violence policy recommendation on workplace violence (adopted 2002). *Issues in Mental Health Nursing, 24,* 599–604.

Swanson, J. W., Van Dorn, R. A., Swartz, M. S., Smith, M., Elbogen, E. B., & Monahan, J. (2008). Alternative Pathways to Violence in Persons with Schizophrenia. *The Role of Childhood Antisocial Behavior, 32*(3), 228–240.

The Joint Commission. (July, 2008). Behaviors that undermine a culture of safety. Retrieved February 2, 2009, from http://www.jointcommission.org/SentinelEventAlert/sea_40.htm

U.S. Department of Labor. (2004). *Guidelines for preventing workplace violence for health care & social service workers* (OSHA 3148-01R). Washington, DC: Occupational Safety and Health Administration.

Chapter Conclusion

This book on politics and policy requires an understanding of how to build support and adapt to change. If we are to be effective advocates, we must be responsive to broader societal needs. Building support is not done simply by presenting the facts. This toolkit is designed to help readers know what it takes in a political environment to build a case and adapt when necessary. A huge mistake in advocacy is to simply believe that the facts are on our side, and if we just continue to list the facts, everyone will believe! In reality, values and political issues are at the core of successful change. Our tasks as political advocates for change are to:

1. Believe we can convince others to adapt
2. Adapt ourselves to handle broader political value issues
3. Learn to mobilize our expert power as one of the largest group of stakeholders in the healthcare field

Chapter References

Fottler, M. D., Blair, J. D., Whitehead, C. J., Laus, M. D., & Savage, G. T. (1989). Assessing key stakeholders: Who matters to hospitals and why? *Hospitals and Health Services Administration, 34*(4), 525–546.

Wilson, J. Q. (1989). *Bureaucracy: What government agencies do and why they do it.* New York: Basic Books.

Index

A

A, 24, 84, 93
academic medical centers
    costs, 131, 155, 178, 202, 220
    power and influence, 137
    staffing, 144, 190, 205
accountability, 2, 49, 122
adult nurse practitioner (ANP), 71
advanced practice nurses (APNs)
    in collaborative relationships, 69
    responsibilities of, 42, 91
advanced practice nurses (APRNs)
    case study, 130, 160, 102, 216, 219
    demand for, 126, 173, 187
    licensure, 134, 225-226
    regulation, 126, 148, 197, 217, 234
advanced practice registered nurse
        (APRN)
    Consensus Work Group
        assumption, 74
allied health professionals
    education, 129-130, 149, 193-194,
        208, 225-226
    statistics, 152, 177, 211, 234
Altruism, 54
altruistic motivations, 52
ambulatory care
    managed care and, 194, 211
    prevalence, 168, 194
American College of Surgeons, 136
American Journal of Nursing, 39
American Nurses Association (ANA),
        190
    codes of ethics of, 53
    on goals of nursing, 68
American Pragmatist School, 13
animal ethics, 5-6
applied ethics in health care
    defined, 35, 65, 105
    philosophy and, 65, 104-105
assent, child
    issues, 88-90
autonomy
    beneficence and, 29
    EOL decision making and
        problems of, 18
Autonomy
    ethical principle of, 21
autonomy
    personal, 20-21, 61-62
    philosophical theories of, 21
    principle of, 17
    professional autonomy, 56
    trust and, 40-41, 55

B

Baby Doe Rules"
    application of, 10, 46
Baucus, Max, 189

beneficence
    nonmaleficence, 18, 81
Bentham, Jeremy, 15
bioethical dilemmas, 43
Bioethics, 5-7, 43, 97
black Americans
    health beliefs, 210
    health disparities, 158, 209-211
    mortality rates, 169

C

Cancer
    cervical cancer, 170-171
    lung cancer, 170
cancer
    policy issues, 172, 235
    prevention, 154, 234
Cancer
    prostate cancer, 158
cancer
    research, 137, 154
Cancer
    risk factors, 155
care
    concept of, 108
    effective, 118-119
    models of, 87
care coordination, 202-204
Carmona, Richard, 170
case studies
    breast cancer, 78
    ethical decision making, 10, 70
    professional advocacy, 111
catastrophic coverage, 180
categorical imperative, 17, 104
Chan, Margaret, 147
childhood asthma, 157
children
    health insurance coverage, 181
    infant mortality, 216
    protection, 147-148, 230
Chiropractors, 184
Chronic Care Model (CCM), 212
chronic disease/illness
    environmental factors, 154
    incidence of, 157
    poverty and, 149
Civilian Health & Medical Program for
        Uniformed Services
        (CHAMPUS), 176
clinical nurse specialists (CNSs), 44
Clinton, Bill, 187, 216
Clinton Health Plan, 185
Cochrane, Archie, 206
Cochrane Library, 207
Code of Ethics for Nurses (ICN)
    International Council of Nurses, 40,
        43, 92
Codman, Ernest, 204
cognitive processes

decision making and, 72
    research and, 75
collaboration
    interdisciplinary work, 59
communication skills
    and APNs, 25
communities
    inner-city, 216
    megacommunities, 167
community hospitals
    ownership, 185
comparative justice, 30
compassion, 36, 48-49
compensatory justice, 29
complementary and alternative
        medicine (CAM)
    insurance coverage, 144-145, 171,
        181
    practitioners, 126, 153, 194, 206,
        220-221
Comstock, Anthony, 228
Comstock law, 228-229
consent. See also informed consent
    verbal, 109
    written, 100
Consolidated Omnibus Budget
        Reconciliation Act (COBRA),
        177
Consumer advocacy, 140
contemporary developments in
        nursing, 64
contemporary professions, 42
cost-containment initiatives, 55
Covey, Steven, 166
craftsmen's guilds, 51
critical human goods, 102
culture/race/ethnicity
    health inequality, 209

D

decision making
    autonomy and, 35, 71
    considerations, 7, 79-81
    example of, 7, 45, 104
    feminist ethics and, 35, 71
    framework, 24, 66, 92
    moral action and, 76-77
    nuances in, 36
    process, 19, 46, 93
Delaware Cancer Treatment Program,
        172
democratic societies, 60, 99-101
deontology
    theories, 12-14, 102
Department of Health and Human
        Services, 167, 179, 240
deprofessionalization, 55
Disability insurance, 177
disabled persons, 178
disciplinary knowledge development,

64
disease burden, 153
distributive justice and anesthesia
    practice
    principle of justice, 29
Doctor of Nursing Practice (DNP)
    degree, 19, 63
Douglass, Frederick, 122
dual federalism, 130

E
Ebola, 156
eco- or environmental ethics, 6
education
    pharmacists, 172
electronic prevention record system,
    162
e-mail, 237
emergency department visits, 203
employer-sponsored health insurance
    quality of, 127, 154, 195, 205
    small employers, 182
    value of, 128, 159, 188, 210,
        238-239
empowering patients, 3
end-of-life (EOL) care
    description, 60, 96-97
    palliative sedation
        case study, 84
Enlightenment, 103-104
environment of practice, 107
Epistemology, 4-6
ethical concerns of APNs
    decision-making capacity, 24-25
    virtue ethics, 20
Ethical principles
    justice, 16, 49, 92
ethical principles
    usefulness and limits of, 19
    veracity and fidelity, 33
ethics
    moral philosophy, 5-6
European Convention on Human
    Rights, 105
evolution of nursing profession
    goals and, 47
    nursing theory and disciplinary
        knowledge development,
        64

F
Facebook, 196
family nurse practitioner (FNP), 118
Federal Older Americans Act, 232
federalism, 125-126, 223
feminist ethics
    approaches, 11, 67
fidelity
    principles of, 33
Fiduciary relationships, 2, 55
for-profit hospitals, 136, 194

G
gender/sexuality
    gag rule, 218
Global Gag Rule, 215
globalization, 147-148
goals of nursing
    codes of ethics and, 51
good practice

as professional responsibility, 66,
    109
government
    health insurance regulation, 183
Grants-in-aid programs, 130
grassroots patient organizations, 118

H
habits of critique, 44-46
health
    as a right, 129
    biological factors, 229
    defined, 128, 152, 180, 209, 226
    social determinants, 149
    status, 139-140, 154, 178, 211, 229
health care. See also access to care
    justice in, 31, 49, 98
    right to, 20-23, 49, 93
health insurance
    cost, 126, 160, 177, 201, 229
    duality, 129
    employer-sponsored health, 181
    for contraception, 217
    history, 127, 147-149, 176-177, 209,
        227
    indemnity plans, 178
    moral hazard, 183
    national health insurance, 137, 220
    point-of-service plans, 186
    private, 128, 159-160, 176-179, 207,
        228
    public health insurance option, 189
    reform, 127-128, 176-177, 220
    universal, 129, 161, 185, 209
Health Insurance Portability and
        Accountability Act (HIPAA),
        177
health maintenance organizations
        (HMOs)
    features, 176
health policies, 121
health policy
    advocacy, 126-127, 147-149,
        196-198, 219-220
    community-based, 131
    essential elements, 125, 190, 220
    focus, 147, 183, 202, 223
    implementation, 125-128, 148, 180,
        205, 221
    long-term care, 131, 181
    policy-making process, 125-126
    politicization of, 215
    public health, 130, 147-152, 189,
        204, 227
    stakeholders, 126, 159, 176, 202,
        219-220
health policy field, 135
health resources, 140, 183, 209
Health Security Act, 190
health services research
    evidence-based practice, 159, 202
    quality improvement, 127, 160,
        204-205
healthcare delivery system
    fragmentation, 131
    improvement, 127, 160, 198-199,
        202
    integrated, 198, 204
healthcare practitioners/providers
    health policy advocacy, 166
    medical errors, 202, 220

patient-centered care, 198, 202
    representation, 159
healthcare system
    access to care, 127, 156, 186
    consumers, 125, 159, 177, 204
    equality of care, 208
    finance-driven, 138
    financing, 130, 160, 182-183, 202
    national health spending, 181
    supply and demand, 227
Healthy People 2010, 156
Healthy Places, 158
hepatitis C, 156
historical development
    of nursing, 4, 47-48, 95
    of social justice, 96
Hobbes, Thomas, 96
hospitals
    competition, 127, 178
    finances, 239
    for-profit, 136, 178
    history of, 132, 176-177
    lobbyists, 189
    nonprofit, 142, 177-178, 240
    public, 127-129, 176, 204-206, 224
    standard of care, 204
Human capital, 147
human papilloma virus (HPV), 170
human rights
    contemporary understanding of, 12
    health care and, 48-49, 107
    history of, 41, 69
human subjects research
    definitions, 6, 92
    historical development of, 96
humanization, 43

I
Illegal immigrants, 187
income, 131-132, 158, 177-178, 209,
    224
individuals and society, tensions
        between
    democratic societies and, 60, 99
    types of societies, 99
inflation, 182-183
information technology
    infrastructure, 138, 152
    Internet-based, 162
informed consent
    limits of, 66
Institute of Medicine (IOM), 171

J
Johnson, Lyndon, 178, 230
Joint Commission, 137, 198-199, 206,
    243
justice. See also injustice
    aspects of, 11-12, 55, 92
    distributive, 30, 97
    in democratic societies, 60

K
knowledge producers, 135

L
Lavizzo-Mourey, Risa, 191
leadership
    levels of, 66
legislation, 38

length of stay (LOS)
    average, 145, 180
licensure
    advanced practice nurses, 226
long-term care
    hospital-based, 134
Long-term care
    insurance, 127-129, 170-172, 176,
        208-210, 233
long-term care
    overview, 125, 147-148, 176, 201
    planning for, 228
    services, 126-128, 147-148, 176,
        201-205, 226

M

Magna Carta, 103
managed care
    impact, 125, 155, 176, 203
    market-based reform, 185
Managed care
    strategies, 147, 185-186, 201
McCarran-Ferguson Act, 183
measles, mumps, and rubella (MMR)
    vaccine
        effects of, 2, 99
Medicaid
    creation, 129, 169, 205
    reimbursement, 139, 172-173, 177,
        206, 235
medical errors
    categories, 136, 208, 226
    causes, 157, 209, 231
    deaths, 155
    human error, 205
    management, 144-145, 159, 185,
        204-205, 221
    nurses and, 137, 191, 220
    reporting, 166, 201-202
Medical ethics, 192
medical supply industry, 135
Medicare
    contracts, 186
    entitlement, 132, 180
    for chronically ill, 163
mental health care management
    deinstitutionalization, 241
    organizations, 126-127, 159,
        185-186, 202, 220
    policy, 125-131, 147-148, 177,
        201-202, 220-221
Mental Health Parity Act, 187
mental illness/disorders
    long-term, 135-136, 186, 225
    populations, 153-154, 183, 202,
        232-233
    treatment, 136, 163, 202, 232-233
mental/behavioral health care
    barriers to, 144, 166, 202, 236
    delivery system, 126
    professionals, 125-128, 161, 184,
        204, 226-227
    providers, 125, 159, 184-186,
        203-208, 230-234
Mexico City policy, 215
midwives, 180, 235
Mill, James, 15
moral action
    and interfering factors, 76-77
    processes of, 73-74
moral distress, 3, 70, 121-122

moral predictability, 71
moral reasoning
    moral theory and, 35
moral rights
    human rights as, 103
moral theories
    normative moral theories, 15
mortality rates
    racial disparities, 214
multispecialty group practices, 186
MySpace, 162

N

narrative ethics, 36
National League for Nursing, 192
neonatology/neonatal issues
    technology and, 50
new federalism, 131
nurse anesthesia practice
    ethical issues in, 11, 90
nurse workforce, 173
nurse–patient relationship
    advocacy and, 115-116
    care and, 3, 48-49, 107
    characteristics of, 47, 92
    importance of, 35, 42, 119
nurses
    patient advocacy, 195-196
    professionalism, 139, 225-226
    salaries, 134
    shortage, 142, 172-173
nursing education, 62, 123
    certification, 160, 234-235
    diploma, 226
    enrollment, 191
    schools, 164, 208, 235
nursing ethics, 4-7, 42-43, 121-124
nursing faculty, aging
    retaining, 164
nursing knowledge and practice
    philosophical perspectives, 20
nursing profession
    evolution, 53
    societal importance, 54
    status of, 57, 105
nursing shortage
    in California, 169
nursing specialties
    clinical nurse specialists, 235
    nurse anesthetists, 235
nursing theory, 64
Nursing's Agenda for Health Care
    Reform, 190

O

Obama, Barack, 139, 190
obstacles to ethical care
    interfering factors, 76-77
older population
    medical expenses, 153
ontology, 6, 67
organizations
    expert power, 225
    political power, 139
orphan drug program, 134

P

palliative care
    programs, 63
paternalism, 27-28

Patient Self-Determination Act (PSDA)
    of 1991
    advance directives and, 84
patients
    high risk, 178, 218
    safety, 133, 172, 190, 201-202, 231
personal ethics, 7
philosophical inquiry, 4-6
philosophical theories
    of autonomy, 17, 124
    of justice, 29-31, 97-98
philosophy
    applied ethics, 5-6
    family tree, 4
    subareas of, 8
physician payment
    fee-for-service, 186
physician-dominated system, 138
physicians
    accountability, 186-187, 229
    dominance, 138, 194
    practice patterns, 138, 186
    shortages of, 63
    supply, 135, 173, 227
Planned Parenthood Federation, 230
Plato, 12
power imbalances, 79
power pyramid, 222
presenteeism, 163
President's Commission (1982), 24
preventative medicine era, 149
preventive ethics, 36-37, 70
Primary care physicians, 136
private hospitals
    revenues, 133, 171, 188
professional advocacy
    for individual patients, 111
    nurse–patient relationship and, 65
    obstacles to, 4, 69, 107
    practice environments and, 6
professional ethics, 1, 121
professional goals, 11, 47, 109
professional licensure, 53
professional responsibility
    and nursing ethics, 4, 46
professions, characteristics of
    nursing possesses, 60
proxy decision making
    advance directives, 84
psychiatric advanced nursing practice
    difficulties, 3, 116
    ethics in, 11, 61, 121-122
public administration, 164, 220-221
public health
    accreditation, 137, 147-148, 190,
        205-206
    deficit in spending, 163
    emergency preparedness, 139, 147
    global public health strategies, 161
    healthcare delivery system, 126
    paradigms, 148
    security, 130-131, 152-153, 177-178,
        240-241
Public Health Accreditation Board, 160
public health professionals, 161-162
public insurance programs, 178
purchase of services, 126

Q

quality of care
    evaluating, 164, 193, 205, 236

measures, 126, 150, 195, 202-206
trilogy, 205

women's health (cont.)
    trust, 29, 85, 111
Women's rights, 227-228

R
Rawls, John, 30
Registered nurses, 234
responsibilities of APNs
    ethics and, 4, 51, 123
    moral rights and, 103
    professional, 1, 42-44, 91
Rest, James, 73
Rest's theory of moral action, 74
retributive justice, 29
risk, 20, 59, 109
risk assessment
    occupational, 150, 240

S
Sanger, Margaret, 227
Second-hand smoke, 170
senses of nursing ethics, 43
Shattuck, Lemuel, 152
Shorr, Daniel, 162
smoking
    cessation, 169-170
social cohesion, 147
social contract, 96-97
social injustices, 17, 116
social justice
    assumptions, 18-19, 79, 91-92
    solutions, 39, 92-93
social policy, 126, 208
social status, 210, 229
Social work, 164
societal obligation, 107
specialty areas of APN
    specific ethical issues
        adult health, 114
status of nursing profession
    ambiguity of, 108
    concerns, 4, 47, 91
    multiple levels of entry and, 60
Stone, Hannah, 228

T
Technology Informatics Guiding
        Education Reform (TIGER)
    collaboration, 161, 208-209, 234
therapeutic relationships
    advocacy in, 123
tobacco
    taxes, 170-171
transparency, 20, 111

U
underlying assumptions, 13, 45, 92
uninsured persons
    insurance coverage for, 185
    medical care, 133, 177, 232-233
    penalties for, 189
Universal Declaration of Human Rights,
    23, 124

V
value theories, 9

W
Wakefield, Mary, 140
white Americans, 210